FIFTH EDITION

Articulation and Phonological Disorders

John E. Bernthal

University of Nebraska–Lincoln

Nicholas W. Bankson

James Madison University

PEARSON

Boston   New York   San Francisco
Mexico City   Montreal   Toronto   London   Madrid   Munich   Paris
Hong Kong   Singapore   Tokyo   Cape Town   Sydney

Executive Editor and Publisher: *Stephen D. Dragin*
Senior Editorial Assistant: *Barbara Strickland*
Marketing Manager: *Tara Whorf*
Composition and Prepress Buyer: *Linda Cox*
Manufacturing Manager: *Andrew Turso*
Cover Administrator: *Kristina Mose-Libon*
Editorial-Production Service: *Matrix Productions Inc.*
Electronic Composition: *Publishers' Design and Production Services, Inc.*

For related titles and support materials, visit our online catalog at www.ablongman.com

Between the time Website information is gathered and then published, it is not unusual for some sites to have closed. Also, the transcription of URLs can result in unintended typographical errors. The publisher would appreciate notification where these errors occur so that they may be corrected in subsequent editions.

Library of Congress Cataloging-in-Publication Data

Articulation and phonological disorders / [edited by] John E.
    Bernthal, Nicholas W. Bankson.—5th ed.
        p.   cm.
    Rev. ed. of: Articulation and phonological disorders / John E.
Bernthal, Nicholas W. Bankson. 4th ed. ©1998
    Includes bibliographical references and indexes.
    ISBN 0-205-34790-8
    1. Articulation Disorders.   I. Bernthal, John E.   II. Bankson,
Nicholas W.
    [DNLM: 1. Articulation Disorders.   2. Voice Disorders.
    3. Phonetics   WM 475 A792 2003]
    RC424.7.B47   2003
    616.85'8—dc21
    DNLM/DLC
    for Library of Congress   2003101684

Printed in the United States of America
10   9   8   7   6   5   4   3   2   1   08   07   06   05   04   03

CONTENTS

PREFACE

This edition reflects our ongoing efforts to teach students about the nature and treatment of disorders of the speech sound system. Since submission of our last edition for publication, new ideas, concepts, and issues have been advanced in the area of clinical phonology, and we have tried to reflect some of them in this edition.

This book presents both theoretical and practical information, recognizing that elements of both are essential to the understanding of the literature and to clinical practice. We have attempted to organize and synthesize the literature so that students view clinical phonology from a broad perspective. We have again adopted an "eclectic" perspective relative to the nature and treatment of phonological disorders because our readers have indicated that this is of value as they acquire the foundation of knowledge necessary for more advanced study in the area. In the assessment and intervention chapters, you will again see some of our own biases regarding clinical management; however, in general we have deferred to clinician's judgment in deciding which assessment and management tools may be most useful. We have, however, added a case study that reflects how we would handle a specific client with a phonological disorder. Throughout the text, we have attempted to identify unresolved issues regarding the topics discussed.

Although it would be impossible to acknowledge everyone who has contributed either directly or indirectly to the writing of this book, we note several people who have contributed immeasurably: Of special assistance have been the revisions of several chapters: Chapter 1 by Ray Kent; Chapters 2 and 3 by Marilyn Vihman; and Chapter 8 by Brian Goldstein and Aquiles Iglesias. A new chapter on phonological awareness, co-authored by Laura Justice and C. Melanie Schuele, has been added to this edition. Given the expanding role of clinicians in the literacy development of children and the fact that clinicians are often called upon to use their knowledge of phonology to develop and/or implement programs of phonological awareness (a precursor to decoding words), it seemed appropriate to include a chapter on the topic in a book of this nature.

The advice and suggestions we have received from the users and reviewers of our previous work have been invaluable, and we hope that this effort reflects a step forward in the presentation of information on clinical phonology. We express our appreciation to the following reviewers: Lauren E. Bland, Jackson State University; Martha A. Boose, The College of St. Rose; M. Adelaida Restrepo, The University of Georgia; and Lee Ann Setzer, Brigham Young University.

We also wish to express our deep gratitude for the efforts of Evie Reiners, our primary editorial assistant, for this and other editions of this text. Her diligence, patience, and sheer competence were critical, and we stand in her debt. We assume all responsibility for errors, oversights, and misconceptions that may appear in this book.

We hope that you find this book helpful as you learn about and practice clinical phonology.

INTRODUCTION

This book has the same goal as the four previous editions, which is to present a comprehensive review of information important to the study of clinical phonology. It includes coverage of the normal aspects of speech sound articulation, normal phonological development, factors related to the presence of phonological disorders, the assessment and remediation of phonological disorders, phonology as it relates to language and dialectal variations, and phonological awareness. Discussion questions are presented with each chapter, and a case study is included in the assessment and remediation chapters.

As in past editions, this text is primarily concerned with those phonological disorders not etiologically associated with known or obvious sensory, structural, or neuromotor deficits. Such disorders traditionally have been labeled *functional* articulation disorders, a category that has come to be viewed clinically as a catch-all, frequently including all individuals with phonological errors of unknown cause. It is recognized, however, that a phonological disorder of unknown etiology may be caused by one or more subtle organic, learning, or environmental factors.

Those acquainted with previous editions of this text will notice some changes in organizational structure, as well as updated information concerning topics covered in previous editions, plus a new chapter on phonological awareness. Once again we have attempted to synthesize the literature and present it in a manner meaningful to students studying clinical phonology.

This book has been divided into nine chapters (as was the last edition; however, there are some changes in topics and organization of material related to assessment and treatment). Chapter 1 reviews normal aspects of articulation and provides an introduction to the phonological system of American English. This information is typically covered in courses other than clinical phonology; however, for those who lack such course work or, as is frequently the case, need review, this content is presented.

Chapters 2 and 3 focus on early and later phonological development in children and review the development of production and perceptual skills at both the prelinguistic and linguistic levels. Because speech-language pathologists must distinguish delayed or deviant phonological development from normal development, they must recognize and understand normal phonological development. These chapters reflect basic concepts, as well as an update of the literature related to phonological acquisition.

Chapter 4 reviews various factors that have been studied in terms of their relationship to the presence and/or maintenance of disordered phonology. The literature related to potential etiological variables associated with impairments of the speech and hearing mechanism is reviewed. Because this text is primarily focused on disorders of unknown or functional etiology, review of the literature related to cognitive-linguistic as well as psychosocial factors as they relate to phonological disorders is also presented.

Chapter 5 addresses procedures for phonological sampling and interpretation. Screening procedures, a battery for doing a comprehensive phonological assessment, and related assessment procedures are reviewed and discussed; included are selected computer programs that may assist in this process. In addition, the chapter reviews how one can determine the need for intervention and how target behaviors are selected. A case study is presented in which topics covered in the chapter are applied to a specific client.

Chapter 6 reviews basic considerations related to treatment, including the framework of intervention sessions, intervention scheduling, treatment style, and how generalization is related to treatment.

Chapter 7 continues the discussion of intervention and focuses on procedures for traditional motor-oriented therapy and linguistic-based approaches to intervention. A discussion of oral-motor activities as part of articulation instruction is presented, along with intervention for children with developmental verbal dyspraxia. A case study is presented, focusing on the same client discussed in the assessment chapter, with an emphasis on how treatment approaches presented in the chapter might be applied to the child.

Chapter 8 presents information critical to increasing our competence in serving a multicultural society and focuses on the influence of other languages and dialects on the development of the linguistic systems of our clients. Common dialectical variations found in our society are reviewed, including African American English, Spanish- as well as Asian-influenced English, and Eastern, Southern Appalachian, and Ozark English.

Chapter 9 is concerned with phonological awareness, including its description, assessment, and intervention. This chapter is included because of the increasing role that speech-language pathologists are playing in the literacy development of children. Phonological awareness is an important early skill related to children who are learning to decode words. Because the education of speech-language pathology students provides them with a unique body of knowledge related to the structure of the sound system, including sound perception, clinicians working with children have been shown to play a very helpful role in developing and promoting phonological awareness assessment and instructional programs in preschool and school programs. Given this increasing role of clinicians in the area of literacy and the advice of reviewers to include such information, it seems appropriate to include a separate chapter on phonological awareness.

1

Normal Aspects of Articulation

RAY KENT

University of Wisconsin—Madison

Introduction

Speech has been defined as a *system that relates meaning with sound*. Meaning itself arises in **language**. A *language is an arbitrary system of signs or symbols used according to pre-scribed rules to convey meaning within a linguistic community*. Of course, once an arbitrary association of symbol with meaning has been made, the users of that language must be consistent in this association if they want to communicate with one another. The word *dog* has a meaning in the English language, but this word can be communicated to other users of English by speaking, by writing, or by signing it with the symbols used by the deaf. Speech is but one modality for the expression of language; however, speech has special importance because it is the primary, first-learned modality for hearing language users. Speech is a system in the sense that it consistently and usefully relates the meanings of a language with the sounds by which the language is communicated.

Not all sound variations in speech are related to meaning. When a person suffers from a cold, he or she has a different way of talking, but so long as the cold is not so severe as to make speech unintelligible, the relation of sound to meaning is basically the same as when the person is healthy. The acoustic signal of speech—that is, the vibrations of air molecules in response to the energy source of human speech—carries more information than just the expression of meaning. As we listen to a speaker, we often make judgments not only about the intended meaning but also about the speaker's age and sex (if the speaker isn't visible), the speaker's mood, the speaker's state of health, and perhaps even the speaker's dialectal background. Thus, on hearing a simple question—"Could you tell me the time, please?"—we might deduce that the speaker is a young southern woman in a hurry, an elderly British gentleman in a cheerful mood, or a young boy quite out of breath.

Structure of Language

To derive a speaker's meaning, the listener is basically concerned with the phonemes in the speech message. From a linguistic perspective, phonemes are sound units related to decisions about meaning. In the list, *cat hat mat bat sat fat that chat,* each word rhymes with every other word because all end with the same sound. However, the words differ in their initial sounds, and these differences can change the meaning of the syllables. In fact, the linguist identifies the phonemes in a given language by assembling lists of words and then determining the sound differences that form units of meaning. The layman usually thinks of words as the units of meaning, but the linguist recognizes a smaller form called the **morpheme**. For example, the linguist describes the words *walked* and *books* as having two morphemes: *walk + past tense* for *walked*, and *book + plural* for *books*. If two sounds can be interchanged without changing word meaning, or if they never occur in exactly the same combination with other sounds, then they are not different phonemes. Hence, phonemes are the minimal sound elements that represent and distinguish language units (words or morphemes).

A **phonemic transcription** (which is always enclosed in virgules / /) is less detailed than a **phonetic transcription** (which is enclosed in brackets [ ]). A phonetic transcription is sensitive to sound variations within a phoneme class. An individual variant of this kind is called an *allophone*. Thus, a phoneme is a family of allophones. Phonemes are the minimal set of sound classes needed to specify the meaningful units (words or morphemes) of the language. Allophones are a more numerous set of distinct sounds, some of which may belong to the same phoneme family. As a very simple example, the word *pop* begins and ends with the same phoneme but often begins and ends with a different allophone. If the final /p/ is produced by holding the lips together after they close, then this sound is the unreleased allophone of the /p/ phoneme. However, the initial /p/ must be released before the vowel is formed, so this sound is the released allophone of the /p/ phoneme. The /p/ phoneme also includes a number of other allophones, though perhaps not as obvious as these two.

To understand more clearly the difference between phonemes and allophones, say the following word-pairs to yourself as you try to detect a difference in the production of the italicized sounds.

> *k*eep - *c*oop   (phoneme /k/)
> m*a*n - b*a*t   (phoneme /æ/)
> te*n* - te*n*th   (phoneme /n/)

In the first pair of words, the phoneme /k/ is articulated toward the front of the mouth in the first word and toward the back of the mouth in the second. Despite the differences in the place of tongue contact, the two sounds are heard by speakers of English to be the same phoneme. Speakers of other languages, such as Arabic, may hear the two sounds as different phonemes. The tongue-front and tongue-back versions are allophones of the /k/ phoneme.

In the next pair of words, *man* and *bat*, the pertinent difference might be more easily heard than felt through articulation. In the word *man*, the vowel is nasalized (produced with sound transmission through the nose) owing to the influence of the surrounding nasal consonants. But in the word *bat*, the vowel /æ/ is not normally nasalized. The phonetic environment of the vowel—that is, its surrounding sounds—determines whether or not the vowel is nasalized. The nasal and nonnasal versions of the vowel are allophones of the /æ/ phoneme.

Finally, in comparing /n/ in the words *ten* and *tenth*, you might notice that your tongue is more toward the front (just behind the upper front teeth) in the word *tenth*. The final *th* sound exerts an articulatory influence on the preceding /n/, causing it to be dentalized or produced at the teeth. Again, the two types of /n/ are simply allophones of the /n/ phoneme.

Allophonic variation is of two types: *complementary distribution* and *free variation*. In complementary distribution, two (or more) allophones never occur in exactly the same phonetic environment, so that the occurrence of one is complementary (nonoverlapping) to the occurrence of the other. For example, the front and back /k/ discussed above are in complementary distribution. The front /k/ occurs in the environment of vowels made in the front of the mouth and the back /k/ occurs in the environment of vowels made in the back of the mouth. Similarly, the nasal and nonnasal allophones of /æ/ are in complementary distribution, determined by the presence or absence of nasals in the phonetic environment. The nasalized /æ/ occurs only when this vowel is preceded or followed by nasal sounds. Allophones are said to be in free variation when they can occur in the same phonetic context. For example, the released /p/ and the unreleased /p/ are in free variation in word-final position in words like *pop* or *map*. As indicated above, the final /p/ can be released audibly with a small burst as the lips open or it can be unreleased if the lip closure is maintained.

The discipline of linguistics is concerned primarily with the structure of language. The disciplines of psychology and speech-language pathology are concerned primarily with the processing of language—with its formulation and its reception. The linguistic study of language structure has influenced the study of language processing, and, to some degree, the reverse is true as well. Descriptions of language processing often use terms, such as syntax, semantics, phonology, and phonetics, that denote traditional areas of linguistic study. These terms have come to have a duel usage, one referring to structure and another to processing.

Figure 1.1 is a diagram of an information processing model of verbal formulation and utterance production. The diagram attempts to show how different types of information are processed in the act of speaking. The cognitive level is where a thought is initiated. This is a prelinguistic, propositional level that involves decisions such as the identification of participants and actions. For example, the cognitive processing that preceded formulation of the sentence, *the dog chased the cat*, involved the identification of a dog and a cat as participants and chasing or pursuit as an action. However, the words *dog*, *cat*, and *chased* were not actually selected. Rather, propositions or relations associated with these words were established.

Information from the cognitive level is used to make decisions at the syntactic and semantic levels. Syntax involves the ordering of words in a sentence and semantics involves the selection of words. Research on verbal formulation indicates that syntactic and semantic processing are interactive (hence, the arrows between them in the diagram). Deciding upon a particular syntactic structure for a sentence can influence word selection, and selection of particular words can limit or direct syntactic decisions. The semantic level is sometimes called lexicalization, or the choice of lexical units. Lexicalization appears to

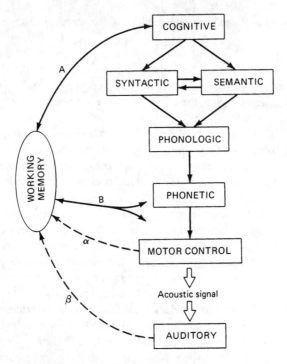

FIGURE 1.1   Information processing model of verbal formulation and utterance production.

Adapted from J. K. Bock, "Toward a cognitive psychology of syntax: Information processing contributions to sentence formulation." *Psychological Review*, 89 (1982): 1–47.

be a two-stage process. The first stage is selection of a lexical concept, not a phonologically complete word. Phonologic specification, that is, specification of the word's sound pattern, is accomplished in the second stage of the process. The phonologic level in Figure 1.1 is the level at which the evolving sentence comes to have phonologic structure. Various decisions are made at this level to ensure that a sound pattern accurately represents the syntactic and semantic decisions made earlier. The phonologic information then directs decisions at the phonetic level, where the details of the sound pattern are worked out. We might think of the phonetic level as producing a detailed phonetic representation of the utterance.

The output of the phonetic level is sufficient to specify the phonetic goals to be satisfied in speech production. Actual motor instructions are determined by a motor control level. This level selects the muscles to be activated and controls the timing and strength of the muscle contractions. This is no small task. Speech requires rapid changes in the activation of about 100 muscles. Once the muscles have done their work, the acoustic speech signal is produced. This signal is then processed by the speaker and the listener(s) as auditory information. For the speaker, the auditory processing completes a feedback loop.

One component that remains to be explained in Figure 1.1 is working memory and its connections to other parts of the diagram. Working memory is a speaker's operational memory, the memory that is used to keep track of the information involved in sentence production. But this memory is limited, so it is in the interest of efficient processing to minimize demands on it. Therefore, the theory goes, two kinds of processing are involved in utterance production. One is **controlled processing**; this kind makes demands on working memory. The other is **automatic processing**, which does not require allocation of working memory. Verbal formulation is performed with both controlled processing and automatic processing. Controlled processing can be identified in Figure 1.1 by the arrows labeled A and B. Note that syntactic, semantic, and phonologic processing are automatic; that is, the speaker does not have direct access to these operations. It is for this reason that slips of the tongue are not detected until they are actually spoken.

Feedback is provided by two channels, labeled α and β in Figure 1.1. Channel α represents information from touch and movement. Channel β represents auditory feedback.

Researchers have concluded that when we ordinarily produce a sentence, we don't make all of the syntactic, semantic, and phonologic decisions before beginning to speak. Rather, it is likely that we will utter a few words and then formulate the remainder of the utterance.

According to this view of verbal formulation, producing a sentence involves highly interactive levels of processing and a complex time pattern for this processing. It would not be surprising, then, to discover that articulation is affected by syntactic, semantic and phonologic variables.

The following discussion of articulatory phonetics presents basic information on speech sound production. For the student who has had a course in phonetics, this chapter should be a summary review. The student without such background should be able to acquire at least the basics of articulatory phonetics. The topics to be discussed are these:

The Speech Mechanism
Vowels
　　Monophthongs (single vowels)
　　Diphthongs
Consonants
　　Stops
　　Nasals
　　Fricatives
　　Affricates
　　Liquids
　　Glides
Suprasegmentals
Coarticulation
Aerodynamics
Acoustics
Afference
Sensory Information
Phonology

Fundamentals of Articulatory Phonetics

The Speech Mechanism

The anatomy of the speech production system is not within the scope of this chapter, but some general anatomical descriptions are needed to discuss the fundamentals of articulatory phonetics. The basic aspects of speech production can be understood by an examination of six principal organs or subsystems, illustrated in Figure 1.2. The *respiratory system*, consisting of the lungs, airway, rib cage, diaphragm, and associated structures, provides the basic air supply for generating sound. The *larynx*, composed of various cartilages and muscles, generates the voiced sounds of speech by vibration of the vocal folds, or it allows air to pass from lungs to the vocal tract (the oral and nasal cavities) for voiceless sounds. The *velopharynx*—the soft palate (or velum) and associated structures of the velopharyngeal port—joins or separates the oral and nasal cavities so that air passes through the oral cavity, the nasal cavity, or both. The *tongue*, primarily a complex of muscles, is the principal articulator of the oral cavity; it is capable of assuming a variety of shapes and positions in vowel and consonant articulation. For articulatory purposes, the tongue is divided into five major parts: the tip or apex, the blade, the back or dorsum, the root, and the body. These divisions are illustrated in Figure 1.3. The *lips*, along with the jaw, are the most visible of the articulators; they are involved in the production of vowels and consonants. The *jaw*, the

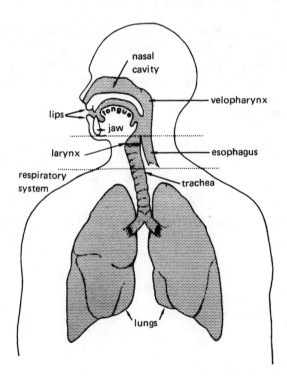

FIGURE 1.2   Organs of speech production.

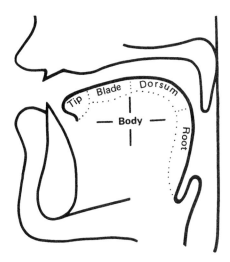

FIGURE 1.3   Divisions of tongue into five functional parts for speech articulation.

massive bony structure and its associated muscles, supports the soft tissues of both tongue and lower lip. It participates in speech production by aiding tongue and lip movements and by providing skeletal support for these organs.

Other anatomical features shown in Figure 1.2 provide general orientation or are relevant in a significant way to the processes of speech and hearing.

The respiratory system and larynx work together to provide the upper airway with two major types of air flow: a series of pulses of air created by the action of the vibrating vocal folds (for voiced sounds like the sounds in the word *buzz*), and a continuous flow of air that can be used to generate noise energy in the vocal tract (for voiceless sounds like the *s* in *see*). The basic function of the respiratory system in speech is to push air into the airway composed of the larynx and the oral and nasal cavities. The basic function of the larynx is to regulate the air flow from the lungs to create both voiced and voiceless segments. The upper airway, often called the vocal tract, runs from the larynx to the mouth or nose and is the site of what is commonly called speech articulation. For the most part, this process is accomplished by movements of the *articulators*: tongue, lips, jaw, and velopharynx. The vocal tract may be viewed as a flexible tube that can be lengthened or shortened (by moving the larynx up and down in the neck or by protruding and retracting the lips) and constricted at many points along its length by actions of tongue, velopharynx, and lips. Speech articulation is thus a matter of lengthening, shortening, and constricting the tube known as the vocal tract.

This entire process is controlled by the nervous system, which must translate the message to be communicated into a pattern of signals that run to the various muscles of the speech mechanism. As these muscles contract, a variety of things can happen: Air may be pushed out of the lungs, the vocal folds may start to vibrate, the velopharynx may close, the jaw may lower, or the lips may protrude. The brain has the task of coordinating all the different muscles so that they contract in the proper sequence to produce the required phonetic result. The margin for error is small; sometimes an error of just a few milliseconds in the timing of a muscle contraction can result in a misarticulation.

It is appealing to suppose that speech production is controlled at some relatively high level of the brain by discrete units, such as phonemes. However, a major problem in the description of speech articulation is to relate the discrete linguistic units that operate at a high level of the brain to the muscle contractions that result in articulatory movements. For example, to say the word *stop*, a speaker's brain must send nerve instructions, in the proper sequence, to the muscles of the respiratory system, larynx, tongue, lips, and velopharynx. The full understanding of speech production therefore involves a knowledge of **phonology** (the study of how sounds are put together to form words and other linguistic units), **articulatory phonetics** (the study of how the articulators make individual sounds), **acoustic phonetics** (the study of the relationship between articulation and the acoustic signal of speech), and **speech perception** (the study of how phonetic decisions are made from the acoustic signal).

Vowel Articulation: Traditional Phonetic Description

A vowel sound is usually formed as sound energy from the vibrating vocal folds escapes through a relatively open vocal tract of a particular shape. Because a syllable must contain a vowel or vowel-like sound, vowels sometimes are called *syllable nuclei*. Each vowel has a characteristic vocal tract shape that is determined by the position of the tongue, jaw, and lips. Although other parts of the vocal tract, like the velum, pharyngeal walls, and cheeks, may vary somewhat with different vowels, the positions of the tongue, jaw, and lips are of primary consequence. Therefore, individual vowels can be described by specifying the articulatory positions of tongue, jaw, and lips. Furthermore, because the jaw and tongue usually work together to increase or reduce the mouth opening (Figure 1.4), for general

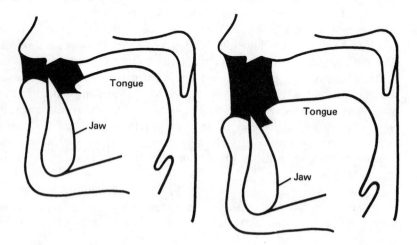

FIGURE 1.4   Variations in mouth opening (darkened area) related to lowering of jaw and tongue.

phonetic purposes vowel production can be described by specifying the positions of just two articulators, tongue and lips. Usually, the vocal folds vibrate to produce voicing for vowels, but exceptions, such as whispered speech, do occur.

The two basic lip articulations can be demonstrated with the vowels in the words *he* and *who*. Press your finger against your lips as you say first *he* and then *who*. You should feel the lips push against your finger as you say *who*. The vowel in this word is a rounded vowel, meaning that the lips assume a rounded, protruded posture. Vowels in English are described as being either rounded, like the vowel in *who*, or unrounded, like the vowel in *he*. Figure 1.5 illustrates the lip configuration for these two vowels.

The tongue moves in essentially two dimensions within the oral cavity, as shown in Figure 1.6. One dimension, front-back, is represented by the motion the tongue makes as you alternately say *he, who* or *map, mop*. The other dimension, high-low, is represented by the motion the tongue makes as you say *heave-have* or *who-ha*. With these two dimensions of tongue movement, we can define four extreme positions of the tongue within the oral cavity, as shown in Figure 1.7. The phonetic symbols for these four vowels also are shown in the illustration. With the tongue high and forward in the mouth, the high-front vowel /i/ as in *he* is produced. When the tongue is low and forward in the mouth, the low-front vowel /æ/ as in *have* is produced. A tongue position that is high and back in the mouth yields the high-back vowel /u/. Finally, when the tongue is low and back in the mouth, the vowel is the low-back /ɑ/. The four vowels, /i/, /æ/, /u/, and /ɑ/, define four points which establish the *vowel quadrilateral*, a four-sided figure against which tongue position for vowels can be described. In Figure 1.8, the vowels of English have been plotted by phonetic symbol and key word within the quadrilateral. As an example, notice the vowel /ɪ/ as in *bit* has a tongue position that is forward in the mouth and not quite as high as that for /i/. The tongue position for any one vowel can be specified with terms such as low-high, front for /ɪ/ as in *bit*, low-mid, front for /ɛ/ as in *bet*, mid-central for /ɝ/ as in *Bert*, and low-mid, back for /ɔ/ as in *bought*.

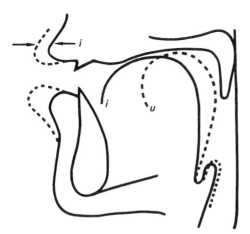

FIGURE 1.5   Vocal tract configurations for /i/ and /u/. Note lip rounding for /u/.

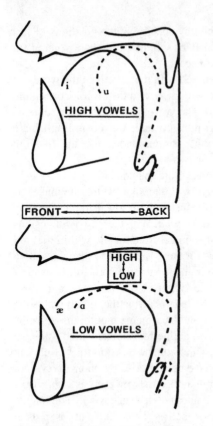

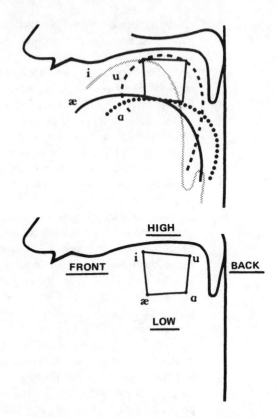

FIGURE 1.6   The two major dimensions of tongue position, front-back and high-low.

FIGURE 1.7   The four corner vowels /i/, /u/, /ɑ/, and /æ/ are shown at the top as tongue positions in the oral cavity and at the bottom as points of a quadrilateral.

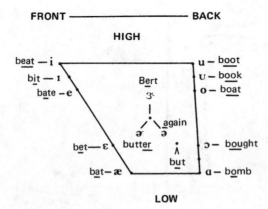

FIGURE 1.8   English vowels, identified by phonetic symbol and key word and plotted within vowel quadrilateral.

The vowels of English can be categorized as follows with respect to tongue position:

Front vowels:	/i/	/ɪ/	/e/	/ɛ/	/æ/
Central vowels:	/ɝ/	/ʌ/	/ɚ/	/ə/	
Back vowels:	/u/	/ʊ/	/o/	/ɔ/	/ɑ/
High vowels:	/i/	/ɪ/	/u/	/ʊ/	
Mid vowels:	/e/	/ɛ/	/ɝ/	/ʌ/	/ɚ/ /ə/ /o/ /ɔ/
Low vowels:	/æ/	/ɑ/			

The vowels can also be categorized with respect to lip rounding, with the following being rounded: /u/, /ʊ/, /o/, /ɔ/, and /ɝ/. All other vowels are unrounded. Notice that, in English, the rounded vowels are either back or central vowels; front rounded vowels do not occur.

Vowel production is also commonly described as *tense (long)* or *lax (short)*. Tense vowels are longer in duration and supposedly involve a greater degree of muscular tension. Lax vowels are relatively short and involve less muscular effort. One way of demonstrating the distinction between tense and lax is to feel the fleshy undersurface of your jaw as you say /i/ as in *he* and /ɪ/ as in *him*. Most people can feel a greater tension for /i/ (a tense vowel) than for /ɪ/ (a lax vowel). The tense vowels are /i/, /e/, /ɝ/, /u/, /o/, /ɔ/, and /ɑ/. The remaining vowels are considered lax, but opinion is divided for the vowel /æ/ as in *bat*.

In standard production, all English vowels are voiced (associated with vibrating vocal folds) and nonnasal (having no escape of sound energy through the nose). Therefore, the descriptors *voiced* and *nonnasal* usually are omitted. However, it should be remembered that vowels are sometimes devoiced, as in whispering, and nasalized, as when they precede or follow nasal consonants. For phonetic purposes it is usually sufficient to describe a vowel in terms of the three major characteristics of tenseness—laxness, lip configuration, and tongue position. Examples of vowel description are given as follows:

/i/ tense, unrounded, high-front
/o/ tense, rounded, high-mid, back
/ɝ/ tense, rounded, mid-central
/ʊ/ lax, rounded, low-high, back

Closely related to the vowels are the *diphthongs*, which, like vowels, are produced with an open vocal tract and serve as the nuclei for syllables. But unlike vowels, diphthongs are formed with an articulation that gradually changes during production of the sound. Diphthongs are dynamic sounds, because they involve a progressive change in vocal tract shape. An example of the articulation of /aɪ/ is shown in Figure 1.9. Many phoneticians regard diphthongs as combinations of two vowels, one called the *onglide* portion and the other called the *offglide* portion. This vowel + vowel description underlies the phonetic symbols for the diphthongs, which have the *digraph* (two-element) symbols /aɪ/, /aʊ/, /ɔɪ/, /eɪ/, and /oʊ/. Key words for these sounds are as follows:

/aɪ/ *I, buy, why, ice, night*
/aʊ/ *ow, bough, trout, down, owl*

/ɔɪ/   *boy, oil, loin, hoist*
/eɪ/   *bay, daze, rain, stay*
/oʊ/   *bow, no, load, bone*

Whereas the diphthongs /aɪ/, /aʊ/, and /ɔɪ/ are truly phonemic diphthongs, /eɪ/ and /oʊ/ are not; they are variants of the vowels /e/ and /o/, respectively. The diphthongal forms /eɪ/ and /oʊ/ occur in strongly stressed syllables, whereas the monophthongal (single-vowel) forms /e/ and /o/ tend to occur in weakly stressed syllables. For example, in the word *vacation*, the first syllable (weakly stressed) is produced with /e/ and the second syllable (strongly stressed) is produced with /eɪ/. Stressed syllables tend to be long in duration and therefore allow time for the articulatory movement of the diphthong. The diphthongs /aɪ/, /aʊ/, and /ɔɪ/ do not alternate with monophthongal forms. To produce a recognizable /aɪ/, /aʊ/, or /ɔɪ/, a speaker must use a diphthongal movement.

As shown in Figure 1.10, the onglide and offglide segments of the diphthongs are roughly located by the positions of the digraph symbols on the vowel quadrilateral. For example, in diphthong /aɪ/, the tongue moves from a low-back to nearly a high-front position. However, it should be noted that these onglide and offglide positions are only approximate and that substantial variation occurs across speakers and speaking conditions.

Vowel Articulation: Description by Distinctive Features

The phonetic descriptions considered to this point are one method of classifying vowel sounds. An alternative is a method relying on *distinctive features*, as defined by the linguists Noam Chomsky and Morris Hallé (1968). The distinctive features are a set of binary (two-valued) features designed to describe the phonemes in all languages of the world. A convenient example of a binary feature is nasality. In general terms, a given speech sound

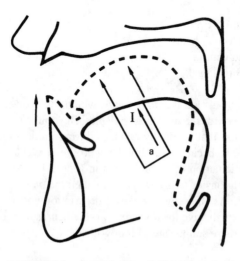

FIGURE 1.9   Articulation of diphthong /aɪ/ (as in *eye*), represented as onglide (/a/) and offglide (/ɪ/) configurations.

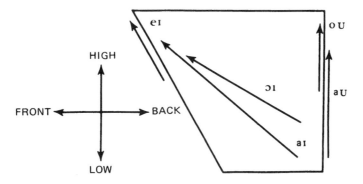

FIGURE 1.10   Diphthong articulation shown as onglide to offglide arrows in the vowel quadrilateral.

is either nasal or nonnasal, meaning that sound energy is transmitted through the nose (nasal) or is not (nonnasal). If nasality is described as a binary feature, then sounds can be classified as +nasal (indicating the nasal transmission of sound) or −nasal (indicating the absence of nasal transmission). Hence, a positive value (+nasal) means that the property is present or is relevant to description of the sound. In some ways, distinctive feature analysis is similar to the guessing game of Twenty Questions in which the participants have to identify an object by asking questions that can be answered with only yes or no. Chomsky and Hallé proposed a set of 13 binary features, which, given the appropriate yes (+) or no (−) answers, can describe all phonemes used in the languages of the world.

In the Chomsky-Hallé system, the voiced vowels are specified primarily with the features shown in Table 1.1. First, notice the three major class features of *sonorant, vocalic,*

TABLE 1.1   Distinctive Features for Selected Vowel Sounds. The Class Features Distinguish Vowels from Various Consonants; Therefore, All Vowels Have the Same Values for These Features.

CLASS FEATURES	i	ɪ	ɛ	æ	ʌ	ɝ	u	ʊ	ɔ	ɑ
Sonorant	+	+	+	+	+	+	+	+	+	+
Vocalic	+	+	+	+	+	+	+	+	+	+
Consonantal	−	−	−	−	−	−	−	−	−	−
CAVITY FEATURES										
High	+	+	−	−	−	−	+	+	−	−
Low	−	−	−	+	−	−	−	−	+	+
Back	−	−	−	−	−	−	+	+	+	+
Rounded	−	−	−	−	−	+	+	+	+	−
Nasal	−	−	−	−	−	−	−	−	−	−
MANNER OF ARTICULATION FEATURE										
Tense	+	−	−	+	−	+	+	−	+	+

and *consonantal*. A sonorant sound is produced with a vocal cavity configuration in which spontaneous voicing is possible. Essentially, the vocal tract above the larynx is sufficiently open so that no special laryngeal adjustments are needed to initiate voicing. For nonsonorants, or *obstruents*, the cavity configuration does not allow spontaneous voicing. Special mechanisms must be used to produce voicing during the nonsonorant sounds. Vocalic sounds are produced with an oral cavity shape in which the greatest constriction does not exceed that associated with the high vowels /i/ and /u/ and with vocal folds that are adjusted so as to allow spontaneous voicing. This feature, then, describes the degree of opening of the oral cavity together with the vocal fold adjustment. Finally, consonantal sounds have a definite constriction in the *midsagittal*, or midline, region of the vocal tract; nonconsonantal sounds do not. Vowels are described as +sonorant, +vocalic, and −consonantal. Taken together, these three features indicate that vowels are produced with a relatively open oral cavity, with no severe constriction in the midsagittal plane, and with a vocal fold adjustment that allows for spontaneous vocal fold vibration.

Vowels are also described with respect to cavity features and manner of articulation features, some of which are shown in Table 1.1 (the others will be discussed with respect to consonants later in this chapter). The cavity features of primary concern in vowel description are:

Tongue Body Features: High-Nonhigh; Low-Nonlow; Back-Nonback (see Figure 1.11a, b, c).

High sounds are produced by raising the body of the tongue above the level that it occupies in the neutral (or resting) position, as shown in Figure 1.11a.

Low sounds are produced by lowering the body of the tongue below the level that it occupies in the neutral position; see Figure 1.11b.

Back sounds are produced by retracting the body of the tongue from the neutral position, as shown in Figure 1.11c.

Rounded–Nonrounded. Rounded sounds have a narrowing or protrusion of the lips.

Nasal–Nonnasal. Nasal sounds are produced with a lowered velum, so that sound energy escapes through the nose.

Table 1.1 shows that most vowels can be distinguished using the cavity features. For example, /i/ and /u/ differ in the back and rounded features, and /æ/ and /i/ differ in the high and low features. Most other distinctions can be made by referring to a manner of articulation called tense–nontense. Tense sounds are produced with a deliberate, accurate, maximally distinct gesture that involves considerable muscular effort. The tense–nontense distinction is best illustrated with the vowel pairs /i/–/ɪ/ and /u/–/ʊ/. Vowels /i/ and /u/ are tense vowels because they are lengthened and are produced with marked muscular effort. As mentioned earlier, the difference in muscular effort can be felt by placing your fingers in the fleshy area just under the chin, saying alternately /i/–/ɪ/. A greater tension occurs during production of the tense vowel /i/ than during the nontense vowel /ɪ/.

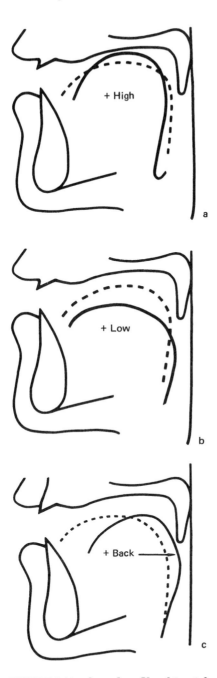

FIGURE 1.11 a, b, and c   Vocal tract drawings illustrating the tongue body features high, low, and back relative to the neutral tongue position (broken line).

Consonant Articulation: Traditional Phonetic Description

The consonants generally differ from the vowels in terms of the relative openness of the vocal tract and the function within the syllable. Vowels are produced with an open vocal tract; most consonants are made with a complete or partially constricted vocal tract. Within a syllable, vowels serve as a nucleus, meaning that a syllable must contain one and only one vowel (the only exceptions to this rule are the diphthongs, which are like vowels plus vowel glides, and certain syllabic consonants to be discussed later). Consonants are added to the vowel nucleus to form different syllable shapes, such as the following, where V represents a vowel and C represents a consonant.

VC shape:	*on, add, in*
CV shape:	*do, be, too*
CVC shape:	*dog, cat, man*
CCVC shape:	*truck, skin, clap*
CCVCC shape:	*screams, squint, scratched*

Consonants are described by degree or type of closure and by the location at which the complete or partial closure occurs. The *manner* of consonant articulation refers to the degree or type of closure, and the *place* of consonant articulation refers to the location of the constriction. In addition, consonants are described as *voiced* when the vocal folds are vibrating and *voiceless* when the vocal folds are not vibrating. Thus, an individual consonant can be specified by using three terms: one to describe *voicing*, one to describe *place*, and one to describe *manner*. Tables 1.2 and 1.3 show combinations of these terms used to specify the consonants of English.

Table 1.2 contains four columns, showing place of articulation, phonetic symbol and key word, manner of articulation, and voicing. The terms for place of articulation usually signify two opposing structures that accomplish a localized constriction of the vocal tract. Notice in the following definitions the two structures involved for the place terms.

Bilabial: two lips (*bi = two* and *labia = lip*)

Labial/velar: lips, and also a constriction between the *dorsum* or back of the tongue and the velum

Labiodental: lower lip and upper teeth

Linguadental or interdental: tip of tongue and upper teeth (*lingua = tongue*)

Lingua-alveolar: tip of tongue and the *alveolar ridge*

Linguapalatal: blade of tongue and palatal area behind the alveolar ridge

Linguavelar: dorsum or back of tongue and roof of mouth in the velar area

Glottal: the two vocal folds

Each of these places of articulation is discussed more fully below. To get a feeling for these different places of consonant articulation, concentrate on the first sounds in each word as you say the sequence: *pie, why, vie, thigh, tie, shy, guy, hi*. Notice from Figure 1.12 on p. 18 that the initial sounds constitute a progression from front to back in place of articulation.

TABLE 1.2 Classification of Consonants by Manner and Voicing within Place

Place of Articulation	Phonetic Symbol and Key Word	Manner of Articulation	Voicing
Bilabial	/p/ (pay)	Stop	−
	/b/ (bay)	Stop	+
	/m/ (may)	Nasal	+
Labial/velar	/ʍ/ (which)	Glide (semivowel)	−
	/w/ (witch)	Glide (semivowel)	+
Labiodental	/f/ (fan)	Fricative	−
	/v/ (van)	Fricative	+
Linguadental	/θ/ (thin)	Fricative	−
(interdental)	/ð/ (this)	Fricative	+
Lingua-alveolar	/t/ (two)	Stop	−
	/d/ (do)	Stop	+
	/s/ (sue)	Fricative	−
	/z/ (zoo)	Fricative	+
	/n/ (new)	Nasal	+
	/l/ (Lou)	Lateral	+
	/ɾ/ (butter)	Flap	+
Linguapalatal	/ʃ/ (shoe)	Fricative	−
	/ʒ/ (rouge)	Fricative	+
	/tʃ/ (chin)	Affricative	−
	/dʒ/ (gin)	Affricative	+
	/j/ (you)	Glide (semivowel)	+
	/r/ (rue)	Rhotic	+
Linguavelar	/k/ (back)	Stop	−
	/g/ (bag)	Stop	+
	/ŋ/ (bang)	Nasal	+
Glottal (laryngeal)	/h/ (who)	Fricative	−
	/ʔ/ —	Stop	+(−)

Table 1.3 provides a breakdown of English consonants by place and voicing within manner classes. The manner of production associated with complete closure is the *stop*, which is formed when two structures completely block the passage of air from the vocal tract, building up air pressure behind the closure. Usually, when the closure is released, the air pressure built up behind the constriction causes a burst of escaping air. The burst is audible in words like *pie* and *two*.

Fricatives, like the initial sounds in *sue* and *zoo*, are made with a narrow constriction so that the air creates a noisy sound as it rushes through the narrowed passage.

Affricates, as in *church* and *judge*, are combinations of stop and fricative segments; that is, a period of complete closure is followed by a brief fricative segment. The stop + fricative nature of the affricates explain why these sounds are represented by the digraph symbols /tʃ/ and /dʒ/.

TABLE 1.3   Classification of Consonants by Place and Voicing within Manner

Manner	Place	Voiced	Voiceless
Stop	Bilabial	b	p
	Alveolar	d	t
	Velar	g	k
	Glottal	------ ʔ -------------------	
Fricative	Labiodental	v	f
	Linguadental	ð	θ
	Alveolar	z	s
	Palatal	ʒ	ʃ
	Glottal		h
Affricative	Palatal	dʒ	tʃ
Nasal	Bilabial	m	
	Alveolar	n	
	Velar	ŋ	
Lateral	Alveolar	l	
Rhotic	Palatal	r	
Glide	Palatal	j	
	Labial/Velar	w	ʌ

Nasals, as in the word *meaning* /minɪŋ/, are like stops in having a complete oral closure (bilabial, lingua-alveolar, or linguavelar) but are unlike stops in having an open velopharyngeal port so that sound energy passes through the nose rather than the mouth.

The *lateral* /l/ as in *lay* is formed by making a lingua-alveolar closure in the midline but with no closure at the sides of the tongue. Therefore, the sound energy from the vibrating folds escapes laterally, or through the sides of the mouth cavity.

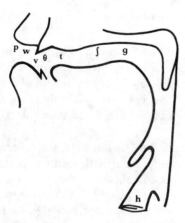

FIGURE 1.12   Places of articulation are marked by location of the phonetic symbols for the initial sounds in *pie, why, vie, thigh, tie, shy, guy, hi*.

The *rhotic* (or *rhotacized*) /r/ as in *ray* is a complex phoneme sometimes called *retroflex* in the phonetic literature. Retroflex literally means *turning* or *turned back* and refers to the appearance of the tongue tip, as viewed in X-ray films, for some /r/ productions. But in other productions of /r/, the tongue has a bunched appearance in the center or near the front of the mouth cavity. Because /r/ is produced in at least these two basic ways, the general term *rhotic* (Ladefoged, 1975) is preferable to the narrower term *retroflex*. This issue is discussed in more detail below.

The /ʍ/, /w/, and /j/ sounds are said to have a *glide* (semivowel) manner of production. These sounds are characterized by a gliding, or gradually changing, articulatory shape. For example, in /ʍ/ and its voiced counterpart /w/, the lips gradually move from a rounded and narrowed configuration to the lip shape required by the following vowel simultaneously with a change in tongue position from high-back (like that for /u/) to the position for the following vowel. The glides always are followed by vowels.

In the following summary, manner of articulation is discussed for different places of articulation, proceeding from front to back.

Bilabial Sounds

In American English, the only consonant phonemes produced with a complete or partial closure (bilabial production) are the voiceless and voiced stops /p/ as in *pay* and /b/ as in *bay*, the nasal /m/ as in *may*, and the voiced and voiceless glides /w/ as in *witch* and /ʍ/ as in *which*. The vocal tract configurations for /p/, /b/, and /m/ are shown in Figure 1.13. These three sounds share a bilabial closure but differ in voicing and nasality. The stops /p/ and /b/

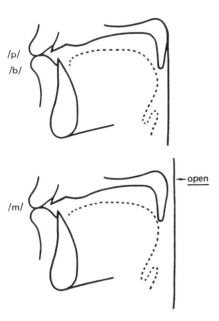

FIGURE 1.13   Vocal tract configurations for /p/, /b/, and /m/. Note labial closure for all three sounds and the open velopharynx for /m/.

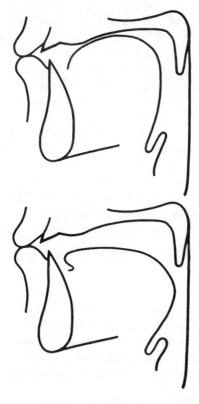

FIGURE 1.14   Variation in tongue position during a bilabial closure. Top: tongue position during *pea*; bottom: tongue position for *pa*.

are called voiced and voiceless *cognates*, which means that they differ only in voicing. The production of these bilabial sounds is usually marked by a closed jaw position because the jaw closes somewhat to assist the constriction at the lips. The tongue is virtually unconstrained for /p/, /b/, and /m/, so that these bilabial sounds often are made simultaneously with the tongue position for preceding or following vowels. In other words, when we say words like *bee*, *pa*, and *moo*, the tongue is free to assume the required shape for the vowel during the closure for the bilabial, as illustrated in Figure 1.14.

The glides /w/ and /ʍ/ have a specified tongue position, roughly like that for the high-back vowel /u/, so these sounds cannot interact as freely with preceding or following sounds. Students (and even some practicing clinicians) sometimes fail to appreciate the importance of tongue articulation for /w/ and /ʍ/; for these sounds, both the tongue and lips execute gliding movements, as shown for the word *we* in Figure 1.15.

Labiodental Sounds

The voiceless and voiced *fricatives* /f/ as in *fan* and /v/ as in *van* are the only labiodental sounds in American English. The articulation is illustrated in Figure 1.16. Frication noise

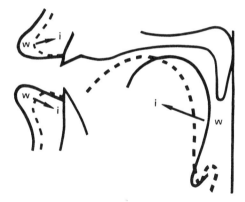

FIGURE 1.15   Illustration of gliding motion of tongue and lips for the word *we* **(/wi/).**

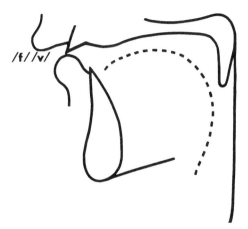

FIGURE 1.16   Vocal tract configuration for /f/ and /v/. Note labiodental constriction.

is generated by forcing air through the constriction formed by the lower lip and the upper teeth, principally the incisors. The noise is quite weak, very nearly the weakest of the fricatives. Like the labial sounds /p/, /b/, and /m/, the labiodentals allow the tongue to assume its position for preceding or following sounds. The jaw tends to close to aid the lower lip in its constricting gesture.

Interdental Sounds

There are only two interdentals, both fricatives: the voiceless /θ/ (e.g., *thaw*) and voiced /ð/ (e.g., *the*). They are illustrated in Figure 1.17. The frication noise is generated as air flows through the narrow constriction created by the tongue tip and the edge of the incisors. The weak frication noise is not much different from that for /f/ or /v/. The weak intensity of

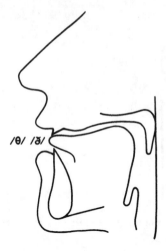

/θ/ /ð/

FIGURE 1.17   Vocal tract configuration for /θ/ and /ð/. Note linguadental constriction.

these sounds should be remembered in articulation testing, and the clinician should include both visual and auditory information in evaluating this pair of sounds. Jaw position for /θ/ and /ð/ usually is closed to aid the tongue in making its constriction. These sounds may be produced with either an interdental projection of the tongue or tongue contact behind the teeth.

Alveolar Sounds

The alveolar place of production is used for two stops: the voiceless /t/ (e.g., *too*) and the voiced /d/ (e.g., *do*); a nasal: /n/ (e.g., *new*); a lateral: /l/ (e.g., *Lou*); and two fricatives: the voiceless /s/ (e.g., *sue*) and the voiced /z/ (e.g., *zoo*). Not surprisingly, given the frequent and diverse movements of the tongue tip in the alveolar region, motions of the tongue tip are among the fastest articulatory movements. For example, the major closing and release movement for the stops /t/ and /d/ is made within about 50 milliseconds, or a twentieth of a second. For /t/ and /d/, an airtight chamber is created as the tongue tip closes firmly against the alveolar ridge and the sides of the tongue seal against the lateral oral regions. The site of tongue tip closure actually varies to a limited degree with phonetic context. When /t/ or /d/ are produced before the dental fricatives /θ/ and /ð/, the stop closure is made in the dental region. This context-dependent modification of alveolar consonant production is termed *dentalization* and is illustrated for /t/ in Figure 1.18.

The nasal /n/ is similar in basic tongue shape and movement to the stops /t/ and /d/. But /n/ differs from both /t/ and /d/ in having an open velopharyngeal port, making /n/ nasalized. But /n/ further differs from /t/ in that /n/ is voiced; /t/ is not. Because /n/ and /d/ are very similar in lingual articulation and voicing, failure to close the velopharyngeal port for /d/, as might happen with some speech disorders, results in /n/. Like /t/ and /d/, /n/ is dentalized when produced in the same syllable and adjacent to a dental sound like /θ/; compare, for example, the /n/ in *nine* /naɪn/ with the /n/ in *ninth* /naɪnθ/.

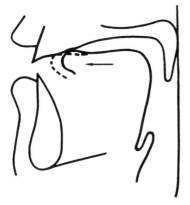

FIGURE 1.18   Dentalization of /t/. The normal alveolar closure is shown by the solid line and the dental closure is shown by the broken line.

The lateral /l/ is a *liquid* formed with midline closure and a lateral opening, usually at both sides of the mouth (see Figure 1.19). Because of the midline closure made by the tongue tip against the alveolar ridge, sound energy escapes through the sides of the oral cavity. Although /l/ is the only lateral sound in English, there are at least two major allo-

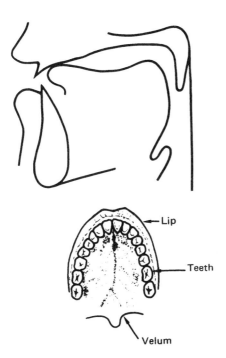

FIGURE 1.19   Articulation of /l/, shown in side view of a midline section (top) and as regions of tongue closure (shaded areas) against roof of mouth.

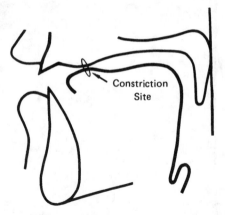

Constriction Site

FIGURE 1.20   Vocal tract configuration for /s/ and /z/. Note lingua-alveolar constriction.

phones. Historically, these allophones are termed *light* and *dark*, but phoneticians disagree as to exactly how these allophones are formed. Wise (1957a, 1957b) explained that the light /l/ is made with linguadental contact whereas the dark /l/ is made with a lingua-alveolar contact. However, Kantner and West (1960) contend that the light /l/ has a greater lip spread and a lower and flatter tongue position than the dark /l/. An important feature of /l/, presumably, is a raising of the tongue toward the velum or palate. Giles (1971) concluded from X-ray pictures of speech that for allophonic variations of /l/, the position of the tongue dorsum falls into three general groups regardless of phonetic context: prevocalic, postvocalic, and syllabic (with syllabic being similar to postvocalic /l/). The postvocalic allophones had a more posterior dorsal position than the prevocalic allophones. Tongue tip contact occasionally was not achieved for the postvocalic allophones in words like *Paul*. Otherwise, the only variation in tongue tip articulation was dentalization influenced by a following dental sound. Apparently, then, /l/ can be produced with either a relatively front (light /l/) or back (dark /l/) dorsal position, but the light and dark variants are perhaps just as well termed prevocalic and postvocalic. Lingua-alveolar contact is not essential at least for /l/ in postvocalic position, which explains why postvocalic /l/ in words like seal may sound like /o/ or /ʊ/. The fricatives /s/ and /z/ are made with a narrow constriction between the tongue tip and the alveolar ridge (Figure 1.20).

Palatal Sounds

The palatal sounds include the voiceless and voiced fricatives /ʃ/ (e.g., *shoe*) and /ʒ/ (e.g., *rouge*), the voiceless and voiced affricates /tʃ/ (e.g., *chin*) and /dʒ/ (e.g., *gin*), the glide /j/ (e.g., *you*), and the rhotic or retroflex /r/ (e.g., *rue*). For these sounds, the blade or tip of the tongue makes a constriction in the palatal region, the area just behind the alveolar ridge (see Figure 1.21).

The fricatives /ʃ/ and /ʒ/, like /s/ and /z/, are sibilants associated with intense noisy energy. For /ʃ/ and /ʒ/, this noise is generated as air moves rapidly through a constriction

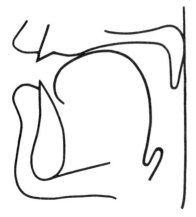

FIGURE 1.21   Vocal tract configuration for /ʃ/ and /ʒ/. Note linguapalatal constriction.

formed between the blade of the tongue and the front palate. Similarly, the affricates /tʃ/ and /dʒ/ are made in the palatal area as stop + fricative combinations. The airstream is first interrupted during the stop phase and then released during the fricative phase that immediately follows. In English, the only affricates are the palatal /tʃ/ and /dʒ/.

The glide /j/ is similar to the high-front vowel /i/ (as in *he*). The tongue is initially far forward and high in the mouth and subsequently moves toward the position for the following vowel. The similarity between /j/ and /i/ can be demonstrated by saying the biblical pronoun *ye* while noting the tongue position. Because the glide /j/ must be followed by a vowel, its articulation involves a gliding motion from the high-front position to some other vowel shape. The gliding motion can be felt during articulation of the words *you, yea, ya*.

As mentioned briefly above, the articulation of /r/ is highly variable. It sometimes is produced as a retroflexed consonant, in which case the tongue tip points upward and slightly backward in the oral cavity. But /r/ also can be produced with a bunching of the tongue, either in the middle of the mouth or near the front of the mouth. These basic articulations are illustrated in Figure 1.22. Some speakers also round their lips for /r/, and some

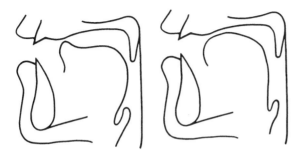

FIGURE 1.22   The two major articulations of /r/: *left,* **the retroflexed articulation;** *right,* **the bunched articulation.**

constrict the lower pharynx by pulling the root of the tongue backward. Because /r/ is variably produced, it seems advisable to use *rhotic* or *rhotacized* (Ladefoged, 1975) rather than *retroflex* as a general articulatory descriptor. Given the complicated articulation of /r/, it is not surprising that it should present a major problem to children learning to talk. The variation in tongue shape and position also complicates a speech clinician's attempts to teach /r/ articulations to a child who misarticulates the sound.

Velar Sounds

A velar constriction, formed by elevation of the tongue dorsum toward the roof of the mouth, occurs for the voiceless and voiced stops /k/ and /g/ and for the nasal /ŋ/. This articulation is illustrated in Figure 1.23, which shows that the constriction can be made with the tongue relatively toward the front or relatively toward the back. The tongue placement is generally determined by the vowel context, with a front placement for velars adjacent to front vowels (e.g., /g/ in *geese*) and a back placement for velars adjacent to back vowels (e.g., /g/ in *goose*). The nasal /ŋ/ has a tongue constriction similar to that for /k/ and /g/ but has an open velopharyngeal port for nasalization. The velar and bilabial places of articulation are similar in that both are used in English only for stops and nasals.

Glottal Sounds

The glottis, or chink between the vocal folds, is primarily involved only with two sounds, the voiceless fricative /h/ and the stop /ʔ/ (a stoppage of air at the vocal folds). The frica-

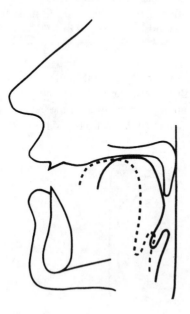

FIGURE 1.23   Vocal tract configurations for velar consonants. Note variation in site of closure.

tive is produced with an opening of the vocal folds so that a fricative noise is generated as air moves at high speed through the glottis. A similar vocal fold adjustment is used in whisper.

It can be seen from Tables 1.2 and 1.3 that more types of sounds are made at some places of articulation than at others. Moreover, some sounds occur more frequently in the English language than others, contributing to a further imbalance in the use of places of articulation. Actual data on the frequency of occurrence of English consonants, grouped by place of articulation, are shown in Figure 1.24. In this circle graph, based on data from Dewey (1923), the relative frequencies of occurrence of different places of articulation are shown by the relative sizes of the pieces of the graph. Notice that alveolar sounds account for almost 50 percent of the sounds in English. The rank order of frequency of occurrence for place of articulation, from most to least frequent, is: alveolar, palatal, bilabial, velar, labiodental, interdental, and glottal. Within each place-of-articulation segment in Figure 1.24, the individual consonants are listed in rank order of frequency of occurrence. For example, /n/ is the most frequently occurring alveolar consonant (in fact, it is the most frequently occurring of all consonants). Because of the differences in frequency of occurrence of consonants, a misarticulation affecting one place of articulation can be far more conspicuous than a misarticulation affecting another place. Therefore, statistical properties of the language are one consideration in the assessment and management of articulation disorders.

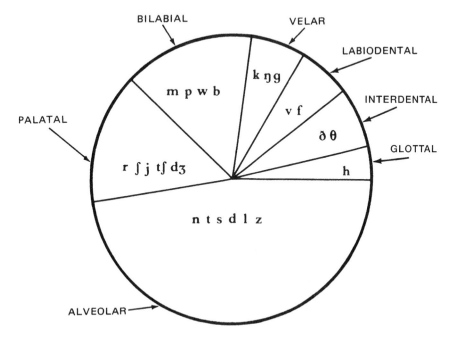

FIGURE 1.24   Circle graph showing relative frequency of occurrence of consonants made at different places of articulation. Based on data from Dewey (1923).

Consonant Articulation: Description by Distinctive Features

Distinctive features, discussed earlier with respect to vowels, can be used as an alternative to the place-manner chart to describe consonants. One simple example is the feature of voiced: All voiced consonants can be assigned the feature value of +voiced, and all voiceless consonants can be assigned the value of −voiced. Some important features for consonants are defined briefly below and are used for consonant classification in Table 1.4. These definitions are based on Chomsky and Hallé (1968).

> *Consonantal* sounds have a radical or marked constriction in the midsagittal region of the vocal tract. This feature distinguishes the "true" consonants from vowels and glides.
>
> *Vocalic* sounds do not have a radical or marked constriction of the vocal tract and are associated with spontaneous voicing. The voiced vowels and liquids are vocalic; the voiceless vowels and liquids, glides, nasal consonants, and obstruents (stops, fricatives, and affricates) are *nonvocalic* (that is, −vocalic).
>
> *Sonorant* sounds have a vocal configuration that permits spontaneous voicing, which means that the airstream can pass virtually unimpeded through the oral or nasal cavity. This feature distinguishes the vowels, glides, nasal consonants, and lateral and rhotacized consonants from the stops, fricatives and affricates (the class of obstruents).

TABLE 1.4   Distinctive Feature Classifications for Selected Consonants

Consonants

Feature	p	b	m	t	d	n	s	l	ø	k
Consonantal	+	+	+	+	+	+	+	+	+	+
Vocalic	−	−	−	−	−	−	−	−	−	−
Sonorant	−	−	+	−	−	+	−	+	−	−
Interrupted	+	+	−	+	+	−	−	−	−	+
Strident	−	−	−	−	−	−	+	−	−	−
High	(−)	(−)	(−)*	−	−	−	−	−	−	+
Low	(−)	(−)	(−)	−	−	−	−	−	−	−
Back	(−)	(−)	(−)	−	−	−	−	−	−	+
Anterior	+	+	+	+	+	+	+	+	+	−
Coronal	−	−	−	+	+	+	+	+	+	−
Rounded	−	−	−	−	−	−	−	−	−	−
Distributed	+	+	+	−	−	−	−	−	+	−
Lateral	−	−	−	−	−	−	−	+	−	−
Nasal	−	−	+	−	−	+	−	−	−	−
Voiced	−	+	+	−	+	+	−	+	−	−

*Feature values enclosed in parentheses indicate that the feature in question may not be specified for this sound. For example, tongue position for /p/, /b/, and /m/ is not really specified, as it is free to assume the position required for the following vowel.

Interrupted sounds have a complete blockage of the airstream during a part of their articulation. Stops and affricates are +interrupted, which distinguishes them from fricatives, nasals, liquids, and glides. Sometimes the feature *continuant* is used rather than interrupted, with opposite values assigned, that is, +continuant sounds are − interrupted and vice versa.

Strident sounds are those fricatives and affricates produced with intense noise: /s/, /z/, /ʃ/, /ʒ/, /tʃ/, /dʒ/. The amount of noise produced depends on characteristics of the constriction, including roughness of the articulatory surface, rate of air flow over it, and angle of incidence between the articulatory surfaces.

High sounds are made with the tongue elevated above its neutral (resting) position (see Figure 1.11a).

Low sounds are made with the tongue lowered below its neutral position (see Figure 1.11b).

Back sounds are made with the tongue retracted from its neutral position (see Figure 1.11c).

Anterior sounds have an obstruction that is farther forward than that for the palatal /ʃ/. Anterior sounds include the bilabials, labiodentals, linguadentals, and linguaalveolars.

Coronal sounds have a tongue blade position above the neutral state. In general, consonants made with an elevated tongue tip or blade are +coronal.

Rounded sounds have narrowed or protruded lip configuration.

Distributed sounds have a constriction extending over a relatively long portion of the vocal tract (from back to front). For English, this feature is particularly important to distinguish the dental fricatives /θ/ and /ð/ from the alveolars /s/ and /z/.

Lateral sounds are coronal consonants made with midline closure and lateral opening.

Nasal sounds have an open velopharynx allowing air to pass through the nose.

Voiced sounds are produced with vibrating vocal folds.

The feature assignments in Table 1.4 are for general illustration of the use of features. The features should be viewed with some skepticism, as several different feature systems have been proposed, and any one system is subject to modification. It should be understood that distinctive features are one type of classification system. It should also be realized that distinctive features have an intended linguistic function that may not always be compatible with their application to the study of articulation disorders. The issue is beyond the scope of this chapter, but the interested reader is referred to Walsh (1974) and Parker (1976).

The relationship between the traditional place terms of phonetic description and the distinctive features is summarized below. For each traditional place term, the associated features are listed. As an example, a bilabial stop is +anterior, −coronal, and +distributed. (The placement of both features within brackets indicates that they are considered together in sound description.)

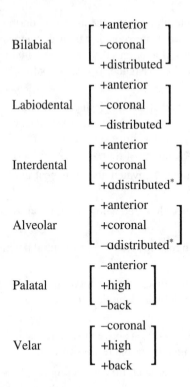

Bilabial $\begin{bmatrix} +\text{anterior} \\ -\text{coronal} \\ +\text{distributed} \end{bmatrix}$

Labiodental $\begin{bmatrix} +\text{anterior} \\ -\text{coronal} \\ -\text{distributed} \end{bmatrix}$

Interdental $\begin{bmatrix} +\text{anterior} \\ +\text{coronal} \\ +\alpha\text{distributed}^* \end{bmatrix}$

Alveolar $\begin{bmatrix} +\text{anterior} \\ +\text{coronal} \\ -\alpha\text{distributed}^* \end{bmatrix}$

Palatal $\begin{bmatrix} -\text{anterior} \\ +\text{high} \\ -\text{back} \end{bmatrix}$

Velar $\begin{bmatrix} -\text{coronal} \\ +\text{high} \\ +\text{back} \end{bmatrix}$

Suprasegmentals

The phonetic characteristics discussed to this point are *segmental*, which means that the units involved in the description are the size of phonemes or phonetic segments. *Suprasegmentals* are characteristics of speech that involve larger units, such as syllables, words, phrases, or sentences. Among the suprasegmentals are stress, intonation, loudness, pitch level, juncture, and speaking rate. Briefly defined, the suprasegmentals, also called *prosodies*, or *prosodic features*, are properties of speech that have a domain larger than a single segment. This definition does not mean that a single segment cannot, at times, carry the bulk of information for a given suprasegmental; on occasion, a segment, like a vowel, can convey most of the relevant information. Most suprasegmental information in speech can be described by the basic physical quantities of amplitude (or intensity), duration, and fundamental frequency (f_0) of the voice. Stated briefly, amplitude refers to the perceptual attribute of loudness; duration, to the perceptual attribute of length; and fundamental frequency, to the perceptual attribute of vocal pitch.

---

*The symbol α is a "dummy variable" and is used here to indicate that the Chomsky-Hallé features can distinguish the interdental and alveolar consonants only if they differ with respect to the feature *distributed*. Thus, if interdentals are regarded as −distributed, then alveolars must be +distributed. (See Ladefoged, 1971 for development of this issue.)

Stress

Stress refers to the degree of effort, prominence, or importance given to some part of an utterance. For example, if a speaker wishes to emphasize that someone should take the *red* car (as opposed to a blue or green one), the speaker might say "Be sure to take the *red* car," stressing *red* to signify the emphasis. There are several varieties of stress, but all generally involve something akin to the graphic underline used to denote emphasis in writing. Although underlining is seldom used in writing, stress is almost continually used in speech. In fact, any utterance of two or more syllables may be described in terms of its stress pattern. Because stress has influences that extend beyond the segment, stress usually is discussed with respect to syllables. The pronouncing guide of a dictionary places special marks after individual syllables to indicate stress. For example, the word *ionosphere* is rendered as (i-ɑn′ ə-sfer′), with the marks ′ and ′ signifying the primary and secondary stress for the syllables.

The International Phonetic Alphabet (IPA) uses a different stress notation from that commonly found in dictionaries. In IPA the stress mark precedes the syllable to which it refers, and the degree of stress is indicated by whether *any* stress mark is used and by the *location* of the stress mark in the *vertical* dimension. The strongest degree of stress is indicated by a mark above the symbol line: ′ɑn (rather like a superscript); the second degree of stress is indicated by a mark below the symbol line: ˌaɪ (like a subscript); and the third degree of stress is simply unmarked: ə. The word *ionosphere* is rendered as /ˌaɪ′ ɑn ə ˌsfir/, with three degrees of stress marked.

Acoustically, stress is carried primarily by the vowel segment within a syllable. The acoustic correlates, roughly in order of importance, are fundamental frequency (especially with a rise in fundamental frequency on or near the stressed syllable), vowel duration (greater duration with increased stress), relative intensity (greater intensity with increased stress), sound quality (reduction of a vowel to a weaker, unstressed form, like /ɑ/ to /ə/, vowel substitution, and consonant changes), and disjuncture (pauses or intervals of silence) (Rabiner, Levitt, and Rosenberg, 1969).

Another form of unstressed (or weakly stressed) syllable is the syllabic consonant. This type of consonant, usually an /l/, /m/, or /n/ (but infrequently /r/), acts like a vowel in forming a syllable nucleus. Examples of syllabic consonants are the final sounds in the words *battle* /bæt̩l/, *something* /sʌmʔm̩/, and *button* /bʌtn̩/. The syllabic function of a consonant is designated by a small vertical mark placed under the phonetic symbol. Syllabic consonants are most likely to occur when the consonant is *homorganic* (shares place of articulation) with a preceding consonant because it is economical or efficient simply to maintain the articulatory contact for both sounds. Additional information on stress will be provided following some basic definitions of related terms.

Intonation

Intonation is the vocal pitch contour of an utterance, that is, the way in which the fundamental frequency changes from syllable to syllable and even from segment to segment. Fundamental frequency can be affected by several factors, including the stress pattern of an utterance, tongue position of a vowel (high vowels have a higher f_0), and the speaker's emotional state.

Loudness

Loudness is related to sound intensity or to the amount of vocal effort that a speaker uses. Although loudness is ordinarily thought to be related to the amplitude or intensity of a sound, some evidence suggests that a listener's judgments of loudness of speech are related more directly to the perceived vocal effort, essentially the amount of work that a speaker does (Cavagna and Margaria, 1968). There is some evidence (Hixon, 1971; MacNeilage, 1972) that intensity variations in speech result mostly from respiratory activity, but variations of f_0 are easily accomplished at the level of the vocal folds.

Pitch Level

Pitch level is the average pitch of a speaker's voice and relates to the mean f_0 of an utterance. A speaker may be described as having a high, low, or medium pitch.

Juncture

Juncture, sometimes called "vocal punctuation," is a combination of intonation, pausing, and other suprasegmentals to mark special distinctions in speech or to express certain grammatical divisions. For example, the written sentence "Let's eat, Grandma," has a much different meaning than the same sentence without the comma, "Let's eat Grandma!" A speaker can mark a comma vocally with a short pause and an adjustment in intonation. Juncture is also used to make distinctions between similar articulations, such as between the word *nitrate* and the phrase *night rate*. Intonation and pausing enable a speaker to indicate which alternative he or she wants to express.

Speaking Rate

The rate of speaking is usually measured in words per second, syllables per second, or phonemes per second. As speaking rate increases, segment durations generally become shorter, with some segments affected more than others. The segments most vulnerable to contraction as a speaker talks more rapidly are pauses, vowels, and consonant segments involving a sustained articulation (like fricatives). Apparently, most speakers do not really increase the rate of individual articulatory movement as they increase their rate of speaking. Rather, they reduce the duration of some segments and reduce the overall range of articulatory movement (Lindblom, 1963). As a result, the articulatory positions normally assumed during a slow rate of speaking may be missed at a faster rate. The "missing" of articulatory positions as speaking rate increases is called *undershoot*. This is why a speaker's words are apt to sound less distinct to you as the rate of speaking increases.

Vowel Reduction

Vowels are particularly susceptible to articulatory change as speaking rate is increased or stress is decreased. Such articulatory alterations are termed *reduction* and are schematized in Figure 1.25. The arrows between pairs of vowels show directions of reduction; for exam-

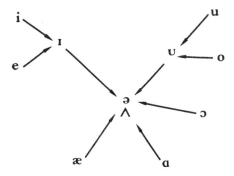

FIGURE 1.25   A scheme of vowel reduction. The arrows between vowel symbols show vowel changes resulting from reduction. For example, /i/ and /e/ reduce to /ɪ/, and /ɪ/ reduces to /ə/, which is the ultimate reduced vowel. Note that these changes occur within the quadrilateral defined by the corner vowels /i/, /æ/, /ɑ/, and /u/.

ple, /i/ reduces first to /ɪ/ and then to /ə/, the ultimate reduced vowel. The scheme shows that, with reduction, all vowels tend toward /ə/ or /ʌ/.

Clear versus Conversational Speech

There is considerable evidence to show that speakers alter their patterns of speech production depending on situation and listener. One variation is clear versus conversational speech. Clear speech is what speakers use when they are trying to be as intelligible as possible. Compared to more casual conversational speech, clear speech is (1) slower (with longer pauses between words and a lengthening of some speech sounds), (2) more likely to avoid modified or reduced forms of consonant and vowel segments (such as the vowel reduction described earlier), and (3) characterized by a greater intensity of obstruent sounds, particularly stop consonants (Picheny, Durlach, and Braida, 1986). When talkers want to be easily understood, they modify their speech to make it slower and more acoustically distinctive. Whereas vowels in conversational speech often are modified or reduced, therefore losing some of their acoustic distinctiveness, these sounds in clear speech are produced in distinctive forms. Similarly, word-final stops in conversational speech frequently are not released, so that the burst cue for their perception is eliminated. But in clear speech, stop consonants (and consonants in general) tend to be released and this feature enhances their perception.

These differences are central to a hypothesis proposed by Lindblom (1990) that speakers vary their speech output along a continuum from *hypospeech* to *hyperspeech* (the H&H hypothesis). The basic idea is that speakers adapt to the various circumstances of communication, to match their production patterns to communicative and situational factors. When a speaker believes that special care is required to be understood, he or she alters articulation accordingly. In Lindblom's view, clear speech (hyperspeech in his H&H hypothesis) is not simply loud speech but reflects an articulatory reorganization (Moon and Lindblom, 1989). Adams (1990), however, reported contrary evidence. He concluded from an X-ray microbeam study of speech movements that changes in speech clarity did not seem to reflect a reorganization of speech motor control. Adams observed that in clear speech, articulatory movements tended to be both larger and faster but there was no general indication that the speech patterns were organized differently than in conversational speech. The important point for clinical purposes is that speech articulation can be controlled by a speaker to enhance intelligibility when conditions warrant such deliberate effort. The primary articulatory change appears to be in the magnitude and speed of movement.

New versus Given Information

New information in a discourse is information that the listener would not be expected to know from the previous conversation or from the situation. Given information is predictable, either from the previous discourse or from the general situation. New information often is highlighted prosodically. For example, Behne (1989) studied prosody in a mini-discourse such as the following:

> "Someone painted the fence."
> "Who painted the fence?"
> "Pete painted the fence."

In this exchange, the new information ("Pete") is lengthened and produced with a higher fundamental frequency. In effect, the speaker uses prosody to highlight the new information.

Contrastive Stress in Discourse

Another discourse-related prosodic effect is *contrastive stress*. Such stress can be given to almost any word, phrase, or clause which the speaker considers to contradict or contrast with one that was previously expressed or implied. For instance, a speaker who wants to emphasize that she took the red ball rather than the green or blue one, might say, "I took the *red* ball" (where the italicized word receives contrastive stress). Contrastive stress is sometimes used clinically to give prosodic variation to an utterance or to elicit a stressed form of a target element.

Phrase-Final Lengthening

At the syntactic level, juncture and pause phenomena are used to mark multiword units. For example, in English, *phrase-final lengthening* operates to lengthen the last stressable syllable in a major syntactic phrase or clause. For example, if we contrast the following two sentences:

1. Red, green, and blue are my favorite colors.
2. Green, blue, and red are my favorite colors.

the word *blue* will be longer in (1) than in (2) because in the former this word is at the end of the subject noun phrase and is therefore subject to phrase-final lengthening. This regularity can be exploited clinically to obtain durational adjustments for a target word. In addition, Read and Schreiber (1982) showed that phrase-final lengthening is helpful to listeners in parsing (that is, to recognize the structure of) spoken sentences. They also suggested that children rely more on this cue than adults do, and, moreover, that prosody assists the language-learner by providing structural guides to the complex syntactic structures of language.

Declination

Another effect at the syntactic level is *declination*, or the effect in which the vocal fundamental frequency contour typically declines across clauses or comparable units. Why this tilt in the overall fundamental frequency pattern occurs is a matter of debate (Cohen, Collier, and t'Hart, 1982), but it is a robust feature of prosody at the sentence or clause level. This pattern is helpful to listeners in recognizing the structure of discourse, such as in identifying sentence units.

Lexical Stress Effects

These effects operate at the level of the word. For example, English has many noun–verb pairs like *'import* versus *im'port*, or *'contrast* versus *con'trast*, in which the difference between the members of a pair is signaled primarily by stress pattern. Another common effect at the word level occurs with a distinction between compounds and phrases. For example, the compound noun *'blackbird* contrasts with the noun phrase *black 'bird* (a bird that is black).

Although the lay listener often thinks stress in English is just a matter of giving greater intensity to part of an utterance, laboratory studies have shown that stress is signaled by duration, intensity, fundamental frequency, and various phonetic effects (Fry, 1955). It is important to remember that stress affects segmental properties such as the articulation of vowels and consonants (Kent and Netsell, 1972; de Jong, 1991). Segments in stressed syllables tend to have larger and faster articulatory movements than similar segments in unstressed syllables. For this reason, stressed syllables often are favored in some phases of articulation therapy.

Because suprasegmentals like stress and speaking rate influence the nature of segmental articulation, some care should be taken to control suprasegmental variables in articulation tests and speech materials used in treatment. Vowels carry much of the suprasegmental information in speech, but stress, speaking rate, and other suprasegmentals can influence consonant articulation as well. The suprasegmental features of speech have been discussed by Crystal (1973), Lehiste (1970), and Lieberman (1967), and the reader is referred to these accounts for a more detailed consideration of this complex area.

Coarticulation: Interactions Among Sounds in Context

Convenient though it might be to consider phonemes as independent, invariant units that are simply linked together to produce speech, this simplistic approach does not really fit the facts. When sounds are put together to form syllables, words, phrases, and sentences, they interact in complex ways and sometimes appear to lose their separate identity. The influence that sounds exert on one another is called *coarticulation*, which means that the articulation of any one sound is influenced by a preceding or following sound. Coarticulation makes it impossible to divide the speech stream into neat segments that correspond to phonemes. Coarticulation implies nonsegmentation, or, at least, interaction of the presumed linguistic segments. Hockett (1955) provided a colorful illustration of the transformation from phoneme to articulation:

> Imagine a row of Easter eggs carried along a moving belt; the eggs are of various sizes, and variously colored, but not boiled. At a certain point, the belt carries the row of eggs between the two rollers of a wringer, which quite effectively smashes them and rubs them more or less into each other. The flow of eggs before the wringer represents the series of impulses from the phoneme source. The mess that emerges from the wringer represents the output of the speech transmitter (210).

Although this analogy makes the process of articulation sound completely disorganized, in fact the process must be quite well organized if it is to be used for communication. Phoneme-sized segments may not be carried intact into the various contractions of the speech muscles, but some highly systematic links between articulation and phonemes are maintained. Research on speech articulation has provided a clearer understanding of what the links are although the total process is far from being completely understood.

It often is possible to describe coarticulation in terms of articulatory characteristics that spread from one segment to another. Examine the following examples of coarticulation:

1a. He sneezed   /h i s n i z d/ (unrounded /s/ and /s/)
1b. He snoozed   /h i s n u z d/ (rounded /s/ and /n/)
2a. He asked   /h i æ s k t/ (nonnasal /æ/)
2b. He answered /h i æ n s ɝ d/ (nasal /æ/)

The only phonemic difference between the first two items is the appearance of the unrounded vowel /i/ in 1a and the appearance of the rounded vowel /u/ in 1b. The lip rounding for /u/ in *He snoozed* usually begins to form during the articulation of the /s/. You might be able to feel this *anticipatory lip rounding* as you alternately say *sneeze* and *snooze* with your finger lightly touching your lips. In articulatory terms, the feature of lip rounding for the vowel is assumed during the /sn/ consonant cluster as the consequence of anticipating the rounding. The contrast between *sneeze* and *snooze* shows that the /sn/ cluster acquires lip rounding only if it is followed by a rounded vowel. This example of sound interaction is termed *anticipatory lip rounding* because the articulatory feature of rounding is evident before the rounded vowel /u/ is fully articulated as a segment.

Another form of anticipatory coarticulation occurs in 2b. Perhaps you can detect a difference in the quality of the /æ/ vowel in the phrases *He asked* and *He answered*. You should be able to detect a nasal quality in the latter because the vowel tends to assume the nasal resonance required for the following nasal consonant /n/. In this case, we can say that the articulatory feature of velopharyngeal opening (required for nasal resonance) is anticipated during the vowel /æ/. Normally, of course, this vowel is not nasalized. The contrasts between 1a and 1b and between 2a and 2b illustrate a type of coarticulation called *antici-patory*. Another type, *retentive*, applies to situations in which an articulatory feature is retained after its required appearance. For example, in the word *me* the vowel /i/ tends to be nasalized because of a carry-over velopharyngeal opening from the nasal consonant /m/. The essential lesson to be learned is that coarticulation occurs frequently in speech, so frequently in fact that the study of articulation is largely a study of coarticulation.

Phonetic context is highly important in understanding allophonic variation. For example, you should be able to detect a difference in the location of linguavelar closure for the /k/ sounds in the two columns of words below.

keen	*coon*
kin	*cone*
can	*con*

The point of closure tends to be more to the front of the oral cavity for the words in the first column than it is for the words in the second column. This variation occurs because, in English, the velar stops /k/ and /g/ do not have a narrowly defined place of articulation; all that is required is that the dorsum, or back, of the tongue touch the ceiling of the mouth. Therefore, the tongue is simply elevated at the position needed for the following vowel. When the tongue is in the front of the mouth (note that the vowels in the left column are front vowels), the dorsal closure is made in the front of the mouth, and when the tongue is in the back of the mouth (as it would be for the vowels in the right column), the point of closure is to the back of the velar surface.

Coarticulation arises for different reasons, some having to do with the phonology of a particular language, some with the basic mechanical or physiological constraints of the speech apparatus. Hence, some coarticulations are learned and others are the inevitable consequences of muscles, ligaments, and bones of the speech apparatus that are linked together and unable to move with infinite speed. Consider, for example, the closing and opening of the velopharyngeal port. This articulatory gesture is rather sluggish (compared to movements of the tongue tip), so it is not surprising that the velopharyngeal opening for a nasal consonant carries over to a following vowel, as in the word *no*. The extent of this carryover nasalization, however, varies with the phonologic characteristics of a particular language. In French, vowel nasalization is phonemic (that is, it can make a difference in meaning), but in English, vowel nasalization is only allophonic. Some aspects of coarticulation reflect universal properties of the human speech mechanism and hence affect all languages. Other coarticulations are governed by the phonemic structure of a particular language and are therefore learned with that language. Many coarticulatory effects are assimilatory in that a feature from one segment is adopted by an adjacent segment. For example, the nasalization of vowels by neighboring nasal consonants is nasal assimilation. Such effects may make speech production easier and faster because articulatory movements can be adapted to a particular phonetic and motor sequence. Assimilation is a general process in spoken language and will be taken up later in discussions of phonology.

Another aspect of coarticulation is the overlapping of articulations for consonants in clusters. Quite often, the articulation for one consonant is made *before* the release of a preceding consonant in any two-consonant cluster. For example, in the word *spy* /spaɪ/, the bilabial closure for /p/ is accomplished shortly (about 10 to 20 msec) before the release of the constriction for /s/. This overlapping of consonant articulations makes the overall duration of the cluster shorter than the sum of the consonant durations as they occur singly; that is, the duration of /sp/ in *spy* is shorter than the sum of the durations of /s/ in *sigh* /s aɪ/ and /p/ in *pie* /p aɪ/. The overlapping of articulation contributes to the articulatory flow of speech by eliminating interruptions. The temporal structure of an /spr/ cluster, as in the word *spray*, is pictured schematically in Figure 1.26. Notice that the constrictions for /s/ and /p/ overlap by 10 to 20 milliseconds and that the closure for /p/ overlaps with the tongue position for /r/ by a similar amount. Because consonants in clusters frequently present special difficulties to children (and adults) with articulation disorders, clinicians must know how such clusters are formed. Because clusters have overlapping articulations of the constituent consonants, in general, the cluster is a tightly organized sequence of articulatory gestures. The articulation of clusters is further complicated by allophonic variations, such as those listed in Table 1.5. In English, unaspirated released stops occur only when stops follow /s/, as in the words *spy*, *stay*, and *ski*. Otherwise, released stops are aspirated, meaning that the release is followed by a brief interval of glottal frication (an /h/-like noise). Similarly, the devoiced /l/ and /r/ normally occur only after voiceless consonants, as in the words *play* and *try*.

The examples of context-dependent articulatory modifications in Table 1.5 show the variety of influences that sounds exert on adjacent sounds. For a given sound, place of articulation, duration, voicing, nasalization, and rounding may vary with phonetic context, and these variations are noted with the special marks shown in Table 1.5.

Some aspects of coarticulation can be understood by knowing the extent to which individual sounds restrict the positions of the various articulators. Table 1.6 summarizes degrees of restriction on lips, jaw, and parts of the tongue for the different places of consonant articulation. A strong restriction is indicated by an X, a slight to moderate restriction by a –, and a minimal restriction by an O. Because this table shows which parts of the vocal tract are free to vary during articulation of a given consonant, it can be used to predict certain aspects of coarticulation. For example, because bilabial sounds do not restrict the tongue as long as it does not close off the tract, Os are indicated for all parts of the tongue. Jaw position is shown as moderately restricted for most places of articulation because some degree of jaw closing usually aids consonant formation. The ability of jaw movement to aid tongue movement declines as place of articulation moves back in the mouth, so a velar con-

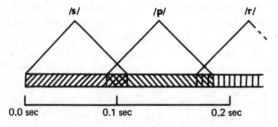

FIGURE 1.26   Schematic drawing of the articulatory organization of a /spr/ consonant cluster (as in the word *spray*), showing overlapping of consonantal articulations. Based on data from Kent and Moll (1975).

TABLE 1.5 Examples of Context-Dependent Modifications of Phonetic Segments

Modification	Context Description
Nasalization of vowel	Vowel is preceded or followed by a nasal, e.g., [ɔ̃n]—*on* and [mæ̃n]—*man*
Rounding of consonant	Consonant precedes a rounded sound, e.g., [kʷwin]—*queen* and [tʷru]—*true*
Palatalization of consonant	Consonant precedes a palatal sound, e.g., [kiʃ ju]—*kiss you*
Devoicing of obstruent	Word-final position of voiced consonant, e.g., [dɔg̥]—*dog* and [liv̥]—*leave*
Devoicing of liquid	Liquid follows word-initial voiceless sound, e.g., [pl̥eɪ]—*play* and [tr̥i]—*tree*
Dentalization of coronal	Normally alveolar sound precedes a dental sound, e.g., [wɪd̪ə]—*width* and [naɪn̪ə]—*ninth*
Retroflexion of fricative	Fricative occurs in context of retroflex sounds, e.g., [harʂɚ]—*harsher* and [pɝʂɚ]—*purser*
Devoicing of sound	Consonant or vowel in voiceless context, e.g., [sɪ̥stɚ]—*sister*
Lengthening of vowel	Vowel preceding voiced sound, especially in stressed syllable, e.g., [ni : d]—*need*
Reduction of vowel	Vowel in unstressed (weak) syllable, e.g., [tæbjuleɪt] [tæbjeleɪt]—*tabulate*
Voicing of sound	Voiceless in voiced context, e.g., [æbs̬ɝd]—*absurd*
Deaspiration of stop	Stop follows /s/, e.g., [sp = aɪ]—*spy* vs. [pʰaɪ]—*pie*

sonant may not restrict jaw position as much as more frontal articulation (Kent and Moll, 1972). The only sound that allows essentially unrestricted coarticulation is the glottal /h/. Thus, /h/ usually is made with a vocal-tract configuration adjusted to an adjacent sound, such as the following vowel in the words *he* /hi/, *who* /hu/, *ham* /hæm/, and *hop* /hɑp/.

Investigators of speech articulation (Daniloff and Moll, 1968; Moll and Daniloff, 1971; Kent and Minifie, 1977) have shown extensive overlapping of articulatory gestures across phoneme-sized segments, causing debate about the size of unit that governs behavior. Some investigators propose that the decision unit is an allophone, others argue for the phoneme, and still others for the syllable. A popular syllable-unit hypothesis is one based on CV (consonant-vowel) syllables, with allowance for consonant clustering (CCV, CCCV, and so on). This hypothesis states that articulatory movements are organized in sequences of the form CV, CCV, CCCV, and the like, so that a word like *construct* would be organized as the articulatory syllables /kɑ/ + /nstrʌkt/. Notice the odd assembly of the second syllable. This issue is of more than academic importance. Discovery of the basic decision unit would have implications for speech remediation; for example, enabling a speech clinician to choose the most efficient training and practice items for correcting an error sound. In addition, syllabic structures may explain certain features of speech and language development as discussed by Branigan (1976).

TABLE 1.6 Coarticulation Matrix, Showing for Each Place of Consonant Articulation Those Articulators That Have Strong Restrictions on Position (Marked with X), Those That Have Some Restriction on Position (Marked with —), and Those That Are Minimally Restricted (Marked with O). For Example, the Bilabials /b/, /p/, and /m/ Strongly Restrict the Lips, Moderately Restrict the Jaw, and Leave the Tongue Essentially Free to Vary. The Glides /w/ and /ʌ/ Are Not Included Because They Involve Secondary Articulations. Lip Rounding, as Often Occurs for /r/, Has Been Neglected.

| | | | *Tongue* | | | |
Place	Lip	Jaw	Tip	Blade	Dorsum	Body
Bilabial /bpm/	X	—	O	O	O	O
Labiodental /vf/	X	—	O	O	O	O
Interdental /ðθ/	O	—	X	X	—	—
Alveolar /dtzsln/	O	—	X	X	—	—
Palatal /ʃ ʒ dʒ tʃ j r/	O	—	—	X	X	X
Velar /gkŋ/	O	O	O	—	X	X
Glottal /h/	O	O	O	O	O	O

Coarticulation also has clinical relevance, in that a sound might be more easily learned or more easily produced correctly in one context than in others. In other words, the phonetic context of a sound can facilitate or even interfere with correct production of the sound. The effect of phonetic context could explain why misarticulations are often inconsistent, with correct production on certain occasions and incorrect productions on others. By judiciously selecting the phonetic context where an error sound is initially corrected, the clinician can sometimes enhance the efficiency of speech remediation. Such examples show why a thorough knowledge of articulatory phonetics is important to decisions in the management of articulation disorders.

There is considerable theoretical controversy about how speech is organized as a motor behavior. Figure 1.27, which illustrates the controversy, depicts three levels of speech organization. (Actually, some contributors to the debate do not agree that these three levels are required; however, since most writers recognize them, they are used here.) The highest level is a sequence of units. This sequence may take the form of a psychological network of conceptual dependencies, a surface-structure representation of words (as suggested by Chomsky), or a syntagma (a rhythmic organization of syllables).

Most experts (it is hard to think of an exception) recognize the existence of some basic speech unit, the second level of Figure 1.27, but they disagree about the nature of this

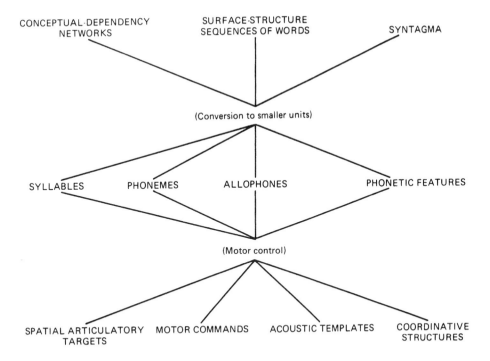

FIGURE 1.27 **Some alternative representations at three levels of organization of speech production. The top level is one of networks or strings, the middle level refers to a basic unit of speech production, and the third level pertains to the direct motor control of speech.**

unit. Some prefer the syllable, others the phoneme, others the allophone, and still others the phonetic feature. Moreover, some think all of these units are involved in a hierarchical organization, with syllables branching into phonemes, phonemes into allophones, and allophones into features.

The third level is motor control—the level at which the basic unit described above is converted into instructions that tell the muscles of speech what to do. One candidate for this level is a spatial articulatory target, a kind of snapshot of what the total vocal tract configuration should be. A second candidate is the motor command, presumed to be identical for each occurrence of the basic control unit (whatever that may be!). For those experts who believe the speech system tries to produce patterns that fit the acoustic goals of speech, the third candidate is an acoustic template. And finally, a relatively recent view identifies this level as a coordinative structure, an assembly of elementary movements that defines a basic unit of action. Obviously, there is no lack of theory!

Aerodynamic Considerations in Speech Production

Because the production of speech depends on the supply and valving of air, a knowledge of air pressure, flow, and volume is essential to an understanding of both normal and disordered speech. Many abnormalities of speech production are caused by irregularities or deficiencies in the supply and valving of air, and a number of clinical assessment techniques rely on measures of air pressure, flow, or volume. To understand the regulation of air pressures and flows in speech, it is important to recognize that (1) air flows only in one direction—from a region of greater pressure to one of lesser pressure; and (2) whenever the vocal tract is closed at some point, the potential exists for the buildup of air pressure behind the closure.

English speech sounds are normally *regressive*, meaning that, in sound production, air flows from the inside (usually the lungs) to the outside (the air around us). The basic energy needed to produce sound is developed in the lungs. After air is inspired by enlargement of the lung cavity, the muscle activation changes so that the lung cavity returns to a smaller size. If the airway above is closed, the same volume of air is enclosed in a smaller space. Because the same amount of air is contained in a smaller cavity, the air pressure within the lungs increases. This overpressure (relative to atmosphere) in the lungs is the source of the regressive air flow for all speech sounds. It is a fact of clinical importance that the air flow requirements for speech are not much greater than the requirements for ordinary breathing; that is, the volume of air inspired and expired in speaking is not much different from that in quiet respiration.

The regulation of air pressure and flow for speech is diagrammed in Figure 1.28, a simple model of the vocal tract. This model, in the form of the letter F, shows the three general areas where constriction (narrowing or closure) can occur: the laryngeal, oral, and nasal sections. The first site of constriction for egressive air is in the larynx. If the vocal folds close tightly, no air can escape from the lungs. If the folds are maximally open, then air passes through the larynx readily. If the folds are closed with a moderate tension, then the buildup of air pressure beneath them eventually blows them apart, releasing a pulse of air. After the folds are blown apart, they quickly come together again through the action of various physical restoring forces. This alternation of closed and open states, occurring many times per second, is called voicing. Successive pulses of air from the vocal folds are a source of acoustic energy for all voiced sounds, such as vowels.

The F-shaped vocal tract model shown in Figure 1.28a illustrates the air flow for vowel sounds. The vocal folds are shown as being partly closed to represent the vibratory pattern of opening and closing. The nasal tube is tightly closed because vowels in English are nonnasal unless they precede or follow nasal consonants. The oral tube is widely open to represent the open oral cavity in vowel articulation. Because the nasal tube is closed, the acoustic energy from the vibrating vocal folds passes through the oral tube.

The configuration of the vocal tract for a voiceless stop like /p/, /t/, or /k/ is diagrammed in Figure 1.28b. The constriction at the larynx is shown as completely open because air from the lungs passes readily through the larynx and into the oral cavity. The constriction at the velopharynx is shown as closed to indicate that no air flows through the nasal tube. The oral constriction is closed to represent the period of stop closure. After this period, the oral constriction opens rapidly to allow a burst of air to escape from the oral pressure chamber. Assuming a stop closure of suitable duration, the air pressure developed within the oral cavity can be nearly equal to that in the lungs because the open vocal folds permit an equalization of air pressure in the airway reaching from the lungs up to the oral cavity. Therefore, voiceless stops have high intraoral air pressures. Also, it should be noted

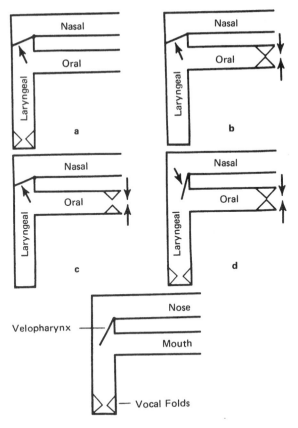

FIGURE 1.28   Simple models of vocal tract for major sound classes: a—vowels, liquids, and glides; b—voiceless stops; c—voiceless fricatives; d—nasals. The major parts of the model are shown at the bottom of the figure.

that children may use *greater* intraoral air pressures than adults (Subtelny, Worth, and Sakuda, 1966; Bernthal and Beukelman, 1978; Netsell, Lotz, Peters, and Schulte, 1994).

The model for voiceless fricatives in Figure 1.28c is like that for voiceless stops, but instead of a complete oral constriction, the model has a very narrow constriction, required for fricative noise. Because the velopharyngeal constriction is tightly closed and the laryngeal constriction is open, voiceless fricatives like /s/ and /ʃ/ have high intraoral air pressures. The voiceless stops and fricatives are sometimes called *pressure consonants*.

Voiced stops and fricatives differ from voiceless stops and fricatives in having vibrating vocal folds. Therefore, the models in Figures 1.28b and 1.28c would have a partial laryngeal constriction to represent voicing of these sounds. Because a certain amount of air pressure is lost in keeping the vocal folds vibrating (that is, pressure across the glottis drops), the voiced stops and fricatives have smaller intraoral air pressures than their voiceless cognates.

Finally, the model for nasal consonants is depicted in Figure 1.28d. A partial constriction at the larynx represents the vibrating vocal folds, and a complete oral constriction
represents the stop-like closure in the oral section of the vocal tract. For nasal consonants,
the acoustic energy of voicing is directed through the nasal cavity. Very little air pressure
builds up within the oral chamber.

Liquids and glides can be modeled in essentially the same way as vowels (Figure
1.28a). Because the oral constriction for these sounds is only slightly greater than that for
vowels, there is very little intraoral air pressure buildup.

Pressures and flows can be used to describe the function of many parts of the speech
system. For example, a normal efficient operation of the larynx can often be distinguished
from inefficient pathological states by the excessive air flow in the latter conditions. This
excessive flow, or air wastage, may be heard as breathiness or hoarseness. Velopharyngeal
incompetence can be identified by recording air flow from the nose during normally nonnasal segments. Frequently, velopharyngeal incompetence is signaled both by inappropriate nasal air flow (for example, air flow during stops or fricatives) and by reduced levels of
intraoral air pressure. Sometimes, more than one pressure or flow must be recorded to
identify the problem. For example, reduced levels of intraoral air pressure for consonants
can be related to at least three factors: (1) respiratory weakness, resulting in insufficient air
pressure; (2) velopharyngeal dysfunction, resulting in a loss of air through the nose; or (3)
an inadequacy of the oral constriction, allowing excessive air to escape.

Clinically, aerodynamic assessment is especially important when dealing with a
structural defect (such as cleft palate) or a physically based control problem as in cerebral
palsy, vocal fold paralysis, and other neurologic disorders). As noted above, young children
may use greater intraoral air pressure than adults for constant production, so normative
pressure data obtained from adults should be used with caution in clinical evaluation of
children. Moreover, the higher pressures in children's speech mean that children must close
the velopharyngeal port even more tightly than adults to prevent nasal loss of air during
stop or fricative consonants. Speech and language clinicians who do not possess equipment
for aerodynamic recordings of speech should nonetheless be aware of the pressure and flow
requirements in speech production. These requirements have important implications for the
diagnosis and evaluation of communicative problems and for the design of remediation
programs.

Acoustic Considerations of Speech

It is far beyond the scope of this chapter to consider in any detail the acoustic structure of
speech sounds, but it is possible to draw here a few major conclusions about the acoustic
signal of speech. Acoustic signals can be described in terms of three fundamental physical
variables—frequency, amplitude, and duration. *Frequency* refers to the rate of vibration of
a sound. Generally, the faster the rate of vibration, the higher the pitch heard. In other
words, frequency is the most direct physical correlate of pitch. *Amplitude* refers to the
strength or magnitude of vibration of a sound. The higher the magnitude of vibration, the
louder the sound heard. Amplitude is the most direct physical correlate of loudness.

Because the actual amplitude of vibration is minute and, therefore, difficult to measure, sound intensity or sound pressure level is used instead when making actual speech measurements. *Duration* refers to the total time over which a vibration continues. Duration is the most direct physical correlate of perceived length.

Virtually all naturally occurring sounds, speech included, have energy at more than a single frequency. A tuning fork is designed to vibrate at a single frequency and is one of the very few sound sources with this property. The human voice, musical instruments, and animal sounds all have energy at several frequencies. The particular pattern of energy over a frequency range is the *spectrum* of a sound. Speech sounds differ in their *spectra*, and these differences allow us to distinguish sounds perceptually.

Table 1.7 is a summary of the major acoustic properties of several phonetic classes. The table shows the relative sound intensity, the dominant energy region in the spectrum, and the relative sound duration for each class. Vowels are the most intense speech sounds, have most of their energy in the low to mid frequencies, and are longer in duration than other sounds (although the actual duration of vowel sounds may range from about 50 milliseconds to half a second). Because vowels are the most intense sounds, they typically determine the overall loudness of speech. The most intense vowels are the low vowels and the least intense, the high vowels.

The glides and liquids are somewhat less intense than the vowels and have most of their energy in the low to mid frequencies. The duration of the glides /w/ and /j/ tends to be longer than that of the liquids /l/ and /r/.

The strident fricatives and affricates (/s, z, ʃ, ʒ, tʃ, dʒ/) are more intense than other consonants but considerably weaker than vowels. The stridents have energy primarily at the high frequencies and, therefore, are vulnerable to high-frequency hearing loss. A good tape recording of the stridents requires a recorder with a wide frequency response. Stridents tend to be relatively long in duration, especially compared to other consonants, and fricatives typically are longer than affricates.

The nasals are sounds of moderate intensity, low-frequency energy, and brief to moderate duration. The nasals have more energy at very low frequencies than do other sounds.

The stops are relatively weak sounds of brief duration. The burst that results from release of a stop closure can be as short as 10 milliseconds. The primary energy for stops

TABLE 1.7 Summary of Acoustic Features for Six Phonetic Classes

Sound Class	Intensity	Spectrum	Duration
Vowels	Very strong	Low frequency dominance	Moderate to long
Glides and liquids	Strong	Low frequency dominance	Short to moderate
Strident fricatives and affricates	Moderate	High frequency dominance	Moderate
Nasals	Moderate	Very low frequency dominance	Short to moderate
Stops	Weak	Varies with place of articulation	Short
Nonstrident fricatives	Weak	Flat	Short to moderate

varies over a wide range of frequencies—from low to high; bilabials have relatively low-frequency energy, while velars and alveolars have most of their energy in, respectively, the mid and mid to high frequencies.

The nonstrident fricatives /f, v, θ, ð/ are weak sounds of typically moderate duration. They tend to have a flat spectrum, meaning that the noise energy is distributed fairly uniformly over the frequency range. Of all sounds, /θ/ usually is the weakest-so weak that it can barely be heard when produced in isolation at any distance from a listener.

Finally, two points should be made concerning acoustic implications for clinical assessment and management. First, the absolute frequency location of energy for speech sounds varies with speaker age and sex. Men have the lowest overall frequencies of sound energy, women somewhat higher frequencies, and young children the highest frequencies. This relationship follows from the acoustic principle that an object's resonance frequency is inversely related to its length. The longest pipe in a pipe organ has a low frequency (or low pitch) and the shortest pipe a high frequency (high pitch); similarly the adult male vocal tract is longer than a woman's or a child's and therefore has resonances of lower frequency. This difference has practical implications. Most acoustic data have been collected for men's speech; much less is known about women's or children's speech, and the data for men may not be directly applicable to either. Moreover, the recording and analysis of women's and children's speech requires a wider frequency range than that suitable for men's speech. This issue can be particularly important for fricatives and affricates.

Second, because speech sounds vary widely in intensity, dominant energy region, and duration, they are not equally discriminable under different listening situations. The acoustic differences summarized in Table 1.7 should be kept in mind when testing articulation or auditory discrimination.

Sensory Information in Speech Production

As speech is produced, a number of different kinds of sensory information is generated. The types of information include tactile (touch and pressure), proprioceptive (position sense), kinesthetic movement sense), and auditory. The total sensory information is genuinely plurimodal, that is, available in several modalities. Most authorities agree that the rich sensory information associated with speech production is particularly important in speech development and in the management of some speech disorders, as when a child must learn a new articulatory pattern. A clinician therefore should be knowledgeable about the kinds and characteristics of sensory, or afferent, information.

The major characteristics of the sensory systems in speech were reviewed by Hardcastle (1976) and more recently by Kent, Martin, and Sufit (1990). Tactile receptors, which consist of free nerve endings and complex endings (for example, Krause end-bulbs and Meissner corpuscles), supply information to the central nervous system on the nature of contact (including localization, pressure, and onset time) and direction of movement. Remarkably, the oral structures are among the most sensitive regions of the body. The tongue tip is particularly sensitive and can therefore supply detailed sensory information. Tactile receptors belong to a more general class of receptors called mechanoreceptors (which respond to mechanical stimulation). These receptors respond not only to physical contacts of articulatory structures but also to air pressures generated during speech.

The proprioceptive and kinesthetic receptors include the muscle spindles, Golgi tendon organs, and joint receptors. Muscle spindles provide rich information on the length of muscle fibers, degree and velocity of stretch, and the direction of movement of a muscle. Golgi receptors relay information on the change of stretch on a tendon caused by muscular contraction or by other influences, including passive movement. Joint receptors, located in the capsules of joints, inform the central nervous system on the rate, direction, and extent of joint movement. Even a relatively simple movement, such as closing the jaw and raising the tongue, supplies a variety of afference to the central nervous system.

The auditory system supplies information on the acoustic consequences of articulation. Because the purpose of speech is to produce an intelligible acoustic signal, auditory feedback is of particular importance in regulating the processes of articulation. Interestingly, when an adult suffers a sudden and severe loss of hearing, speech articulation usually does not deteriorate immediately, but only gradually. The other types of sensory information are probably sufficient to maintain the accuracy of articulation for some time.

Many tactile receptors are comparatively slow acting because the neural signals travel along relatively small fibers in a multisynaptic pathway (a pathway composed of several neurons). Much of the tactile information is available to the central nervous system after the event to which it pertains. This information is particularly important to articulations that involve contact between articulatory surfaces, such as stops and fricatives. Obviously, prolonging an articulation helps to reinforce its sensory accompaniment. When the mucosal surfaces of the articulators are anesthetized, one of the most disturbed class of sounds is the fricatives.

Generative Phonology

Phonology has been defined as the part of linguistics concerned with "putting sounds together" or "putting sounds into words." Somewhat more precisely, Sloat, Taylor, and Hoard define phonology as "the science of speech sounds and sound patterns" (1978; 1). These authors note that each language has its own sound pattern, which is (1) the set of sounds used by a certain language, (2) the acceptable arrangement of these sounds to form words, and (3) the various processes by which sounds are added, deleted, or changed. Thus, the sound patterns of different languages can differ in the sounds available for use, the permissible ordering of these sounds, and the rules or processes that operate on the sounds. Phonological rules are prescriptions that convert abstract phonological representations into phonetic representations. An example from Hyman (1975) is the pronunciation of the verb *miss*. The word is pronounced /mis/ in the phrase *we miss it* but /mɪʂ/ in the phrase *we miss you*. In English, the /s/ often is palatalized when it is followed by a palatal /j/ (which itself may be deleted). Thus, the morpheme *miss* has these two pronunciations determined by the phonology of English.

Phonological processes are operations that affect sound change, both within individual language users and within the history of a particular language. Some examples of processes are cluster reduction: *snow* /snoʊ/ → /noʊ/; deletion of unstressed syllables: *baloney* /bəloʊnɪ/ → /bloʊnɪ/; and final consonant devoicing: *pig* /pɪg/ → /pɪk/. Other examples will be discussed later in this chapter and in other chapters of this book.

Although this chapter is not directly concerned with linguistics, the student should at least recognize the relevance of some phonological principles to the study of normal and disordered articulation. The study of phonology offers many important insights into the interactions among sound segments and the interactions between speech articulation and higher levels of linguistic organization. In a sense, phonological analysis is a key to the door between articulation and the various levels of language structure. Many aspects of articulation—such as the duration of constriction for an /s/, the duration of a vowel sound, the occurrence of palatalization for consonants, or the devoicing of a normally voiced segment—can be understood through the study of phonology.

Some of the interactions among units in the oral expression of language can be described and perhaps even explained through *phonological rules*. A phonological rule is a formal expression of a regularity that occurs in the phonology of a language or in the phonology of an individual speaker. These rules are either *context-free* or *context-sensitive*. A context-free rule is not dependent on a specific context. For example, if a child always substitutes (replaces) stops for fricatives (e.g., *sees* /siz/ becomes /tid/), we can formulate a rule that states simply that fricatives become stops:

Fricative → Stop

In this example, the word *fricative* represents the category of fricatives and the word *stop* represents the category of stops and the arrow means "is replaced by." Thus, the rule means that a fricative unit is replaced by a stop unit. Because this change or replacement always occurs, it is not necessary to state any context restriction on its operation.

On the other hand, assume that a child replaces fricatives with stops only in the initial position of a syllable; for example /si/ (*see*) becomes /ti/ and /zu/ (*zoo*) becomes /du/. The restriction to syllable-initial position is a context restriction, or a constraint on the operation of the rule. To formalize this operation, the following rule can be used:

Fricative → Stop   /   #   ___

This rule states that a fricative unit is replaced by a stop unit if the fricative is in the context such that it initiates a syllable. The slash / means "in the environment such that," the # represents a syllable boundary, and the underline ___ indicates the location of the fricative segment. Hence, the /#___ means that the fricative immediately follows the syllable boundary (that is, begins the syllable).

A general form of a phonological rule is the following:

$X \rightarrow Y$ / a ___ b

This rule expresses a modification in which X becomes Y whenever X occurs following a and preceding b. The rule structure is decomposed as follows:

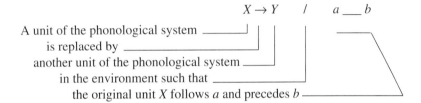

$$X \rightarrow Y \quad / \quad a \underline{\quad} b$$

A unit of the phonological system ⌐
       is replaced by ⌐
   another unit of the phonological system ⌐
      in the environment such that
        the original unit *X* follows *a* and precedes *b*

For example, imagine an allophonic modification in which a vowel is nasalized if it occurs between two nasal consonants (as in the word *man*). A rule of the form given above could be used to describe this change as follows:

Vowel → Nasal vowel   /   Nasal consonant ___ Nasal consonant

But a nasal consonant can be regarded as a sound having the features +nasal and +consonant. When features such as nasal and consonant apply together, it is convenient to place them in brackets so that the rule above becomes:

$$\text{Vowel} \rightarrow \begin{bmatrix} +\text{Nasal} \\ +\text{Vowel} \end{bmatrix} \quad / \quad \begin{bmatrix} +\text{Nasal} \\ +\text{Consonant} \end{bmatrix} \underline{\quad} \begin{bmatrix} +\text{Nasal} \\ +\text{Consonant} \end{bmatrix}$$

Some additional examples of rules are given below. By studying these rules, the student should be able at least to interpret phonological rules, if not to devise them. The basic advantage of a phonological rule is that it expresses in a formal or mathematical fashion a regularity of the phonological system and allows for an accurate, compact description of various context dependencies.

Example of deletion rule: Consonants following nasal consonants are deleted.

$$C \rightarrow \emptyset \qquad / \quad \begin{bmatrix} +\text{Nasal} \\ C \end{bmatrix} \underline{\quad}$$

(Ex.: [ænt] → [æn])

Explanation: As an abbreviatory convenience, *C* stands for consonant, and a nasal consonant is *C* with the feature +nasal. Deletion is represented by the null element O so that the rule literally reads "a consonant is replaced by a null element (nothing) when the consonant follows a nasal consonant."

Example of insertion rule: A schwa vowel is inserted following syllable-final voiced stops.

$$\emptyset \rightarrow /\text{ə}/ \qquad / \quad \begin{bmatrix} +\text{Voiced} \\ +\text{Stop} \end{bmatrix} \underline{\quad} \#$$

(Ex.: [dɔg] → [dɔgə])

Explanation: The rule literally reads "a null element (nothing) is replaced by a schwa vowel when the null element occurs at the end of a syllable following a voiced stop."

Example of feature-changing rule: Syllable-final voiced obstruents are devoiced.

$$\begin{bmatrix} -\text{Sonorant} \\ +\text{Voiced} \end{bmatrix} \rightarrow [-\text{Voiced}] \quad / \quad \underline{\quad} \#$$

(Ex.: [bɪg] → [bɪk])

Explanation: Obstruents are stops, fricatives, and affricates, all of which are represented by the feature −sonorant. Thus, the rule states literally that "voiced nonsonorants (i.e., obstruents) are replaced by their voiceless counterparts at the end of syllables."

Example of feature-assimilation rule: A normally voiceless consonant is voiced when it occurs between two voiced sounds.

$$\begin{bmatrix} \text{C} \\ -\text{Voiced} \end{bmatrix} \rightarrow [+\text{Voiced}] \quad / \quad [+\text{Voiced}] \underline{\quad} [+\text{Voiced}]$$

(Ex.: [æbsɝd] → [æbzɝd])

Explanation: A voiceless consonant becomes voiced if the preceding and following segments are voiced.

Natural Phonology

A topic of considerable interest and importance in phonology is that of naturalness. A natural class, property, process, or rule is one that appears to be preferred or is frequently used in phonologic systems (Sloat et al., 1978; Stampe, 1972; Ingram, 1976). Evidence of naturalness is generally taken from developmental studies (early appearance or acquisition in a child's language), from cross-linguistic studies (universality across languages), or from studies of sound change in a language. One phonological property is more natural than another if the first appears before the second in language development and if the first is attested to in a greater number of languages. *Markedness* is a term sometimes used in this connection. An *unmarked* sound is one that appears to be natural. Unmarked sounds are acquired earlier than marked sounds in children's language, tend to be established in a language before marked sounds can be added, and tend to occur in different languages more frequently than marked sounds. By these criteria, voiceless stops are an example of unmarked (more natural) sounds, whereas voiced obstruents are marked (less natural).

Studies of natural phonology have shown that certain *assimilatory* and *nonassimilatory* processes occur commonly enough to be regarded as natural (Sloat et al., 1978). An assimilatory process is one in which a sound changes to assimilate (become similar) to another sound. A nonassimilatory process does not appear to be based on similarity between sounds.

Examples of Assimilatory Processes

Voicing changes. These are intervocalic voicing and voicing and devoicing of obstruents. In intervocalic voicing, an obstruent (stop, fricative, or affricate) becomes voiced when it occurs between two vowels (hence, intervocalic). For example, *puppy* /pʌpɪ/ becomes /pʌbɪ/. The voiceless obstruent is assimilated to the voiced elements that surround it. The pattern of obstruent voicing or devoicing varies with languages, but one common process is word-final devoicing, in which an obstruent loses its voicing when it occurs at the end of the word. This change sometimes is considered assimilatory because it is thought that the voiced segment is assimilated to the voiceless pause at the end of the word. For example, *dog* /dɔg/ becomes /dɔk/.

Nasalization. As already discussed in this chapter, vowels and, occasionally, other resonants are assimilated to nasal consonants by becoming nasal themselves. Thus, in the word *lamb* /læm/, the vowel often is nasalized.

Nasal assimilation. Nasal consonants tend to assume the place of articulation of a neighboring sound. In English, this process is amply illustrated by the large number of homorganic nasal-stop combinations: *impolite, imbue, improper, indelicate, unturned, endeared, anchor, anger, congress.*

Palatalization. Nonpalatal consonants become palatal when followed by a front vowel or a glide. For example, the /n/ in *news* and the /k/ in *cute* become palatalized when these words are produced with the glide + vowel /ju/ (/njuz/ and /kjut/). As mentioned above, /s/ often is palatalized when it is followed by the glide /j/ in phrases such as *miss you.*

Examples of Nonassimilatory Processes

Deletion or loss of segments. Sometimes a segment or number of segments at the end of a word are dropped in a process known as *apocope*. For example, in the Eastern dialect of English, speakers often drop the /r/ in words such as *car, store,* and *stair*, pronouncing *car* /kar/ as /ka:/. Young children also frequently delete the final consonants of words. Final consonant omission is noted by speech clinicians more often than initial consonant omission. When segments are lost at other than the end of a word, the process is sometimes called *syncope*. Apocope and syncope frequently simplify (or reduce) clusters; *extra*, for example, may become /ɛktrə/ and *asks* may become /æks/.

Insertion of segments. In one type of insertion process, called *prosthesis*, a segment is added in the initial position. In another type, called *epenthesis*, a segment is added elsewhere in the word. Children frequently will break up clusters by inserting vowels (often the schwa /ə/): *blue* becomes /bəlu/ and *clock* becomes /kəlak/.

Metathesis. The order of segments is reversed in this process. For example, a child may say /nets/ for *nest* /nɛst/ and /mjukis/ for music /mjusik/ (the second example also involves final-segment devoicing).

Breaking. By this process, long vowels become diphthongs, as in the examples *fast* /fæɪst/, *pass* /pæɪs/, *bag* /bæɪg/, and *cat* /kæɪt/. Breaking often may be heard in the speech of young children.

Natural phonology offers some valuable perspectives on the acquisition of phonology by children. Some authors believe that natural phonological processes are innate or are acquired early and rather easily by children and that whenever a natural process opposes a phonological property of the language the child is learning, some resistance may be expected. Stampe (1969) viewed natural processes as innate processes that simplify the adult target word. One interesting implication of naturalness is that children tend to exhibit strong biases or preferences in their sound formations and sound sequences. It has been proposed that some such preferences are based on phonetic grounds. For example, obstruent devoicing (or the tendency for stops, fricatives, and affricatives to be devoiced) may be related to the fact that it is difficult to maintain laryngeal vibrations during a period of vocal tract closure. To maintain voicing during closure of the tract, special measures must be taken to enable air flow to continue through the vocal folds. This can be done through an expansion of the oral air chamber (Perkell, 1969; Kent and Moll, 1969), accomplished by expanding the pharynx or by depressing the larynx. However, not all natural processes have a simple phonetic basis, and, most likely, other factors will have to be considered in reaching a full explanation. Whatever this explanation may be, it behooves the speech clinician to be aware that speech and language learning may be influenced by phonological forces that occur commonly enough to be called natural. Such preferences or predispositions in speech production may be a substrate for the process of acquisition. Furthermore, the maintenance of natural processes beyond their usual survival time in learning a particular phonological system could result in articulation disorders.

Nonlinear Phonology

Nonlinear phonology was developed as an alternative to linear generative phonology because the latter was perceived to have certain shortcomings. Some aspects of generative phonology (launched largely through the classic work, *The Sound Pattern of English* by Chomsky and Hallé, 1968) were considered earlier. The basic goals of generative phonologies are to (1) describe phonological patterns in natural languages, (2) formulate the rules that account for these systems, and (3) identify universal principles that apply to phonological systems. A particular reason why nonlinear phonologies were introduced was to account for the influence of stress (as in weak and strong clusters in English stress systems) and the description of tone and stress features in levels of representation independent of the segmental representation. Linear generative phonology was regarded by some to be inadequate in dealing with prosodic effects in general. Early generative phonologies regarded phonological representation as "linear strings of segments with no hierarchical organization other than that provided by syntactic phrase structure" (Clements and Keyser, 1983; 1). This kind of generative phonology was characterized by rules that operated in a domain of linear strings of segments. But this approach encountered some difficulties in regard to the effects of stress and other prosodic variables. More generally, linear generative phonology failed to account satisfactorily for the relationships among various sizes of units because phonological operations were constrained to act on linear sequences.

There are several different versions of nonlinear phonology, but two particularly influential theories are autosegmental theory (Goldsmith, 1976, 1990; Hayes, 1988) and metrical theory (Goldsmith, 1990; Hayes, 1988). Autosegmental theory divides phonological features into parallel tiers of quasi-independent sequences. The tiers are like interconnected but independent levels. The term *autosegment* refers to a unit in a given tier. An autosegment can be realized in one or more ways; for example, a tonal tier may allow realizations such as high, mid, or low tones. The sequences in each tier are time-aligned with association lines that indicate simultaneity across tiers. In this way, stress and segmental representations are coordinated. A detailed discussion cannot be given here for this complex development in phonological theory, but the central idea is fairly simple: Phonological patterns evolve from connections across different representations, and not, as linear generative phonology maintained, from operations across a single linear sequence of phonological units. Nonlinear phonology is a significant break from an earlier theoretical view. It accommodates interactions across various sizes and types of phonological representation.

Metrical theory organizes phonological units into hierarchies, for example, feet, syllables, and segments. Unlike linear generative phonology, metrical theory gives a special definition to stress. Stress patterns arise from rhythm (an alternating prominence, such as strong–weak) and syllable weight. Stress assignments are made across the various levels of the hierarchy (such as syllables, feet, and words). This treatment of stress is very different from that of linear generative phonology.

Hierarchy also is important to theories of feature geometry, another development in nonlinear phonology. Two influential accounts of feature geometry are McCarthy (1988) and Sagey (1986). In systems such as that shown in Figure 1.29, syllable, consonant, and vowel appear as superordinate nodes that govern other nodes specifying laryngeal and

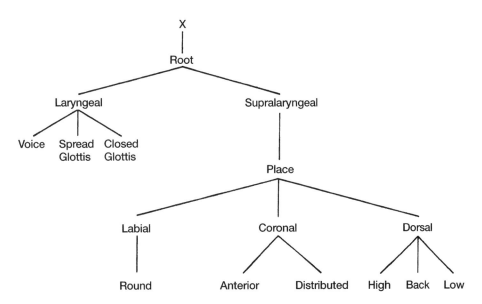

FIGURE 1.29   Hierarchical tree structure for one version of feature geometry. The features under the supralaryngeal node have been defined previously. The features under the laryngeal node refer to vocal fold configurations.

supralaryngeal articulations. That is, the features are arranged hierarchically. Linear phonology, such as that of Chomsky and Hallé (1968), typically specified features in a matrix where orthogonality or independence among features was desirable if not always attainable. In contrast, feature geometry exploits nonorthogonality among features. The hierarchical patterns implied by nonorthogonality become organizing principles in feature geometry.

The three phonological theories reviewed here—autosegmental theory, metrical theory and feature geometry—all represent major departures from what had been the standard phonological theory. Not surprisingly, these new theories are now being considered with respect to phonological development (Schwartz, 1992; Spencer, 1988) and phonological disorders in children (Bernhardt, 1990; Chiat, 1989; Chin and Dinnsen, 1991; Gandour, 1981; Spencer, 1984).

Optimality Theory

Optimality theory is a relatively new and highly influential account of phonology. It resembles some other phonological theories in maintaining that internal (innate) mechanisms govern phonological decisions. In generative phonology, these mechanisms were the distinctive features, which are thought to apply universally across languages. In natural phonology, the innate mechanisms were phonological processes. In optimality theory, the innate mechanisms are *constraints*, which act to select the most optimal output from a set of alternatives. Where do the alternatives arise? These are produced by a mechanism called a *generator* that provides a set of potential output forms for a given input representation. Say, for example, that the input is the word /kæt/. Suppose that the generator supplies the following output forms: /kæt/, kætl/, /æt/, /kæts/. All of these are potential matches to the input representation, but only one should be selected. A mechanism called an *evaluator* uses language-specific constraints to select the most optimal output from the set of outputs supplied by the generator. That is, the evaluator selects the most appropriate (harmonious or optimal) output. Because the ranking of constraints is language specific, a particular ranking reflects learning of a given language. In this way, optimality theory can account for developmental changes in phonology.

Which Phonological Theory to Select?

There is no lack of phonological theories. Only a few have been discussed here, see Ball and Kent (1997) for a more complete discussion. How can we choose among them? This decision depends, in part, on how the theory is to be applied. If the intention is to apply the theory to the development of speech or to phonological/articulatory disorders, the following criteria may guide the selection.

1. Does the theory account for common patterns observed in the development of spoken language in children?
2. Does the theory account for individual differences in the acquisition of speech?

3. Can the theory deal effectively and reasonably with continuity (developmental change)?
4. Is the theory helpful in designing treatment programs for children with phonological/articulatory disorders?
5. Does the theory relate to readily observable events or behaviors?
6. Does the theory provide an index of severity of disorder or disability?
7. Does the theory have elegance and parsimony?

These are questions to consider as you learn more about disorders and phonology. The other chapters in this book will guide your decision process if you accept the challenge of selecting the theory that seems most appealing to you.

Summary of Levels of Organization of Speech

Various levels of organization of speech are shown in Table 1.8, beginning with the syllable and working down to the acoustic sequence that might be seen on a spectrogram or visual representation of sounds. Although *syllable integrity* is the highest level shown, the table could have begun with an even higher level, such as a phrase or a sentence. However, for our purposes here, it is sufficient to consider only the levels presented in the table. The syllable is an organizational unit that consists of one or more phonemes; in this case, the syllable /pa/ includes the phonemes /p/ and /a/. Because phonemes are abstract, a phonemic description does not touch on a number of details of phonetic organization and speech behavior. Some of these details are shown in the level of *phonetic properties*. The phoneme /p/ has as its phonetic representation the aspirated [ph], and the phoneme /a/ has as its phonetic representation the lengthened [a:]. These phonetic representations are, of course, allophones of the /p/ and /a/ phonemes. The English phoneme /p/ is always aspirated in syllable-initial position, and the phoneme /a/ frequently is lengthened when uttered in an open monosyllable (that is, a CV syllable).

Segmental features comprise the next level of the table. These features are phonetic dimensions or attributes by which sounds may be described. For example, the consonant [p] is defined by its inclusion in the classes of *stops, labials*, and *consonantals* and by its exclusion from the classes of *nasals* and *voiced sounds*. These features are similar to the distinctive features discussed earlier in this chapter, but they are intended to be more phonetic in character. Even without rigorous definitions of the features suggested, it should be clear that each feature defines an articulatory property of the sound in question; for example, vowel [a] is a syllable nucleus, is not a consonant, is low-back and unrounded, and is a voiced nonnasal sound.

The features are less abstract than phonemes but still must be interpreted by the motor control system of the brain to provide proper neural instructions to the speech muscles; that is, the features listed for [p] and [a] must be translated into a pattern of muscle contractions that yields the articulatory sequence shown in the next to last level of the table. The −*nasal* feature of [p] requires that the velopharynx be closed, and the −*voice* feature of the same segment requires that the vocal folds be abducted (open). In this way, each feature requirement is given an articulatory interpretation, accomplished by the contraction of muscles.

TABLE 1.8   Levels of Organization of Speech

SYLLABIC INTEGRITY:	/p a/ SYL
PHONEMIC COMPOSITION:	/p/ + /a/
PHONETIC PROPERTIES: Note: stop /p/ is aspirated and vowel /a/ is lengthened	[pʰa:]

SEGMENTAL FEATURES:	[p] — +Stop
	        +Labial
	        +Consonantal
	        –Nasal
	        –Voice
	[a] — +Syllabic
	        –Consonantal
	        –Front
	        +Low
	        –Round
	        –Nasal
	        +Voice

ARTICULATORY SEQUENCE:	Closure of velopharynx Abduction of vocal folds Adjustment of tongue for /a/ Closure of lips Opening of lips and jaw Adduction of vocal folds Final abduction of vocal folds
ACOUSTIC SEQUENCE:	Silent period during /p/ closure Noise burst for /p/ release Aspiration period as folds close Voiced period after folds close, with distinct resonant shaping

Finally, as the consequence of muscle contractions, a series of speech sounds is uttered. In this *acoustic sequence*, the last level of the table, one can see acoustic segments of the kind visible on a spectrogram. Notice that one acoustic segment does not necessarily correspond to a single phoneme. The phoneme /p/ is associated with at least three acoustic segments: a silent period corresponding to the bilabial closure, a noise burst produced as the lips are rapidly opened, and an aspiration interval related to a gradual closure of the vocal folds in preparation for voicing the following vowel.

Although Table 1.8 is fairly detailed, it represents only part of the complexity of speech. In the linguistic-phonetic organization of speech behavior, we need to consider three major components: the segmental (or phonetic) component, the suprasegmental (*prosodic*) component, and the *paralinguistic* component. The first two already have been discussed in this chapter. The paralinguistic component is similar to the prosodic component in that it might be called nonsegmental. This component includes those aspects of speech represented by terms such as *emotion* and *attitude*. A speaker who plans an utterance must decide not only about phonetic sequencing but also about prosodic structure and emotional and attitudinal content (that is, the "tone of voice"). The segmental component includes words, syllables, phonemes, and features. The suprasegmental or prosodic component includes stress, intonation, juncture, rate, loudness, and pitch level. The paralinguistic component is made up of tension, voice quality, and voice qualifications (Crystal, 1969).

The complexity of speech behavior can be illustrated by listing the various types of information represented in the speech signal. A *partial* listing (mostly from Branigan, 1979) is

1. A set of articulatory targets or goals corresponding to the intended phonetic sequence
2. Assignment of stress to the syllables that make up the sequence
3. Adjustments of syllable duration to stress, phonetic composition, and position of the syllable in the utterance
4. Specification of junctural features, including transitions between elements and terminal juncture at the end of the utterance
5. Internal ordering of words as it reflects syntactic form to convey semantic intentions (meaning)
6. Determination of other prosodic features such as speaking rate, pitch, level, and loudness
7. Use of paralinguistic features to convey emotion or attitude

It is important to remember that even an apparently simple aspect of speech behavior can be influenced by a host of variables. For example, the duration of a vowel is determined by tongue height, tenseness or laxness, consonant context, stress pattern, frequency of occurrence of the word in which the vowel occurs, syntactic ordering of the word in which the vowel appears, and rate of speaking (Klatt, 1976).

Concluding Note on Implications for Speech Acquisition

Speech articulation has its early roots in the vocalizations of infants. Just how the coos and babbles of the first year of life relate to the development of speech is not well understood, but there is growing evidence that early vocalizations prepare the child for acquisition of a phonetic system. The syllable appears to be an important unit in early sound patterns, and the development of syllabic organization of sounds may be a major framework of speech development. If so, it is of interest to chart the way in which syllabic structures develop during the first year of life. The following account is based on several chapters in *Precursors of Early Speech Development*, edited by Bjorn Lindblom and Rolf Zetterström (1986) and *The Emergence of the Speech Capacity* by Oller (2000).

The major phases in syllable development are as follows: (1) Continuous phonation in a respiratory cycle provides the basic phonatory pattern from which refinements in articulation can develop; (2) intermittent phonation within a respiratory cycle breaks the basic pattern of continuous phonation and, thus, is a precursor of syllable units; (3) articulatory (supraglottal) movements interrupting or combined with phonation provide early experience in the control of co-occurring phonation and articulation; (4) marginal syllables (in isolation or in sequence) are early syllabic forms that, while lacking the detailed structure of adult syllables, prefigure the basic syllable shape; (5) canonical syllables (in isolation or in sequence) anticipate important structural properties of adult speech and may be particularly important in relating an infant's perceptions of adult speech with his or her own productive patterns; and (6) reduplicated babble (repeated syllable patterns) gives the infant experience with both prosody (especially rhythm) and sequences of articulations. It is on this vocal bedrock that speech develops. For a time, babbling and early words coexist, sharing some phonetic properties but, perhaps, differing in others.

The CV syllable, occurring in virtually all of the world's languages, has long been recognized as a preferred basic unit of speech articulation. It appears to be an optimal unit for learning perceptual discriminations in infancy. Infants younger than four months can discriminate segments contained in sequences of the form CV, CVC, VCV, and CVCV (Bertoncini and Mehler, 1981; Jusczyk and Thompson, 1978; Trehub, 1973); and an alternating CV pattern seems to enhance the infant's ability to discriminate variations in place, manner, and voicing. Since redundant syllable strings, such as [ba ba ba ba] (Goodsitt, Morse, and Ver Hoeve, 1984), further enhance this performance, we can conclude that the CV syllable train characterizing reduplicated babble is an excellent perceptual training ground for the infant.

The advantage of the CV syllable applies to production as well. This syllable form is one of the earliest syllables to be identified in infant vocalizations; the vocalizations of 1-year-olds are, predominantly, simple V or CV syllables and their elaborations, for example, VCV or CVCV (Kent and Bauer, 1985). Branigan (1976) regarded the CV syllable as a training ground for consonant formation. Most consonants are produced first in the initial position of CV syllables and then, later, in postvocalic (e.g., VC) position.

The importance of the canonical CV syllable as a unit for perceptuomotor integration is indicated by its long-delayed appearance in the vocal development of hearing-impaired infants (Kent, Osberger, Netsell, and Hustedde, 1987; Oller, 1986). There is also evidence that early CV syllable production is linked, in a developmental chain, to the early word production and to the articulation of word-final consonants (Menyuk, Liebergott, and Schultz, 1986).

Speech acquisition is a complex process, one that involves learning a language (its syntax, semantics, and phonology)—a speech code that relates meaning to sound, and a motor skill by which the speech organs are controlled to produce rapid and overlapping movements. The layman often characterizes developing speech in the child by reference to frequently occurring substitutions (as when the child says *wabbit* for *rabbit* or *thee* for *see*) or other common misarticulations. But developing speech differs from adult speech in other ways.

First, children's speech generally is slower than adult speech. For example, McNeill (1974) reported speaking rates of slightly over 3 words per second for adults, about 2.5 words per second for 4- to 5-year-olds, and 1.6 words per second for children of about 2.

Not surprisingly, then, the durations of individual segments are longer in children's speech (Naeser, 1970; Smith, 1978; Kent and Forner, 1980). Smith reported that the durations of nonsense utterances were 15 percent longer for 4-year-olds than for adults and 31 percent longer for 2-year-olds than for adults. Similarly, when Kent and Forner measured durations of phrases and short sentences, they found them to be 8 percent longer for 12-year-olds than for adults, 16 percent longer for 6-year-olds than for adults, and 33 percent longer for 4-year-olds than for adults. Some individual segments, such as the duration of stop closure, were observed by Kent and Forner to be twice as long in children's speech as in adult speech. The speaking rates of children have implications for both the production and perception of speech. It has been shown that children more successfully imitate sentences spoken at a rate nearer their own than at slower or faster rates (Bonvillian, Raeburn, and Horan, 1979).

Second, children's speech differs from adult speech in its variability. When children make the same utterance several times, the duration of individual segments varies more than for adults (Eguchi and Hirsh, 1969; Tingley and Allen, 1975; Kent and Forner, 1980). This difference in reliability of production may be an index of the child's linguistic and neuromotor immaturity. In general, a young child's speech patterns are less well controlled than an adult's, and there is evidence that the control continues to improve until the child reaches puberty (Kent, 1976).

A third difference between the speech of children and adults is in patterns of coarticulation. Data on this difference are not abundant, but Thompson and Hixon (1979) reported that with increasing age, a greater proportion of their subjects showed nasal air flow beginning at the midpoint of the first vowel in /ini/. They interpreted this to mean that anticipatory coarticulation occurred earlier for progressively older subjects. In other words, more mature speakers show increased anticipation in producing a phonetic sequence.

In summary, young children differ from adults not only in their obvious misarticulations, but also in their slower speaking rates, greater variability (error) in production, and reduced anticipation in articulatory sequencing.

QUESTIONS FOR CHAPTER 1

1. Discuss the relationship among the following concepts: *morpheme, phoneme, allophone.* For example, explain why a morpheme is relevant to identifying phonemes and why phonemes are relevant to identifying allophones.

2. This chapter summarized two ways of describing vowel articulation: traditional phonetic description and distinctive features. Discuss the similarities and differences between these two approaches.

3. Using Table 1.2 as a guide, classify all of the consonants in the phrase *Good morning, take a ticket, and get in line,* according to place of articulation, manner of articulation, and voicing. Note that in all of the words containing two or more consonants, the consonants share a phonetic feature. What is this feature for each word?

4. What is coarticulation and why does it occur?

5. Compare and contrast any two of the theories of phonology discussed in this chapter.

REFERENCES

Adams, S. G., "Rate and clarity of speech: An x-ray microbeam study." Ph.D. dissertation, University of Wisconsin–Madison, 1990.

Ball, M. J., and R. D. Kent, *New Phonologies: Developments in Clinical Linguistics*. San Diego, Calif.: Singular Publishing Group, 1997.

Behne, D., "Acoustic effects of focus and sentence position on stress in English and French." Ph.D. dissertation, University of Wisconsin–Madison, 1989.

Bernhardt, B., "Application of nonlinear phonology to intervention with six phonologically disordered children." Unpublished Ph.D. thesis, University of British Columbia, Vancouver, B.C., Canada, 1990.

Bernthal, J. E., and D. R. Beukelman, "Intraoral air pressures during the production of /p/ and /b/ by children, youths, and adults." *Journal of Speech and Hearing Research, 21* (1978): 361–371.

Bertoncini, J., and J. Mehler, "Syllables as units in infant speech perception." *Infant Behavior and Development, 4* (1981): 247–260.

Bock, J. K., "Toward a cognitive psychology of syntax: Information processing contributions to sentence formulation." *Psychological Review, 89* (1982): 1–47.

Bonvillian, J. D., V. P. Raeburn, and E. A. Horan, "Talking to children: The effects of rate, intonation, and length on children's sentence imitation." *Journal of Child Language, 6* (1979): 459–467.

Branigan, G., "Syllabic structure and the acquisition of consonants: The great conspiracy in word formation." *Journal of Psycholinguistic Research, 5* (1976): 117–133.

Branigan, G., "Some reasons why successive single word utterances are not." *Journal of Child Language, 6* (1979): 411–421.

Cavagna, G. A., and R. Margaria, "Airflow rates and efficiency changes during phonation." *Sound Production in Man, Annals of the New York Academy of Sciences, 155* (1968): 152–164.

Chiat, S., "The relation between prosodic structure, syllabification and segmental realization: Evidence from a child with fricative stopping." *Clinical Linguistics and Phonetics, 3* (1989): 223–242.

Chin, S. B., and D. A. Dinnsen, "Feature geometry in disordered phonologies." *Clinical Linguistics and Phonetics, 5* (1991): 329–337.

Chomsky, N., and M. Hallé, *The Sound Pattern of English*. New York: Harper & Row, 1968.

Clements, G. N., and S. J. Keyser, *CV Phonology*. Cambridge, Mass.: M.I.T. Press, 1983.

Cohen, A., R. Collier, and J. t'Hart, "Declination: Construct or intrinsic feature of speech pitch?" *Phonetica, 39* (1982): 254–273.

Crystal, D., *Prosodic Systems and Intonation in English*. Cambridge (UK): Cambridge University Press, 1969.

Crystal, D., "Non-segmental phonology in language acquisition: A review of the issues." *Lingua, 32* (1973): 1–45.

Daniloff, R. G., and K. L. Moll, "Coarticulation of lip rounding." *Journal of Speech and Hearing Research, 11* (1968): 707–721.

Dewey, G., *Relative Frequency of English Speech Sounds*. Cambridge: Harvard University Press, 1923.

Eguchi, S., and I. J. Hirsh, "Development of speech sounds in children." *Acta Orolaryngologica*, Supplement No. 257 (1969).

Fry, D., "Duration and intensity as physical correlates of linguistic stress." *Journal of the Acoustical Society of America, 27* (1955): 765–768.

Gandour, J., "The nondeviant nature of deviant phonological systems." *Journal of Communication Disorders, 14* (1981): 11–29.

Giles, S. B., "A study of articulatory characteristics of /l/ allophones in English." Ph.D. dissertation, University of Iowa, 1971.

Goldsmith, J., "Autosegmental phonology." Ph.D. dissertation, Massachusetts Institute of Technology, 1976 (published by Garland Press, 1979).

Goldsmith, J. A., *Autosegmental and Metrical Phonology*. Oxford: Basil Blackwell, 1990.

Goodsitt, J., P. Morse, and J. Ver Hoeve, "Infant speech recognition in multisyllabic contexts." *Child Development, 55* (1984): 903–910.

Hardcastle, W. J., *Physiology of Speech Production*. London: Academic Press, 1976.

Hayes, B., "Metrics and phonological theory." In F. Newmeyer (Ed.), *Linguistics: The Cambridge Survey. II. Linguistic Theory: Extensions and Implications* (pp. 220–249). Cambridge (UK): Cambridge University Press, 1988.

Hixon, T. J., "Mechanical aspects of speech production." Paper read at Annual Convention of the American Speech and Hearing Association, Chicago, November 17–20, 1971.

Hockett, C. F., "A manual of phonology." *International Journal of American Linguistics (Memoir II)*. Baltimore: Waverly Press, 1955.

Hyman, L. M., *Phonology: Theory and Analysis*. New York: Holt, Rinehart and Winston, 1975.

Ingram, D., *Phonological Disability in Children*. New York: Elsevier, 1976.

Jong, K. J. de, "The oral articulation of English stress accent." Ph.D. dissertation, Ohio State University, Columbus, Ohio, 1991.

Jusczyk, P., and E. Thompson, "Perception of phonetic contrasts in multisyllabic utterances by 2 month old infants." *Perception and Psychophysics*, *23* (1978): 105–109.

Kantner, C. E., and R. West, *Phonetics*. New York: Harper & Row, 1960.

Kent, R. D., "Anatomical and neuromuscular maturation of the speech mechanism: Evidence from acoustic studies." *Journal of Speech and Hearing Research*, *19* (1976): 421–447.

Kent, R. D., and H. R. Bauer, "Vocalizations of one year olds." *Journal of Child Language*, *12* (1985): 491–526.

Kent, R. D., and L. L. Forner, "Speech segment durations in sentence recitations by children and adults." *Journal of Phonetics*, *8* (1980): 157–168.

Kent, R. D., R. E. Martin, and R. L. Sufit, "Oral sensation: A review and clinical prospective." In H. Winitz (Ed.), *Human Communication and Its Disorders: A Review-1990* (pp. 135–191). Norwood, N.J.: Ablex, 1990.

Kent, R. D., and F. D. Minifie, "Coarticulation in recent speech production models." *Journal of Phonetics*, *5* (1977): 115–133.

Kent, R. D., and K. L. Moll, "Vocal-tract characteristics of the stop cognates." *Journal of the Acoustical Society of America*, *46* (1969): 1549–1555.

Kent, R. D., and K. L. Moll, "Cinefluorographic analyses of selected lingual consonants." *Journal of Speech and Hearing Research*, *15* (1972): 453–473.

Kent, R. D., and K. L. Moll, "Articulatory timing in selected consonant sequences." *Brain and Language*, *2* (1975): 304–323.

Kent, R. D., and R. Netsell, "Effects of stress contrasts on certain articulatory parameters." *Phonetica*, *24* (1972): 23–44.

Kent, R. D., M. J. Osberger, R. Netsell, and C. G. Hustedde, "Phonetic development in identical twins differing in auditory function." *Journal of Speech and Hearing Disorders*, *52* (1987): 64–75.

Klatt, D. H., "Linguistic uses of segmental duration in English: Acoustic and perceptual evidence." *Journal of the Acoustical Society of America*, *59* (1976): 1208–1221.

Ladefoged, P., *Preliminaries to Linguistic Phonetics*. Chicago: University of Chicago Press, 1971.

Ladefoged, P., *A Course in Phonetics*. New York: Harcourt Brace Jovanovich, 1975.

Lehiste, I., *Suprasegmentals*. Cambridge, MA: M.I.T. Press, 1970.

Lieberman, P., *Intonation, Perception and Language*. Cambridge, MA: M.I.T. Press, 1967.

Lindblom, B. E. F., "Spectrographic study of vowel reduction." *Journal of the Acoustical Society of America*, *35* (1963): 1773–1781.

Lindblom, B., "Explaining phonetic variation: A sketch of the H&H theory." In W. J. Hardcastle and A. Marchal (Eds.), *Speech Production and Speech Modelling* (pp. 403–439). Amsterdam, The Netherlands: Kluwer, 1990.

Lindblom, B., and R. Zetterström (Eds.), *Precursors of Early Speech Development*. New York: Stockton, 1986.

McCarthy, L., "Feature geometry and dependency: A review." *Journal of Phonetics*, *43* (1988): 84–108.

MacNeilage, P. F., "Speech physiology." In H. H. Gilbert (Ed.), *Speech and Cortical Functioning* (pp. 1–72). New York: Academic Press, 1972.

McNeill, D., "The two-fold way for speech." In *Problèmes Actuels en Psycholinguistique.* Paris: Editions du Centre National de la Recherche Scientifique, 1974.

Menyuk, P., J. Liebergott, and M. Schultz, "Predicting phonological development." In B. Lindblom and R. Zetterström (Eds.), *Precursors of Early Speech* (pp. 79–93). Basingstoke, Hampshire (UK): MacMillan, 1986.

Moll, K. L., and R. G. Daniloff, "Investigation of the timing of velar movements during speech." *Journal of the Acoustical Society of America*, *50* (1971): 678–684.

Moon, S. J., and B. Lindblom, "Formant undershoot in clear and citation-form speech: A second progress report." Royal Institute of Technology (Stockholm, Sweden) Speech Transmission Laboratory, *Quarterly Progress and Status Reports*, *1* (1989): 121–123.

Naeser, M. A., "The American child's acquisition of differential vowel duration." *Technical Report No. 144, Wisconsin Research and Development Center for Cognitive Learning*, University of Wisconsin, Madison, 1970.

Netsell, R., W. K. Lotz, J. E. Peters, and L. Schulte, "Developmental patterns of laryngeal and respiratory function for speech production." *Journal of Voice*, *8* (1994): 123–131.

Oller, D. K., "Metaphonology of infant vocalizations." In B. Lindblom and R. Zetterström (Eds.), *Precursors of Early Speech* (pp. 21–35). Basingstoke, Hampshire (UK): MacMillan, 1986.

Oller, D. K., *The Emergence of the Speech Capacity*. Mahwah, N.J.: Lawrence Erlbaum, 2000.

Parker, F., "Distinctive features in speech pathology: Phonology or phonemics?" *Journal of Speech and Hearing Disorders*, *41* (1976): 23–39.

Perkell, J. S., *Physiology of Speech Production*. Cambridge, Mass.: M.I.T. Press, 1969.

Picheny, M. A., N. I. Durlach, and L. D. Braida, "Speaking clearly for the hard of hearing. II: Acoustic characteristics of clear and conversational speech." *Journal of Speech and Hearing Research*, *29* (1986): 434–446.

Rabiner, L., H. Levitt, and A. Rosenberg, "Investigation of stress patterns for speech synthesis by rule." *Journal of the Acoustical Society of America*, *45* (1969): 92–101.

Read, C., and P. A. Schreiber, "Why short subjects are harder to find than long ones." In E. Wanner and

L. Gleitman (Eds.), *Language Acquisition: The State of the Art*. Cambridge (UK): Cambridge University Press, 1982.

Sagey, E., "The representation of features and relations in non-linear phonology." Unpublished Ph.D. thesis, Mass. Institute of Technology, Cambridge, Mass., 1986.

Schwartz, R. G., "Nonlinear phonology as a framework for phonological acquisition." In R. S. Chapman (Ed.), *Processes in Language Acquisition and Disorders*. Chicago: Mosby-Year Book, 1992.

Sloat, C., S. H. Taylor, and J. E. Hoard, *Introduction to Phonology*. Englewood Cliffs, NJ: Prentice Hall, 1978.

Smith, B. L., "Temporal aspects of English speech production: A developmental perspective." *Journal of Phonetics*, 6 (1978): 37–68.

Spencer, A., "A nonlinear analysis of phonological disability." *Journal of Communication Disorders*, 17 (1984): 325–348.

Spencer, A., "A phonological theory of phonological development" (pp. 115–151). In M. J. Ball (Ed.), *Theoretical Linguistics and Disordered Language*. London: Croon Helm, 1988.

Stampe, D., "The acquisition of phonetic representation." In R. I. Binnick et al. (Eds.), *Papers from the Fifth Regional Meeting of the Chicago Linguistics Society* (pp. 443–453). Chicago: Chicago Linguistics Society, 1969.

Stampe, D., "A dissertation of natural phonology." Ph.D. dissertation, University of Chicago, 1972.

Subtelny, J., J. Worth, and M. Sakuda, "Intraoral pressure and rate of flow during speech." *Journal of Speech and Hearing Research*, 9 (1966): 498–518.

Thompson, A. E., and T. J. Hixon, "Nasal air flow during speech production." *Cleft Palate Journal*, 16 (1979): 412–420.

Tingley, B. M., and G. D. Allen, "Development of speech timing control in children." *Child Development*, 46 (1975): 186–194.

Trehub, S., "Infants' sensitivity to vowel and tonal contrasts." *Developmental Psychology*, 9 (1973): 91–96.

Walsh, H., "On certain practical inadequacies of distinctive feature systems." *Journal of Speech and Hearing Disorders*, 39 (1974): 32–43.

Wise, C. M., *Introduction to Phonetics*. Englewood Cliffs, N.J.: Prentice Hall, 1957a.

Wise, C. M., *Applied Phonetics*. Englewood Cliffs, N.J.: Prentice Hall, 1957b.

2 Early Phonological Development

MARILYN MAY VIHMAN
University of Wales—Bangor

How much does a normally developing child accomplish in the first three or four years of exposure to the native language? In the babbling period, children exposed to different languages sound just about the same. Adults cannot reliably distinguish between babies learning languages as different as English and Spanish (Thevenin, Eilers, Oller, and LaVoie, 1985) or French and Chinese (Boysson-Bardies, Sagart, and Durand, 1984) just by listening to recordings of their babbling and first words. Francescato suggested that "two hypotheses are possible: Either all children, of all languages, at the beginning of their linguistic activity share the 'same' language, or every child, of every language, speaks from the beginning its own language" (1968: 152f.). In some sense both hypotheses are true. Children in different language environments draw on the same "universal" repertoire of syllable shapes and sounds. At the same time, each child creates, out of these universal syllable shapes and sounds, a unique subset of sound preferences and patterns as he or she develops a phonological and communicative system of his or her own. Gradually, these unique or idiosyncratic patterns accommodate to and are replaced by the adult system to which the child is exposed.

In a remarkably short time most children develop intelligible speech. In two to three years they typically come to articulate well enough so that people outside the immediate family can understand what they are saying. At that point, the child can already be recognized as a member of a specific language community by his or her speech patterns; that is, he or she will have acquired the incidental phonetically distinguishing features as well as the system of contrasting sounds of the specific language spoken in his or her environment. In other words, in learning the phonology of American English, the infant also will have learned to pronounce like an American from California or Kansas or New Jersey.

Models of Phonological Development: The Child as an Active Learner

Linguists and psychologists have long sought to explain how children learn to distinguish and produce the sound patterns of the adult language. The earliest studies were largely *diary studies* or descriptions of the investigator's own child; several detailed studies of this sort were available by the 1940s. The first well-articulated model of phonological development—namely, Jakobson's structuralist model—was formulated at that time. Although it continues to be influential today, a number of other models, based on different perspectives and assumptions, have since been proposed (see Ferguson, Menn, and Stoel-Gammon, 1992; Menn and Stoel-Gammon, 1995; Vihman, 1996). In the past 20 years, there has been a shift in thinking about language acquisition. The earlier structuralist model presupposed little initiative on the part of the learner. Today most investigators agree that the child, whose goal is to "sound like the adults around her" (Menn, 1981; 131), is an active participant in the learning process.

Behaviorist Model

In the United States, the prevailing view from the 1950s to the early 1970s was the behaviorist model associated with Mowrer (1960) and Olmsted (1971). This model applied a psychological theory of learning to the human infant and emphasized the role of contingent reinforcement in speech acquisition. The child's babbling was held to be gradually "shaped," through classical conditioning principles, into forms appropriate for the adult speech community in question. In the course of the daily caretaking routines of feeding and changing, the infant was believed to associate the vocalizations of the caretaker, usually the mother, with "primary reinforcement," such as food and comfort; thus, the adult's vocalizations acquire the value of "secondary reinforcement." The child's own vocalizations acquire secondary reinforcing value as well, by virtue of their similarity to the caretaker's vocalizations. The speech sound repertoire is further refined as the caretaker selectively reinforces sounds that resemble those used in the adult language and as the child is "self-reinforced" for producing sounds that match those in the environment. Thus, the behaviorists emphasized continuity between babbling and early speech. The behaviorist paradigm as such is no longer widely accepted today as a model for language acquisition, primarily because it fails to account for the infinite capacity to produce new patterns that is the hallmark of human language (cf. Chomsky's [1959] critique of B. F. Skinner's *Verbal Behavior*). With specific reference to phonology, there is little evidence that caretakers selectively reward (or "shape") the child's sound productions in the prelinguistic period. On the other hand, there is good reason to credit the self-rewarding value of the child's experience of a match between his or her own productions and patterns available in the input (Vihman, 1993; Vihman and Velleman, 2000).

Structuralist Model

In contrast to the behaviorists, who drew on general learning theory for their assumptions about infant phonological development, the linguist Roman Jakobson (1941/68) drew on the structuralist theory of language to account for speech sound development. He hypothesized a discontinuity between babbling, which he saw as a random activity, and the onset of speech production. Jakobson postulated that phonological development follows a universal and innate order of acquisition. The distinctive features of speech sounds, arranged in a hierarchy, "unfold" in a predictable order as the child produces phonemic contrasts embodying them. The child was thought to start with two maximally contrasting sounds: a bilabial stop, /p/, and a low vowel, /a/. The child then begins to differentiate the consonant system by acquiring the contrast between nasal and oral: /p/ (oral) versus /m/ (nasal). The next feature contrast divides both oral and nasal consonants into a labial (/p/, /m/) and a dental pair (/t/, /n/). Jakobson proposed that the child's consonant and vowel systems continue to diversify and differentiate, step by step, as the child learns new feature contrasts. Features needed to differentiate stops, nasals, bilabials, and dentals were held to be acquired earlier than those needed to differentiate fricatives, affricates, and liquids.

Though Jakobson's views provided a vital stimulus to research and are still widely cited, intensive data collection and analyses since that time have tended to weaken several aspects of his position. For one thing, the existence of regularities in prelinguistic (or babbling) vocal patterns has been clearly demonstrated (Ferguson and Macken, 1983) as has the gradual emergence of adult-based word shapes from the babble vocalizations (Vihman, Macken, Miller, Simmons, and Miller, 1985). Thus, the hypothesis of discontinuity between babble and speech appears to be unfounded.

A more basic difficulty is Jakobson's postulation of phonemic contrast as the basis of phonological development in the earliest stages. As Kiparsky and Menn (1977) pointed out, the corpus of words a child begins with is typically too small to provide clear evidence for or against the hypothesized sequence of **phonemic oppositions**. No set order of use of consonants is evident in the early words of the many different children whose data have been carefully recorded and analyzed. More importantly, the order of emergence of phonemic oppositions (nasal vs. oral, labial vs. dental) is extremely difficult to ascertain, and requires an evaluation of the child's system based on the adult phonemes attempted as well as on the phonemic patterns used by the child. The undertaking is further complicated since many children seem to selectively **avoid** attempting words that include certain consonants. In fact, the child is now thought to be targeting *whole-word* rather than individual segments or phonemes (Ferguson and Farwell, 1975; Beckman and Edwards, 2000). Furthermore, in light of the great *variability* seen in the child's early speech productions, the issue of a universal order of acquisition of phonemes has lost much of its support.

Generative Phonology Models

Generative phonology models also emphasize the universal and maturational aspects of phonological acquisition. According to Stampe (1969; cf. Donegan and Stampe, 1979), the child comes innately equipped with a universal set of phonological processes—operations which change, delete, or otherwise simplify phonological units—that reflect the natural limitations and capacities of human vocal production and perception. The child's task is to suppress those processes which do not occur in the particular adult language to which he or she is exposed (Stampe terms this account "natural phonology"). For example, a child may be expected to devoice word-final obstruents (i.e., at first, the English-speaking child would pronounce *bad* as [bæt]), since this is a phonetically natural process found in many languages. In German, where *Hund* ("dog") is pronounced [hunt], the devoicing process accurately reflects adult phonology, and thus, the German-speaking child need not "suppress" it; however, the English-speaking child must suppress the process to match adult pronunciation (eventually producing *bad* as [bæd]).

Smith (1973) developed a generative model of phonological development, based on a formal description of the phonology of his son Amahl, from age 2 to 4. He contrasted two possible descriptions of the child's phonology: (1) the "rule rewriting" description, consisting of a mapping of the adult forms onto the child's (e.g., "/f, v/ become [w] prevocalically," or in other words, "rewrite /f/ or /v/ as [w] . . ." to account for *feet* → [wi:t], *fork* → [wɔ:k], etc.); and (2) an account in which the child's system is viewed in its own right, with the functional units and their interrelations defined and organized differently than in the adult system. Smith found no evidence to support the idea that the child had his own system. The postulated child system seemed to have no bearing on the child's response to unfamiliar adult forms, on his phonological treatment of new forms, or on his reorganization of older forms under the influence of new patterns. Smith postulated instead that there is a set of ordered universal tendencies, such as the use of consonant and vowel harmony and cluster reduction, that are innate or learned very early.

The generative phonology model has been influential in clinical practice with disordered phonology since the 1970s. The model rejects the possibility of the child's developing his or her own phonological system, but rather supports the concept of "innate" or universal child phonological rules or processes—a position which remains controversial, though use of the term *phonological process* and of the re-write or realization rule format has become general in the fields of disordered child phonology (cf. Ingram, 1976; Grunwell, 1981; Edwards and Shriberg, 1983). Finally, the model postulates full, accurate perception from the earliest stages of speech production. That is, the child is assumed to perceive and store or represent speech forms correctly. According to this position, which has been challenged, it is innate constraints on the child's *production* that lead to simplification in the child's output forms.

Cognitive Models

A different perspective on child phonology, which also developed in the 1970s, is the "cognitive" or "problem-solving" model (Menn, 1983; Macken and Ferguson, 1983; Ferguson, 1978, 1986). This model emerged largely out of the speech sound acquisition data rather than being an application of adult models to the child (see especially Ferguson and Farwell, 1975). It was influenced by Waterson (1971), who presented data from her son P to support the idea that it is the *word* rather than the segment that serves as a basic unit of phonological structure in the earliest stages of development. Waterson describes groups of early words as schemas (now more commonly termed "templates") that share certain overall features derived from the adult form, such as accentual pattern, syllable structure, nasality, continuance (presence of fricatives), or voicing (see Velleman and Vihman, 2002). In Waterson's view, the child's perception of the phonetic features of adult words is incomplete or partial at first. For Waterson and others (e.g., Braine, 1976; Maxwell, 1984), both child perception and production are likely to involve imperfect matches with the adult model at first, and therefore, both must undergo development and change before the child can arrive at an adult-like system.

According to the cognitive model, the child uses a variety of individual strategies depending on his or her natural predispositions as well as on a number of external factors (such as the child's birth order and the interactional style of the primary caretakers, in addition to differences in motoric maturation and phonological sensitivity: cf. Lieven, 1997).

Longitudinal studies provided the primary evidence that active (albeit unconscious) hypothesis testing and problem solving play an important role in phonological acquisition as in cognitive development in general (Karmiloff-Smith, 1992). Evidence includes (1) *selectivity in early word choice.* In the early period of rapid vocabulary learning, children seem to selectively attempt to say adult words of certain shapes while avoiding sounds or sound patterns which are outside their repertoire. For example, one child initially used only two-syllable words with open syllables (no final consonants in syllables) beginning with a stop or nasal (*daddy, mommy, doggy, patty(-cake)*, and *bye-bye*: Ferguson, Peizer, and Weeks, 1973). Different children begin by mastering different articulatory patterns and, accordingly, by attempting different (identifiable) adult words. (2) *Mastering long words.* Children develop idiosyncratic strategies to produce long words. For example, Priestly (1977) described the use by his son Christopher of the pattern [CVjVC] to produce a number of polysyllabic words—for example, *Panda* → [pajan], *berries* → [bɛjas], and *tiger* → [tajak]. Though these "exploratory forms" fail to match the adult forms in segmental terms, they accurately, if idiosyncratically, capture the correct syllable count. (3) *"Phonological idioms" and regression.* A child may first produce a complex adult word in a relatively advanced form (e.g., *pretty*, pronounced [prəti]) and only later revert to a simplified form which conforms more closely to the other forms in his or her productive vocabulary (e.g., *pretty* → [bɪdi]; Leopold, 1947). In such cases, the child apparently takes a step backward or regresses since the new form is farther from the adult model. On the other hand, the new form fits into the child's own emerging **phonological system**. Thus, the **regression** seems to reflect *systematization* on the child's part, as it creates a small number of output patterns for the various word forms the child knows.

The cognitive model provides a useful complement to the phonological process-based (segmental) analysis. In particular, this model is able to capture the "gestalt" or the "canonical form" underlying child productions that are highly irregular in terms of segment-by-segment comparison with the adult model. This model focuses primarily on the earliest period of word production, when the child appears to be targeting whole words rather than segments (see also Menyuk, Menn, and Silber, 1986). Waterson's prosodic analyses of one child's data provide rich illustrations of the characteristic **individuality** of early phonological development. However, the cognitive model may be criticized for overemphasizing the individual creative aspects of phonological acquisition. Within the framework of the biologically possible, the child is seen as having considerable space for active exploration, hypothesis-formation, and systematization. Little attention is paid to the **constraints** on learning which may result from maturation, both physiological and psychological, or from the structure of language in general and also from the particular language of the child's environment.

Biological Models

Locke (1983, 1990; Locke and Pearson, 1992) proposed a biological model of the origins of phonological system in the child (cf. also Kent, 1992, Kent and Miolo, 1995). He suggests that innate perceptual biases and dispositions to certain motor action are at the root of phonological acquisition. In babbling, the child's phonetic repertoire is essentially universal, being constrained by biological factors such as the size and shape of the infant vocal tract and the relative complexity of neuromotor control required for various articulations. For example, simply raising and lowering the jaw can result in alveolar stop production at a time when independent manipulation of the tongue has not yet come under voluntary control (Locke, 1993; see also Davis and MacNeilage, 2000). Babbling is critical in that it allows the child to construct auditory-kinesthetic links which can serve as a phonetic guidance system for acquiring language (Fry, 1966; Vihman, 1991). Influence from the language of the child's environment is thought to emerge with the production of first words, and is based on the storage and retrieval of some relatively stable perceived forms of the language.

Biological and linguistic approaches to vocal development have converged in the idea of self-organizing principles. According to Lindblom (1992, 2000), phonetic forms in all languages have evolved to meet the complementary needs of the two participants in vocal communication, the listener and the speaker. The needs of the listener are met when a language uses vowels such as /i/, /a/, and /u/, which are maximally distant from one another and thus easy to discriminate. On the other hand, the needs of the speaker are met when a language uses consonant-vowel sequences which require little tongue movement and are thus *easy to articulate*, such as apico-dental /t/ followed by a front (or "apical") vowel (/i/), or velar /k/ followed by a back vowel (/u/). The compromise between these two sets of **performance** constraints leads to phonetic universals, specifying "core" segments (phonemes) that are used in most languages and "exotic" segments (phonemes) which occur only in languages with large phonetic inventories. In the case of the child learning to speak, a small number of articulatory gestures are used over and over in different combinations to produce word patterns, or articulatory **motor patterns** corresponding to **unitary acoustic patterns**. The overlapping use of the same articulatory gestures to produce different word patterns or syllables (/ti/, /tu/, /ki/, /ku/) will eventually lead to the emergence of a network of phonologically contrastive segments (/t/, /k/, /i/, /u/) by "self-segmentation." The basis of the principle of self-organization is that neither genetic specification nor linguistic input is sufficient to account for the development of a phonological system, but the interaction of the two promotes novelty and complexity in the child's emergent system.

Despite the evidence that problem solving plays a role in phonology, universal biologically or linguistically based constraints undoubtedly set the parameters within which acquisition must occur. Beyond this, both **maturation** (natural biological development and change) and **practice** may be said to influence learning. An apparent difficulty for the biological model is the extent of individual differences that have been reported among children from a single language background in the babbling stage (Vihman, 1993). If the earliest period of linguistic development is under relatively strict biological or maturational control, one might expect greater uniformity across infants at this stage of phonological development. However, genetic variation across individual members of a species is the rule in developmental biology and may account for the early differences in phonetic production (Locke, 1988). On the other hand, some global influence of the specific ambient language has been detected in infant vocalizations as early as 10 months (cf. Boysson-Bardies, Hallé, Sagart and Durand, 1989; Boysson-Bardies and Vihman, 1991), suggesting that phonetic "learning" must begin in the pre-lexical period.

Nonlinear Phonology Models

In the 1980s a new type of model of adult phonology gained widespread attention and acceptance. The term **nonlinear phonology** is used to cover this family of formal models of somewhat different types. They deemphasize rules or processes and linear segmental strings and place a focus on prosodic phenomena. The term *prosodic* refers to two different kinds of phenomena, neither of which is at the level of the individual segment: (1) so-called **suprasegmental phenomena**, such as word-accent involving stress or tone, which take at least a whole word or syllable as their domain, and (2) other whole-word-based phenomena such as *phonotactics* or arrangements of sounds, including the permissibility of particular consonant sequences, vowel sequences, or syllable-final consonants. In these new models, representations are regarded less as a sequence of segmental "beads on a string" than as analogous to an orchestral score in which the synchronization of each instrument with the other instruments is as much a part of the score as the actual notes each is to play. In phonological terms, the "instruments" are the various separable components of the speech apparatus. Other new models which fit under the general rubric nonlinear are autosegmental, metrical and lexical phonology (Goldsmith, 1990) and prosodic phonology (Nespor and Vogel, 1986). The most popular extension of this perspective is optimality theory, in which phonological rules are dispensed with entirely, being replaced by permissible patterns or constraints (Paradis, 1988; Bernhardt and Stemberger, 1998; Kager, Pater, and Zonneveld, in press).

Nonlinear models offer advantages in accounting for developmental data. As Menn (1978) pointed out, two properties of autosegmental formalism are particularly well suited to the description of children's phonological systems: (1) the possibility of specifying domains of application for phonetic features which extend beyond the segment, such as the syllable or the word; and (2) the freedom from sequential ordering of features which results from the nonlinear concept of the sound system being viewed simultaneously from separate tiers, or levels of organization (see Figure 2.1). The separate specification of features that affect only or mainly consonants (glottalization, retroflexion) or only vowels (vowel harmony, nasalization) in adult language provides a natural format for dealing with consonant harmony, a very common pattern in child phonology that is rarely encountered in adult languages. The reordering of adult segments, called metathesis, is often seen in child productions, e.g. *pasghetti* for *spaghetti*. The notion of specifying different features on different tiers provides a useful account for the reordering of heterogeneous segments.

Later applications of nonlinear models to child data have made bolder departures from the generative model. For example, Vihman, Velleman, and McCune (1994) suggested that whole levels of representation may be lacking in the initial stages of phonological organization. Thus the skeletal (CV) level can be considered to be missing at 14 and 15 months in the child whose development is illustrated in Figure 2.2 because all of the child's words have the shape CV, with a single vowel choice, [a]. There is no evidence that lexical representation is broken down into C and V at all in such a case; the word/syllable/CV representations are not distinct. Similarly, a child's representation may lack branching, either at the word level (if only monosyllabic words are produced; see Figure 2.2, 14 and 15 mos.) or at the syllable level (no clusters, diphthongs, or syllable-final consonants are produced; contrast the first and second syllables of *monkey* in Figure 2.1).

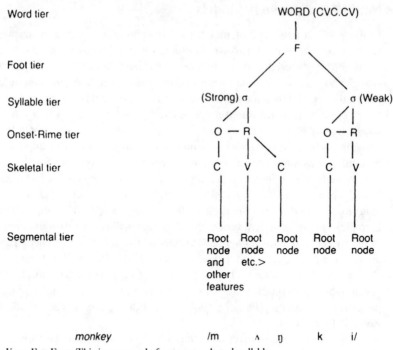

Word tier

Foot tier

Syllable tier

Onset-Rime tier

Skeletal tier

Segmental tier

WORD (CVC.CV)

F

(Strong) σ   σ (Weak)

O — R   O — R

C   V   C   C   V

Root   Root   Root   Root   Root
node   node   node   node   node
and   etc.>
other
features

monkey   /m   ʌ   ŋ   k   i/

Key: F = Foot. This is composed of a strong and weak syllable.
  σ = Syllable.
  O = Onset. This includes all prevocalic consonants (C) in a syllable.
  R = Rhyme/Rime. This includes the vowel (V) and postvocalic
      consonants in a syllable.

FIGURE 2.1 Nonlinear representation of the word *monkey.* **Source: Bernhardt and Stoel-Gammon (1994), reprinted by permission of the American Speech-Language-Hearing Association.**

Planar segregation is a nonlinear concept which has proven highly useful for analyzing child data. The idea is that features can spread only within a plane or tier, so that consonants affect consonants or vowels affect vowels (resulting in consonant or vowel harmony, respectively), with no concomitant C to V or V to C effects. Thus, planar segregation is one way of expressing a relative lack of complexity in the child's initial phonological representations/organization.

Nonlinear models are compatible with the nativist approach to the acquisition of phonology. Following Chomsky's (1981) parameter-setting model of language acquisition, Bernhardt (1994) has proposed a nativist interpretation:

> If a child comes to the language-learning situation with a representational framework and a set of universal principles, "templates" are then available to utilize for decoding and encoding . . . . Exposure to the input language(s) will both confirm the universally-determined representation (e.g., that, as expected, the language has CV units and stop consonants) and also

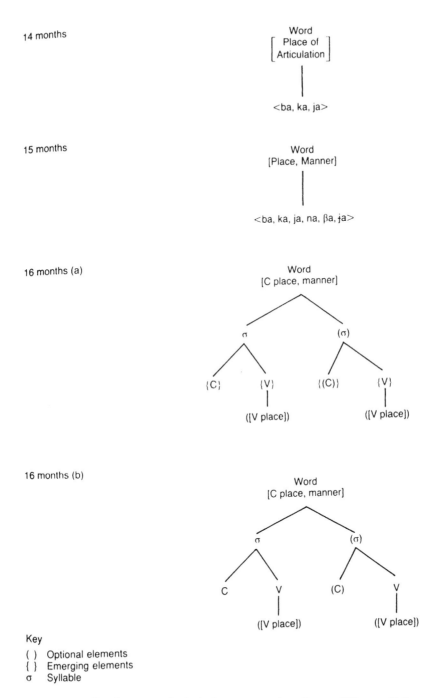

14 months

Word
[Place of Articulation]

<ba, ka, ja>

15 months

Word
[Place, Manner]

<ba, ka, ja, na, βa, ɟa>

16 months (a)

Word
[C place, manner]

σ   (σ)

{C}   {V}   {(C)}   {V}

([V place])   ([V place])

16 months (b)

Word
[C place, manner]

σ   (σ)

C   V   (C)   V

([V place])   ([V place])

Key

( ) Optional elements
{ } Emerging elements
σ   Syllable

FIGURE 2.2. Development of a lexical representation. *Source*: **Vihman, Velleman, and McCune (1994). In Yavas (Ed.),** *First and Second Language Phonology.* **Reprinted with the permission of Singular Publishing Group.**

result in "setting" of parameters where options are available (e.g., that the language has final consonants and that stress is syllable-initial in a given language) . . . (161).

(See also Bernhardt and Stoel-Gammon, 1994; Bernhardt and Stemberger, 1998.)

An alternative functionalist interpretation of the establishment of the expectation of CV syllables and stop consonants is equally plausible and follows quite naturally from the character of vocal development in the first year (see below). However,

"whether phonological acquisition is specified by innate parameters; determined by some characteristics of the language to which the child is exposed; "chosen" by the child based on idiosyncratic perceptual, physiological, or cognitive biases; or some combination of the above is an open and widely debated question. In any case, the course of phonological development includes the addition of complexity to any or all of these aspects of the representation." (Vihman et al., 1994)

Summary

The earlier behaviorist and structuralist models developed out of the prevailing American and European linguistic schools of the midcentury and were, to a great extent, deductive rather than empirically based. Extensive analysis of the vocal productions of children in the past three decades led to the rejection of most aspects of these views. The remaining models all remain influential in phonological acquisition. The generative phonology model emphasizes universal constraints and a systematic, smooth progression toward the adult system; it explicitly denies the development of the child's own system and posits accurate perception of the adult forms from the start. The cognitive model, on the other hand, allows for individual or idiosyncratic child systems, based in part on initially imperfect perception of adult forms. This model emphasizes the active role of the child, involving individual strategies, hypothesis-formation, and problem solving. The biological model complements rather than competes with the cognitive model, reflecting renewed interest in the biological roots of language in humans as well as in the individual child. Finally, the more recent formal models of adult phonology, nonlinear models, provide new perspectives on developing structure which are better adapted to the understanding of the acquisition of child phonology than were earlier, segmentally based generative models.

Infant Perception: Breaking into the Code

Having reviewed the main theories of normal phonological development, we will now present a chronological account of infant perception and production. We begin with speech perception by infants, since perception of the sounds of the adult language would logically seem to precede adultlike sound production. Perception and production are thought to develop in parallel but to interact with each other. Perception and production are treated separately here for purposes of explanation.

The study of infant perception continues as a productive field of inquiry, with exciting new research findings emerging on a regular basis (see Jusczyk, 1997). We know that very young infants are capable of hearing the difference between most of the sounds used contrastively in any language. These perceptual capacities allow the child to make sense of what William James (1890) described as the "blooming buzzing confusion" of the world facing the newborn infant.

Problems Facing the Child

At the outset of our inquiry, we must ask how the child gets started on the difficult task of "learning to pronounce." To begin with, what do we know about how the child hears the sounds of language? The stream of speech is not naturally segmented into separate sounds, but rather consists of a continuous flow of overlapping sounds. This presents a **segmentation** problem for the infant. The adult listener applies his or her knowledge of the language to pick out contrasting syllables and segments as well as words and phrases. But what of the naive ear of the infant? How does the child pick out the sound units of language?

Equally problematic is the question of **perceptual constancy**. How does the child listening to speech decide what counts as the "same sound," despite differences in the physical features of the sound? The acoustic signals produced by males, females, and children are quite different due to significant differences in vocal tract size and configuration. Equally important acoustic differences result from differences in phonetic context (e.g., consonant before /i/ versus /u/), positional context (e.g., word-initial versus word-final), and rate (e.g., the rapid, fluent speech of "small talk" versus the slower, more hesitant production of carefully considered discourse). How does the child recognize as the "same sound" variations associated with different speakers, different contexts, and different rates of speech?

Research Methodology Used to Study Infant Perception

A considerable body of evidence concerning the perceptual abilities of infants is available as a result of the ingenious research methodologies developed in the 1970s and 1980s. These methodologies are based on a simple observation: Infants, like older people, react to changes they perceive in their environment and become bored by ("habituate to") repetitions of the same event.

In 1971, Eimas, Siqueland, Jusczyk, and Vigorito reported a procedure known as the **high-amplitude sucking** paradigm to test infants' discrimination of voiced and voiceless and aspirated and unaspirated stops. This procedure has been used to obtain data on the discriminatory skills of infants from birth to 3 or 4 months of age. It allows the infant to control the presentation of a speech stimulus by the rate of sucking on a pacifier attached to a pressure transducer. Once the infant's baseline sucking rate has been established, a repeating speech stimulus such as [pa pa pa] is presented. The frequency of repetition of the sound is controlled by the infant's sucking rate. The presentation of the speech sound is presumed to serve as "contingent reinforcement" for the infant; increased sucking is interpreted as an expression of awareness of, and interest in, the sound stimulus. After several minutes, the infant's sucking rate typically levels off (called *asymptote*) and then decreases. Decreased sucking is taken to indicate that the infant has habituated and is no longer interested in the stimulus. The stimulus is then changed for the experimental group of infants, who hear a different repeated syllable (e.g., [ba ba ba]), while the infants in the control group continue to hear the sound stimulus first presented.

The sucking responses of the experimental group during this changed-stimulus condition are compared with those of the control group, which receives only a single stimulus throughout the experiment. If, following presentation of the second stimulus, the experimental group increases its sucking response while the control group maintains or slows its sucking rate, it is inferred that the experimental subjects perceived the difference between the two stimuli.

The other procedure most often used to test infant perception is the **visually reinforced head turn**, which is most appropriate for older infants (aged 6 to 12 months). Originally developed for assessing audiometric thresholds, this localization technique typically presents a repeated background sound for a time, follows it with a minimally different stimulus for a few seconds, and then repeats the original background stimulus. A head turn toward the sound source when the second sound is introduced is reinforced with the presentation of a lighted, animated toy that "rewards" the infant for discriminating the new sound from the old. If the infant turns his or her head during **change** trials (in which a new sound is introduced) but not during **control** trials (in which the same sound continues to be presented), it is concluded that the infant is able to discriminate the two contrasting sounds.

There are difficulties in the use of each of these procedures. In particular, since not all infants will habituate, large numbers of subjects must be tested to obtain statistically meaningful results. Nevertheless, several of the findings have been replicated many times over, in different laboratories by different investigators, so the results appear to be consistent.

Categorical Perception

The acoustic cues relevant to speech sounds—such as the cues associated with voicing and aspiration or with place of articulation—may vary along a continuous parameter, but adults respond to these acoustic signals as if sharp boundaries were present at specific points along the continuum. For example, in producing the syllable /pa/ or /ba/, the speaker completely closes off the flow of air through the vocal tract (by bringing his or her lips together) and then releases the closure (by opening his or her mouth) in order to produce the following vowel. The difference between /p/ and /b/ is determined by the timing of the opening of the lips in relation to the onset of vocal-cord vibration for vowel production. If the vocal cords begin to vibrate *before* the release of the oral closure, the stop is "pre-voiced," as in French word-initial /b/ or English intervocalic /b/. If the vocal cords begin to vibrate *at about the same time* that the lips are opened, an English (word-initial) /b/ is heard, but if the vibration of the vocal cords is *delayed*, English (word-initial) /p/ (aspirated [pʰ]) is heard. The parameter just described is referred to as voice onset time, or VOT.

A continuum of VOT possibilities exists beyond those associated with English "pre-voiced" (intervocalic) /b/, word-initial /b/, and word-initial /p/, although most languages seem to make use of one or more of these three in their phonemic system. Using **speech synthesis** (the artificial production of speech sounds), investigators have tested adult perception of the acoustic cues corresponding to the VOT continuum (Lisker and Abramson, 1964). Presented with a series of synthetic speech-like sounds resembling a range of different VOT values, adults generally perceive the stimuli as belonging to one of the phonemic categories distinguished in their own language. Thus, English-speakers hear virtually all stimuli as either /ba/ or /pa/, as if a sharp boundary divided the two; this is known as **categorical perception**. For some years, these findings were assumed to reflect adults' experience with the categories of their language. However, research with infants led to the surprising finding that 2- to 4-month-old babies also differentiate sound categories despite their inexperience with the sounds of any language. Although infants do not discriminate between acoustically different stimuli *within* the adult categories, they are able to discriminate similar acoustic differences *between* adult sound categories.

English /b/ versus /p/ are discriminated by infants as if the two phonemic categories were known to them. This finding was initially attributed to an *innate mechanism* in humans for the recognition of speech categories. Later research showed that not only human infants but also chinchillas and monkeys can distinguish this categorical boundary (Kuhl, 1987). So the argument for an innate human mechanism *specialized for speech perceptions* lacks strong supporting evidence. It is more likely that the phonetic boundary between the English language categories of voiceless and voiced stops happens to correspond to a *naturally salient physical boundary* which is distinguished by infants, whether or not they have been exposed to English, and also by other mammals possessing auditory biases similar to those of humans. Hauser (1996) provides a useful discussion of the close relationship between humans' and other animals' *auditory* mechanisms—in contrast with the uniqueness of the human *speech production* mechanism (which we will consider below).

The human auditory system seems to be especially attuned to **abrupt discontinuities**, or natural breaks, in the acoustic stream, like those created by stop consonants. Such a phonetic predisposition, together with the ability to discriminate continuous acoustic signals in a categorical way, may be crucial in enabling the child to solve the segmentation problem; that is, to break into a code based on overlapping sounds embedded in an ongoing stream of speech.

Universal Perception: Early Abilities

Using the various procedures described earlier, investigators have been able to demonstrate that an infant can discriminate a wide range of phonetic contrasts used in adult languages, regardless of the language of the child's environment (for overviews, see Vihman, 1996; Jusczyk, 1997). Thus, children as young as 2 to 3 months of age can discriminate **place of articulation** in syllable-initial [b], [d], and [g]. Two-month-old infants can also discriminate [d] versus [g] in medial and final position. Only the distinction between contrasting unreleased (C)VC syllables (e.g., *bat* [bæt] and *back* [bæk]), which are not always easily identified by adults (Householder, 1956), were found to exceed infants' perceptual abilities. Investigation of **manner of articulation** contrasts has shown that infants can discriminate stops from nasals as well as from glides and [ra] from [la].

Furthermore, 1- to 4-month-old infants have been found to discriminate the three vowels most commonly contrasted in languages ([a] vs. [i] vs. [u]). Embedding the vowels in a syllable ([pa] vs. [pi]) did not impede discrimination. In addition, infants of this age raised in an English-speaking environment were able to distinguish **oral** versus **nasal** vowels ([pa] vs. [pã)]), even though the oral-nasal contrast is not used phonemically in English vowels (Trehub, 1976). (It does function phonemically in French and Hindi.) Kuhl (1987) reviewed a number of studies in which she and her colleagues tested 1- to 4-month-old infants for perceptual constancy by presenting tokens of the vowels [a] and [i], each produced on monotone and rise-fall **pitches**, with the different pitch-tokens varied randomly. The children were able to discriminate the vowels and disregarded the differences in pitch. However, when the reverse situation was tested, contrasting the two pitch contours with random shifting between [a] and [i] as the vowel carrying the pitch, the infants failed to discriminate the pitch contrast. Similar testing of vowel contrasts produced by adult male versus female and child talkers showed that infants easily discriminate even the acoustically similar vowels /a/ and /ɔ/, regardless of changes in the speaker.

A few contrasts have been reported as difficult to discriminate in the early months. Thus the child must learn such contrasts as voicing and place in fricatives, for example ([sa] vs. [za], [fa] vs. [θa], [fi] vs. [θi]) (Eilers and Minifie,1975; Eilers, 1977). These results are interesting because the /f/ versus /θ/ distinction is a notoriously difficult one for children, even as late as age 3 or 4 (cf., e.g., Locke, 1980b), and it can prove difficult for adults as well, especially in noisy listening conditions. However, other studies have shown that when computer-synthesized tokens are used instead of naturally produced syllables, 2- to 3-month-olds can discriminate [fa] versus [θa] (Jusczyk, Murray, and Bayly, 1979).

Another type of discrimination that may exceed infants' perceptual capacities is that between different stops embedded in multisyllabic vocalizations with relatively short syllables (less than 300 milliseconds: [ataba] vs. [atapa]) (Trehub, 1973). This observation is interesting in light of children's use of syllable deletion and multisyllabic words well into the third year, which reflects the difficulty that the production of multisyllabic words poses for them. These production problems associated with multisyllabic words may result from perceptual as well as articulatory difficulties. In other words, relatively short syllables embedded in long words may be difficult to perceive and store even when the child is successfully producing one- and two-syllable words. Later studies have shown that the difficulty of making discriminations within a "long word" context can be reduced by adding exaggerated stress to the contrasting syllable, as caretakers typically do in speaking to children (Fernald and Simon, 1984; Karzon, 1985).

In summary, in the first few months of life, infants are capable of distinguishing between consonants that differ in place and manner of articulation, and also between some vowels. Distinguishing among certain fricatives and between stops embedded in longer, multisyllabic vocalizations is more problematic for young children.

The Role of Linguistic Experience

Some investigators have suggested that *linguistic experience* within the first six months of life may influence the child's perceptual capacities, particularly with respect to voicing and aspiration contrasts in stops. Children exposed to languages with pre-voiced stops were found to discriminate pre-voiced from voiced (unaspirated) stops, whereas infants exposed only to English did not make this discrimination. However, exposure to the speech of a given language does not ensure that a specific phonemic category or contrast will be perceived (MacKain, 1982). Pre-voiced stops occur in English, though only in intervocalic position. Thus, the child exposed to English does "experience" pre-voiced stops, though they are not contrastive. It is unclear how the young child's exposure to the different phonemic categories in particular languages leads to differential categorical perception of speech at this early stage of development.

On the other hand, recent work investigating "implicit" or "incidental" learning has provided new insight into the way that infants may acquire knowledge of the segmental properties of the native language. This kind of learning is related to frequency of occurrence of phonological events in the environment. It requires no attention to speech per se, but merely exposure to it. For example, adults or children focusing on a drawing task were found to develop knowledge of the sequences of segments ("possible co-occurrences") represented in a recording of uninterrupted strings of consonant + vowel syllables that was playing in the background, although most of the participants in the experiment subsequently reported paying no conscious attention to the auditory stimuli (Saffran, Newport, Aslin, Tunick, and Barrueco, 1997). Implicit learning, unlike the explicit learning of specific forms or structures of language, does not appear to change with development. That is, it becomes neither better nor worse in older individuals. Furthermore, such learning has been demonstrated in prelinguistic infants (Saffran, Aslin and Newport, 1996).

The Role of Prosody

In the 1990s research on infant perceptual capacities began to focus on larger speech units (sequences of sentences, clauses, and phrases rather than isolated syllables) and on other influences affecting infant attention to the speech signal (own mother or own language vs. other mother, other language; speech directed to infants, or "motherese," vs. speech directed to adults). Such studies have provided evidence that infants are strongly attracted to the sound of their own language, especially when spoken by the mother and especially when she uses the wide pitch contours characteristic of motherese. The attraction of prosodically varied speech is thought to be related to its emotional tone; it is part of the process of bonding between mother and infant. In add   the infant's close attention to the caretaker's speech most likely plays an importan'   ʼ⁻ beginning to identify the relevant **units** of the adult language. Specifi⁄   ⁻⁻sitive to the perceptual unity of **clauses** by 6 months of age;
verb) appear to be detectible by 9 months (Jusczyk
ond half of the first year, however, infants appear
marily to prosodic contours, or the "melody of sp
as well (Vihman, Nakai, and DePaolis, 2000).
natural basis for the explicit word learning that
of life.

Summary

What perceptual capabilities are infants bɾ
flow of speech? And which capabilities de

language used around them? Researchers report that during the first months of life, infants respond differentially to different speech stimuli and treat some sounds varied along a continuum as if they belonged to categories of sounds used in the adult language. These discriminations probably reflect inherent biases in the auditory systems of mammals, including humans. Certain natural boundaries between sounds appear to be universally salient to infants, whether or not the natural boundary is matched by a phonemic contrast in the adult language to which the child is exposed. These built-in biases make it possible for the infant to begin finding recognizable patterns in the stream of overlapping sounds that constitute speech.

Many contrasts used in language are discriminable from an early age, including the differences among place of consonant articulation (labial/dental/velar) or manner of articulation (stops vs. nasals or glides, /ra/ vs. /la/); other contrasts, especially distinctions among different fricatives, unreleased final stops, and those embedded in multisyllabic utterances, may be discriminated only later, as they require maturation and increased exposure to language. Attempts to demonstrate the effects of experience with different phonemic systems during the first few months of life remain inconclusive. Prosodic characteristics of speech also play an important role, especially in the earliest stages of development of perceptual knowledge of the native language.

Infant Production: Interaction of Maturation and Experience

The problem facing the infant learning to produce speech sounds can be broken down into a series of increasingly complex tasks, ranging from vocal production per se to communicative use in the context of adult-based sound patterns, or *words* (Menyuk et al., 1986). These tasks include (1) learning to produce a variety of vocal sounds, (2) matching sound patterns produced by adults to some of the well-practiced vocal patterns in the infant's repertoire, (3) associating certain adult sound patterns with situations where they are often produced (situation-bound word use), (4) achieving the understanding that sound-pattern production can be used as a means to share a focus of attention or to make a request, and (5) utilizing adult-based words to serve communicative goals in novel settings (the referential and symbolic use of words).

The tasks outlined above identify the cognitive challenges in learning to speak. Mastery of the articulatory gestures alone will take five years or more; perceptual development presumably plays a role in this process as well. When the process of phonological acquisition is barely underway, the child has already begun work on other aspects of communicative development, including the problem of apprehending the significance of regular and recurrent form-meaning correspondences (i.e., developing comprehension of words and of communicative gestures, such as pointing, clapping, or waving). As outlined above, the cognitive problems for the would-be language user involve matching his or her own productive capacities to the sound patterns of the adult language, developing the ability to them at will, and developing the skills to use language to refer to events outside the situational context. We begin our account of vocal production with the first task, ce a variety of vocal sounds.

Learning to Produce a Variety of Vocal Sounds

The infant's vocal tract is not simply a miniature or smaller version of the adult's (see Figure 2.3). Differences include: (1) a much shorter vocal tract; (2) a relatively shorter pharyngeal cavity; (3) a tongue mass placed relatively farther forward in the oral cavity; (4) a gradual, rather than a right-angle, bend in the oropharyngeal channel; (5) a high larynx; and (6) a close approximation of the velopharynx and epiglottis (Kent and Murray, 1982). The differences in anatomical structure affect the nature of infant vocal productions. For example, the close relationship of laryngeal and velopharyngeal cavities leads to nasal breathing and early nasal vocalizations by the infant; it is only after the velum and epiglottis grow farther apart, when the infant is about 4 to 6 months old, that nonnasal vocal sounds first appear in significant quantities.

Early Stages of Production

Oller (1980) and Stark (1980) have provided similar descriptions of vocal production over the first year of life. **Reflexive** vocalizations (i.e., vocalizations arising as automatic

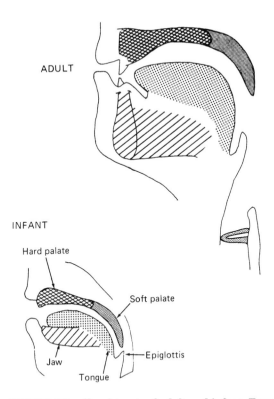

FIGURE 2.3. Vocal tracts of adult and infant. From R.D. Kent and A.D. Murray, "Acoustic Features of Infant Vocalic Utterances at 3, 6, and 9 Months." *JASA*, 72 (1982): 353–365. Used with permission.

responses to internal or external stimulation, such as hunger or discomfort) have typically been separated in the literature on infant vocal production from other aspects of speech and language. One aspect of reflexive vocalization should be noted as it appears to be of some consequence in the transition to language. This is the "grunt," a brief glottal-initial sound with no supraglottal constriction that first occurs as the product of physiological changes associated with effort (McCune, Vihman, Roug-Hellichius, Delery, and Gogate, 1996). Stark (1993) has described such grunts as a result of physical effort involved for the infant in maintaining the head erect. The same involuntary vocal production has been noted in association with other postural adjustments, such as reaching (Trevarthan and Hubley, 1978) or crawling (Stark, Bernstein, and Demorest, 1993). "Grunting" can be seen as a foundational sound-meaning link in production (i.e., a precursor to language), though unlike true language production, it is not intentional, communicative, or arbitrary.

Oller (1980) divides the first six months into three sequential stages, which he terms the *phonation stage*, the *cooing stage*, and the *expansion stage*. He also identifies two babbling stages, in the second half of the first year, of *canonical and variegated babbling*. There is considerable overlap between stages, and the ages assigned to each stage are only approximations. Furthermore, although the appearance of canonical babbling is a landmark event, variegated babbling has been found to be difficult to distinguish as a chronologically separate "stage."

1. In the **phonation** stage (0–1 month), speech-like sounds are rare. The largest number of nonreflexive, nondistress sounds are the "quasi-resonant nuclei," which Oller (1980) characterizes as vocalizations with normal phonation but limited resonance, produced with a closed or nearly closed mouth. These elements give the auditory impression of a syllabic nasal.
2. In the **goo** or **cooing** stage (2–3 months), velar consonant-like sounds are produced with some frequency, but the rhythmic properties of adult syllables and the timing of the articulatory gestures for adult consonants have not yet been mastered. Acoustically, the cooing sounds are similar to rounded back vowels such as [u].
3. In the **expansion** stage (4–6 months), the child appears to gain increasing control of both laryngeal and oral articulatory mechanisms. He or she explores the vocal mechanism through the playful use of squealing, growling, yelling, and "raspberry" vocalizations (bilabial trills). "Fully resonant nuclei" (adultlike vowels) begin to be produced in this period, as does "marginal babbling," in which consonantlike and vowel-like features occur but lack the mature regular-syllable timing characteristics of canonical babbling.

Stark (1978) emphasized the interrelationship of earlier and later vocal behaviors in the first six months of life. The emergence of cooing is dependent on increased control over voicing, which is first found only in crying. The new co-occurrence of voicing, egressive breath direction, and consonant-like closures results from the overlap between the maturation in voluntary laryngeal control and continuing reflexive activity of the vocal tract. The acquisition of control over this new behavioral combination is probably derived from the interaction of maturation and the experience of exercising the new behavior. The modified combination is then ready to begin to form new combinations with other more primitive behaviors. Thus, cooing or comfort sounds are expanded through the use of vocal play, which allows the infant to gain greater control over the activity of the tongue, lips, and jaw.

Beginnings of Adultlike Production: The Emergence of Consonants

The first probable evidence of adult language influence on production is manifested by the emergence of canonical babbling (Oller's Stage 4; also known as reduplicated babbling), typically at about 6 to 8 months. The sudden appearance of genuine syllabic production involving a true consonant and a "fully resonant nucleus" or vowel, often (though not exclusively) chained in repeated sequences such as [bababa], [dadada], or [mamama], constitutes the chief production milestone in the first year. The onset of this stage is easily recognized by parents, who report the child to be babbling or even "talking," although few, if any, consistent sound-meaning relations are likely to be observed.

Canonical babbling has been viewed primarily as the outgrowth of physiological maturation, uninfluenced by exposure to the adult language. However, Oller and his colleagues have reported that deaf children do not produce canonical babbling within the first year (Oller and Eilers, 1988; cf. also Stoel-Gammon and Otomo, 1986), whereas such babbling typically occurs in hearing babies by 10 months at the latest. These findings suggest that canonical babbling depends on auditory exposure and, thus, may reflect the influence of the adult language as well as physiological maturation.

The onset of canonical babbling may be viewed as a production discontinuity since it represents the first use of true consonantal articulation. The fact that stops (and nasals, or stops articulated with a lowered velum) are the earliest true consonants to be produced may be related to the natural **perceptual salience** of syllables with a stop onset. Stops present the sharpest possible contrast with vowels and provide the most obtrusive break in the acoustic stream of speech sounds. On the other hand, stop production is also relatively undemanding: syllables such as [ba], [da], [na] may be articulated through mandibular action alone (Kent, 1992). It is likely that this production milestone represents an advance in: (1) motor control, which is maturational or tied to natural physiological development in the first year; (2) the (experience-based) integration of visual and auditory perception of adult sequences of open/closed mouth and voice/silence alternation; and (3) global imitation of adult vocalization. In other words, children see as well as hear stop consonants in adult speech, produce such sounds themselves, and engage in repetitive vocal production or sound play, recreating their impression of adult speech.

Variegated Babbling and Universal Production Patterns

The last babbling stage (Oller's Stage 5) is variegated babbling, in which continued use of adult-like syllables is supplemented by the use of increasingly varied consonants and vowels within a single vocalization (e.g., from the babbling of a 9-month-old girl, [ʔəmae:h], [wətʌ], [te:kæ], [hɛtapa]: Vihman, Ferguson, and Elbert, 1986). Elbers (1982) views bab-

bling in this period as "a systematic, continuous and largely self-directed process of exploration," in which the child constructs a phonetic "spring-board" to speech (45). Variegated
babbling may emerge very soon after the onset of canonical babbling (Smith, Brown-
Sweeney, and Stoel-Gammon, 1989; Mitchell and Kent, 1990). A number of studies have
looked at the sound repertoire found in the variegated babbling of children learning different languages. These segmental repertoires are virtually indistinguishable. Locke (1983)
cited the babbling repertoires for infants (aged 9 to 15 months) acquiring one of 15 languages each. He found that stops and nasals formed the base of each inventory, with a relatively low incidence for most other sounds (see also McCune and Vihman, 2001).
However, direct cross-linguistic comparisons of sound production frequencies in babbling
vocalizations, examined through both instrumental analysis (of vowels) and phonetic
transcription (of consonants), have revealed the first language-specific differences at 10
months, when word production is barely underway or has not yet begun (Boysson-Bardies
et al., 1989; Boysson-Bardies and Vihman, 1991).

Vowel Production in the First Year

So far, we have concentrated mainly on the early development of consonants since it is the
onset of true consonant use that seems to mark the beginning of adultlike vocal production.
However, it is vowel production that dominates infant vocalization throughout the first
year. Vowels have been less extensively investigated, primarily because they are particularly difficult to transcribe reliably and thus difficult to characterize (Davis and Mac-
Neilage, 1990). For example, Lieberman (1980) reported inter-transcriber reliability of 73
percent for the vowels produced by children aged about 3 to 14 months. Lieberman's
reported findings for a single child's vowel productions are summarized below.

Lieberman used spectrographic analysis as a supplement to phonetic transcription
and reported little change in average formant frequency values over the period investigated.
However, the various vowels transcribed for 4 months showed considerable acoustic overlap in formant frequencies. A month later, spectrographic analysis yielded identification of
a rudimentary vowel triangle. The gradual differentiation in the acoustic vowel space could
be seen to continue (based on data from other subjects) until age 3.

The vowels most often perceived over the entire period were lax—[ɛ, ɪ, æ, ʌ, ʊ]—
and were already present at the earliest session. The vowel [ɛ] was heard most frequently
(33 percent of all the vowels transcribed), and the remaining lax vowels each accounted for
11 percent (17 percent of the data). The remaining (tense) vowels each accounted for no
more than 5 percent, with the back rounded [o] and [u] least frequent (1 percent each).

Kent and Murray (1982) investigated the acoustic features of vocalic utterances at 3,
6, and 9 months (seven infants at each age). Their findings were similar to those reported
by Lieberman. The range of F_1 and F_2 frequencies increased somewhat across each age
interval, but the majority of the vowels used by the 9-month-old infants showed roughly the
same formant pattern as did the vowels of the younger subjects. Given the anatomical differences between adults and infants, it is not surprising that the range of possible infant
vowel productions should be more restricted than those of adults. The formant patterns of
infant vowels fit within the range of mid-front or central adult vowels.

Consonant-vowel Interactions

Davis and MacNeilage (1990) reported an interaction of consonant and vowel occurrence in the late babbling and early words of a child whose production they investigated intensively. Alveolars were found to be followed disproportionately by high-front vowels, velars (when used at all) by high-back vowels, and labials by central vowels. These investigators suggested that the alveolars and velars may each tend to be followed by the high vowel closest in articulatory space for mechanical reasons, reflecting a lack of differentiation of articulatory gestures. However, Vihman reported a tendency for these C-V associations to reflect the influence of different adult languages (e.g., /(alveolar) Ci/ is a common sequence in English—*daddy, pretty, lady, dolly,* while /ko/ occurs in many Japanese words used by young children), and suggests that reliance on such sequences may be a strategy particular to word production. Vihman claimed that only the labial/central vowel association appeared to reflect an early physiological basis, in which the tongue remains in a neutral, resting position while the lip gesture is actively recruited for articulation. A later controlled study of nine children acquiring English at 18, 21, and 24 months of age found little evidence of C-V interactions in word production, although velar words with back vowels tended to be preferentially selected, and back vowels tended to be accurately produced after velars (Tyler and Langsdale, 1996). On the other hand, Davis and MacNeilage have continued to report C-V interactions in the vocal production of infants, interactions which they subsequently identified in adult languages as well (Davis and MacNeilage, 1995; MacNeilage and Davis, 2000; MacNeilage, Davis, Kinney, and Matyear, 2000).

Prosodic Development in Early Vocal Production

The development of the stress and intonational patterns of language has received considerably less attention than has the development of segments and segmental contrasts. This reflects, in part, the fact that the prosodic properties of adult languages are also less well understood. Nevertheless, the literature points to a few conclusions. Acoustic analysis of infant vocalizations across the first year of life shows that falling pitch is the most common contour during this period. Kent and Murray (1982) offer a physiological explanation, suggesting that a falling fundamental frequency, or pitch contour, is the natural result of a decline in subglottal pressure in the course of a vocalization. A reduction of vocal fold length and tension as the muscles of the larynx relax at the end of a vocalization could also lead to a falling **pitch contour**. A rising pitch contour requires an increase in vocal fold length or tension at the end of the vocalization, or an increase in subglottal pressure, or both. It seems natural, then, that the development of contrastive, rising pitch contours should develop later than falling pitch contours. It appears that this sequence is a general one, regardless of the language being acquired.

Once the variegated babbling stage has been reached, the child may also produce jargon. This phenomenon results when adult-like pitch movement and rhythm are imposed on rapidly produced multisyllabic strings of variegated babble. In children acquiring English, multisyllabic jargon strings of this kind typically end with a relatively low pitch on the next-to-last syllable followed by a shift to a mid or mid-falling pitch on the last syllable.

Notice that a phrase-final shift in pitch is a characteristic adult English intonation pattern. Jargon seems to represent the child's attempts to reproduce the intonation patterns of speech, that is, of phrases or sentences; the result often impresses the adult listener as conversation without words (cf. Menn, 1976; Peters, 1983; Vihman and Miller, 1988).

Summary

Young children face a series of production tasks on their way to learning the language of their environment. To begin with, they must gain control of laryngeal and articulatory gestures to develop the precision necessary to produce the sounds of language. Developing such control involves both maturation of the laryngeal, articulatory, and perceptual mechanisms and accommodation to the sound patterns of the specific language spoken to the child. Thus, phonological development in the young child involves the interaction of physical maturation and social experience.

During the first six months of life, three stages of voluntary vocal behavior can be distinguished: the phonation stage, the cooing stage, and the expansion stage. Acquisition of control over each new behavioral combination is the result of the interaction of maturation and experience or practice in using the new motor behavior.

Between age 6 and 10 months, canonical babbling begins to be produced. This constitutes the main discontinuity, or sharp qualitative change, in infant production in the first year, and it provides the first concrete evidence of the influence of auditory experience with an adult language. In the last babbling stage, variegated babbling, the child prepares the phonetic ground for his or her first attempts at adult words. At this stage, infant consonantal repertoires are largely indistinguishable across languages, but consonant and vowel production frequencies begin to reflect differences in the child's linguistic experience.

During the first year, infant vowel production shows little change. Adult transcribers typically perceive the primitive vowels as mid-front or central. C-V interactions have been identified, possibly reflecting a biomechanical production bias toward economy of articulatory movements. Falling pitch contours predominate in the children's productions in the first year, perhaps for (universal) physiological reasons. Once the child has begun producing variegated babble, adultlike stress patterns and intonation contours may also be used, giving the surface effect of adult language, but without content or meaning.

The Transition Period: From Babble to Speech

We have reviewed the infant's perception and production of speech during the first year of life. The infant manifests impressive discriminatory abilities for speech sounds at a very early age. However, we have yet to consider how these abilities serve the child in linguistic perception, in identifying and remembering meaningful sound patterns of the adult language. The child also faces a series of tasks in learning to produce meaningful speech. So far, we have only discussed the first of these tasks—learning to produce a variety of vocal sounds. By the end of the first year, the child is babbling or, in other words, producing adultlike sequences of syllables that include a range of different consonants and vowels. Furthermore, the child is no longer restricted to a single consonant or vowel type per vocalization. Some use of rising pitch contours may occur alongside the more common falling pitch.

We turn now to the transition period, when the babbler becomes a talker. The critical development in this period is the linking of sound patterns with meaning, first in comprehension, then in word production. Sporadic signs of understanding may occur in the middle of the first year, so we will have to backtrack slightly in our chronological account to pick up the trail of the child's first steps in the use of meaning and communication.

The transition period is best defined by certain developmental events. It begins with the onset of comprehension of the adult language, and it closes when word use begins to dominate babble, typically some time after the child has produced about 50 different words spontaneously. The age range in which these developments occur is extremely variable. Some normally developing children fail to produce many recognizable words before the age of 2, although they will show evidence of good language comprehension long before this time. For many, and perhaps most, children, the transition to speech will occur during the period from about 9 to 18 months.

Relating Sound Patterns to Meanings

When the child first begins to respond differentially to particular words or phrases of the adult language—that is, begins to show comprehension—he or she has begun to match discriminable differences in sound patterns with differences in the use or function of those patterns. The first reports of language comprehension, found in the diary records kept by linguist parents, noted earliest signs of comprehension at age 4 or 5 months. At 20 weeks, Hans Lindner responded to *Tick-tack* (German for tick-tock) by looking toward the large, loudly ticking wall clock that had often been pointed out to him (Lindner, 1898, reported in Ferguson, 1978). At 6 months, Deville's daughter responded to *bravo* by clapping her hands, and at 7 months she would respond to French *chut* (*quiet!*) by refraining from touching an item of interest (Deville, 1890, 1891, reported in Lewis, 1936). Lewis observed his child's first responses to words at 8 or 9 months: a smile for *Cuckoo!* "uttered in a special tone of voice," recoil from a movement for *No!* and a wave for *Say goodbye!* (Lewis, 1936; 107). In each case, the child had heard the word repeatedly in context, and the expected behavior (e.g., the appropriate gesture for routines involving clapping or waving) had been made clear on numerous occasions. The earliest signs of word recognition may be isolated occurrences. By 10 or 11 months, there is generally considerable evidence of language comprehension although it is difficult to determine precisely how much the child understands from words alone and how much involves familiarity with the situational contexts in which words are used.

Perception in the Transition Period: Entry into the Native Language

The beginnings of comprehension of the adult language, combined with production of the first learned gestures (e.g., clapping, waving), mark a significant new step in the child's development. We assume that at this point children have begun to develop a repertoire of familiar phonetic patterns drawn from the adult language and linked with specific meanings. Until very recently, there was little direct testing of perception of word-patterns in this period. Hallé and Boysson-Bardies (1994) introduced a new perception paradigm, however, by presenting to French infants two lists of words: "familiar words," or words the child could be expected to know from the home environment, and "rare words," which the child could not be expected to have heard. They found that at 11 months, infants looked longer in response to the familiar than to the rare words. Building on this finding, Hallé and Boysson-Bardies (1996) altered the familiar words in various ways to see what the effect would be on infant response. If the infants continued to look longer in response to the familiar words, the change could be taken not to have affected a critical element in the infants' representation of the words. These investigators found that *omission* of the initial consonant blocked word recognition, but *change in the manner of articulation* of the first consonant did not.

Vihman et al. (2000) tested infants acquiring British English, using the same paradigm. They found that the English infants also looked longer in response to familiar words (such as *baby, mummy, thank you*) than in response to rare words (such as *bridle, maiden, fog light*) by 11 months, though at 9 months there was as yet no difference in response. Unlike the French children, the English children's recognition of familiar words was blocked when the initial consonant was changed but not when the medial consonant was changed. It was suggested that the accentual difference between French (consistent final-syllable accent) and English (first-syllable stress on most words used with infants) might be the basis for this difference. Perhaps change to the onset consonant of an accented syllable is particularly salient to infants, and thus sufficient to block recognition, out of context, in this early period of word learning. Furthermore, the English children continued to respond with longer looking times to the familiar words even when the *stress pattern was changed* (i.e., BAby produced as baBY), suggesting that at this age infants are able to disregard the prosody and recognize words on the basis of their segmental pattern alone. (Notice that the accentual pattern of words is not invariable, especially in playful talk to infants: *Byebye*, for example, can be stressed on either syllable.)

Investigations of infant perception at the end of the first year revealed an important shift whose timing coincides with the beginnings of word recognition—or at least with early comprehension of language in well-established contexts. Werker and her colleagues (Werker, Gilbert, Humphrey, and Tees, 1981; Werker and Tees, 1983) set out to discover the point at which the infant's broad capacities for discrimination of phonemic contrasts are replaced by the adult's language-specific responses to speech sounds. They tested adults and 4-, 8-, and 12-year-old children on two contrasts which are phonemic in Hindi but unfamiliar to English-speakers: place of articulation (dental /t/ vs. retroflex /ʈ/) and VOT (voiceless aspirated /th/ vs. breathy voiced /dh/). In addition, they tested a contrast used in an Interior Salish Northwest Indian language, glottalized velar /kʔ/ versus glottalized uvular /qʔ/. Less than half of the adults and children aged 4 or over were able to discriminate these foreign contrasts, whereas most of the 6- to 8-month-old infants tested showed evidence of discrimination. In a critical study, Werker and Tees (1984) tested infants in age groups spanning the last half of the first year (6–8, 8–10, and 10–12 months) on the Hindi and Salishan place of articulation contrasts. The youngest group again showed discrimination, while the oldest group did not. The 8–10-month-olds were relatively successful with the Hindi contrast, but most of them did not discriminate the Salishan contrast.

The apparent decline in "universal" perceptual capacity at the end of the first year is intriguing and has aroused a good deal of interest. Have infants "entered into" the phonemic system of the language to which they are exposed at this time (Werker, 1991), when they are just beginning to attend to language with some sign of understanding of the (arbitrary) association of verbal sounds and (situation-based) meanings? It is difficult to see how the child could have structured perceptual information to that extent at this early stage. Furthermore, the child's earliest word production appears to reveal a broad or holistic phonological base rather than a full-blown set of phonemic (segmental) contrasts. One hypothesis for the apparent reorganization of perception at the onset to speech is that it is mediated by the child's emerging productive (articulatory) abilities (Locke, 1990; Vihman, 1991, 1993). As the child develops articulatory control and familiarity, through self-monitoring, with the sound as well as the feel of a few well-practiced articulatory gestures, we may suppose that certain salient sound patterns of the adult language begin to "stand out" perceptually, since they appear to match those familiar vocal patterns that the child has been repeatedly producing. Since influence from the particular language of the child's environment has just begun to affect the child's babbling at this age, it is possible that such an articulatory filter may serve to alter the child's initial "unbiased" response to speech sounds, replacing the "universal" readiness for any language by a more finely tuned readiness for the language of the child's caretakers (Werker and Pegg, 1992).

Protowords: "Grunts" as Precursors of Word Production

The child develops intentional communication at the same time that he or she is improving articulatory control and increasing in capacity to recognize adult sound patterns. Thus, a child may communicate meaning with gestures before doing so consistently with adult-like words. A number of observers of infants in this age range have noted the use of **protowords**, consistent vocal forms with no apparent adult model with the same or similar range of uses (see the review in Vihman, 1996). Generally, the forms are simple CV shapes, with glottals, [ʔ] and [h], or stops filling the consonant slot. Meanings are simple as well: broad markers of focus of attention or attempts to share interest or make a request (McCune et al., 1996). These minimal vocal expressions are produced quietly, with no apparent communicative intent at first; they appear to be related to the effort grunts observed contemporaneously as well as earlier, and may reflect the "effort of attention." Between about 14 and 16 months a new function may be observed, typically first expressed by grunts or other simple glottal-initial vocalizations. The new function involves the sharing of a focus of attention or interest; a related function is that of request (for an adult to do something for the child or provide something). The child may vocalize and point or show an object, all the while looking at an adult. These simple communicative forms reflect an important shift in the child's understanding of vocal function: Now meanings can be expressed by vocal forms—though the grunt form is not fully arbitrary, since it has its origin in the effort of movement and, secondarily, the effort of attention. Such a shift in understanding appears to be one of the prerequisites for adultlike word use, or the generalized use of words across a range of different situational contexts. Even children who already have a sizable conventional vocabulary may continue to use communicative grunts for some months, frequently together with pointing.

Common Tendencies

Vihman and her colleagues have investigated the extent of common tendencies vs. individual differences in early vocalizations, both across children learning the same language and across different languages (Vihman et al., 1986; Vihman and Greenlee, 1987; Boysson-Bardies and Vihman, 1991; Vihman, 1993). To assess variability across subjects at comparable stages of development, they defined sampling points on the basis of lexical use. Two early points reflected the beginnings of word use (ages ranged from 8 to 15 months), and two later points were taken from half-hour sessions in which 15 or more different words were used spontaneously (in this later period, the children had cumulative vocabularies, as reported by their mothers, of about 30 to 50 words; ages ranged from 12 to 23 months).

These studies found that variability in the phonetic categories analyzed was greatest at the earlier stages; a trend toward uniformity across subjects learning the same language was detected as the children's productive vocabularies increased. The strongest finding for the early lexical period was the considerable differences across subjects learning the same language, both in specific phonetic choices and in the degree of stability of phonetic preferences over time.

We can see the growing influence of the adult language in various ways during the transitional period from babbling to words. A trend toward increased use of consonants begins for all infants with the onset of canonical babbling (Kent and Murray, 1982), although this trend levels off toward the end of the first year if lexical acquisition is proceeding slowly. Repeated use of a growing repertoire of consonants over a period of weeks or months is the best predictor of rapid lexical development (McCune and Vihman 2001). Once lexical acquisition is underway, early words are considerably more likely to include a true consonant (stop, nasal, fricative, or liquid) than are babble vocalizations. This finding suggests that increasing knowledge of the adult language plays a significant role in the continued shift toward the use of consonants in this period.

The use of labials in babbling and words is highly variable in the earlier lexical stages, when the children have 10-word vocabularies at most. In the later stages, however, labials can account for as much as a third of all consonant productions, or even more. McCune and Vihman (2001) reported that labials occur frequently in the word repertoire of early talkers. Labial use is more characteristic of infant words than of babble, yet a study of mothers' speech in English, French, and Swedish showed that mothers used alveolars more frequently than labials in all three groups (Vihman, Kay, Boysson-Bardies, Durand, and Sundberg, 1994).

The advantage of labials for word production can be accounted for in various ways. In purely motoric or "mechanical" terms, first of all, labials are the only supraglottal consonants that are independent of the following vowel, since the tongue is not involved in their use (Davis and MacNeilage, 1990). Secondly, production of labial consonants affords more easily interpretable proprioceptive feedback than do consonants produced in other places (involving different parts of tongue and palate), since the entire surface of the lips is involved in the case of labials (McCune and Vihman, 2001). Finally, and perhaps most importantly, lip movement can be seen, providing an extra cue to production. Being able to see (and clearly feel) the articulatory movement involved in producing the *b* of words like *baby* or *bottle* may well make it easier for the child to gain control of the production of labials than of other consonants. Interestingly, this "overuse" of labials is not found in the early lexicon of blind children (Mulford, 1988) but is particularly characteristic of the vocalizations of the deaf (Stoel-Gammon and Otomo, 1986; see also Donahue, 1993). Furthermore, labials are especially prominent in the first words of late talkers (Rescorla and Bernstein-Ratner, 1996; Thal, Oroz, and McCaw, 1995) and of infants recovering from tracheostomy (Bleile, Stark, and McGowan, 1993). Again, it seems likely that the multiple cues afforded by labials are exploited by these special populations of children.

In short, by the end of the transition period, when the child has a cumulative vocabulary of about 50 words, there are several signs of the influence of the adult language on the segmental shape of the child's vocalizations. Some of the characteristics of the child's vocal patterns reflect characteristics of all adult language, such as the dominance of true consonants. The preference for producing words with labials is also detectable in a range of languages, but it probably reflects characteristics of the learning process—mastering an articulation for which proprioceptive and visual as well as auditory cues are available—rather than the form of adult languages. On the other hand, some early signs of the influence of the specific language environment are also evident by this point. For example, some children learning English, a language particularly rich in word-final consonants, begin to make use of final consonants in babble and especially in words by the end of the transition period (Vihman and Boysson-Bardies, 1994), whereas children learning languages with fewer final consonants make negligible use of them.

Prosodic Advances

Cross-linguistic study of the transition period has revealed the beginnings of prosodic organization by the time the child has produced 50 words or more, at about 18 months, typically (Vihman and Boysson-Bardies, 1994). Theoretical studies have proposed various developmental models for the acquisition of syllabic stress (Allen and Hawkins, 1980; Fikkert, 1994; Gerken, 1994; Archibald, 1995). On the one hand, stress and final syllable lengthening are the two main sources of perceptual salience in early words, based on the syllables children retain when shortening words (Echols, 1993; Vihman, 1996). Children tend to omit syllables *preceding* the stressed syllable (as in *balloon* → [bwun]), but they rarely omit either stressed syllables or (final) syllables *following* the stressed syllable (*potato* → [tʰédo]), since the final syllable is lengthened in English, as in many other languages (Snow, 1998). On the other hand, the source of syllable omissions cannot simply be a failure to perceive the less salient syllables, since segments from those syllables may be retained (as seen with *balloon*, above; cf. Wijnen, Krikhaar and den Os, 1994; Kehoe and Stoel-Gammon, 1997b). Onsetless medial syllables (those preceded by a single sonorant consonant) are most likely to be omitted (yielding a three-syllable production for *crocodile* but a two-syllable production for *dinosaur*).

There is little evidence to support the idea of a universal accent/stress template. Instead, children acquiring a language with a single, homogeneous accentual system, like French, which is consistently iambic (weak-strong pattern), show fairly consistent observance of this pattern in their production quite early (by the 50-word point). On the other hand, disyllables produced by children acquiring English reflect the dual adult English pattern of primarily trochaic (strong-weak) words and iambic (weak-strong) phrases (*a book, the dog*). Adultlike control of the more complex English stress pattern develops more slowly than that seen in the less complex French patterns (cf. Vihman, 1996, ch. 8; Vihman, DePaolis, and Davis, 1998).

Summary

By the beginning of the transition period (ca. age 9 to 18 months), the child has begun to demonstrate understanding of a variety of words, even if only in narrow or routine contexts. At this time children express their growing communicative abilities through the use of gestures and grunts to express attention to and interest in familiar objects and events. By the end of the transition period, the child's experience with a particular language is reflected in both production and perception. Once the child has begun to make intentional efforts to communicate with particular adult sound patterns (form) associated with particular situations (meaning), phonological organization can begin.

The sounds that occur most commonly in a child's babbling are likely to be the sounds the child uses in early words. Both words and babble are characterized at this time by a high proportion of one- and two-syllable forms as well as stops and open syllables. Use of consonants increases with knowledge of the adult language, and relatively extensive use of labials is particularly characteristic of early words. Language-specific phonotactic features, such as final consonants in English, also emerge over this period, and the accentual pattern of the adult language begins to be reflected in child words and babble. The bulk of phonological development takes place over the age range one to three years, at a time when the child is also experiencing an extraordinary growth of word knowledge and embarking on the acquisition of syntax. Yet it seems fair to say that the biggest challenge of all—that of "getting the idea" of what language is all about, apprehending form-meaning correspondences, and learning to match, represent, and access them at will—occurs in the transition stage.

Individual Differences: Profile of Two 1-Year-Old Girls

Although a general sequence of vocal development can be identified for the first year and a half of life, the extent of individual variability is striking. For one thing, children differ greatly in amount of vocalization during this period. In one study, for example, the average number of vocalizations produced by nine infants ranged from 97 to 265 per half-hour session (the children's interaction with their mothers was sampled at monthly intervals) (Vihman et al., 1985).

Individual differences are also apparent in other aspects of phonological development. Infants vary in the sounds they produce (*phonetic preferences*) and in the stability of these sound preferences. Finally, infants may differ in the organization of their phonological systems and in their approaches to learning phonology. These differences can be identified as early as the period of transition from babbling to speech. We will illustrate differences in phonetic preferences and in phonological organization in this period by describing the development of two girls.

Phonetic Preferences and Word Selection

Molly and Deborah are both first-born daughters of well-educated parents with a strong interest in their children's development. Both girls are naturally "talkative" (in fact, they ranked first and third in amount of vocalization among the nine children studied by Vihman et al., 1985), and both developed large vocabularies by the end of the study (50 words or more at 16 months).

Although Molly and Deborah were similar in many respects, they differed substantially in their phonetic preferences and word selection, and on the stability of their word shapes (Vihman et al., 1986; Vihman and Greenlee, 1987). In the early lexical period, Molly showed a striking preference for labials (66 percent: mean use for the group, 44 percent) and nasals (41 percent: group mean, 16 percent), while Deborah more closely resembled the other nine children sampled. In the later period, Molly developed a strong focus on final consonants (23 percent: mean use for the group, 12 percent), while Deborah began using an unexpectedly large proportion of fricatives (26 percent against a mean of 10 percent).

Children select their early words at least partly on phonetic grounds (Ferguson and Farwell, 1975; Schwartz and Leonard, 1982). The word-initial consonant is most likely to be a deciding factor in a child's attempting a particular word, at least in English (Shibamoto and Olmsted, 1978), although overall word shape, prosody, and vowel pattern undoubtedly play a role as well (Vihman, 1981; Stoel-Gammon and Cooper, 1984; Davis and Mac-Neilage, 1990). Deborah's attraction to fricatives is reflected in the words she attempts, which tend to include the sounds [s] and [ts]: *scratchy* [tsi:tsi], *Sesame Street* [si:si] (14 months), while Molly attempts an unusually large number of words with final nasals (*bang, down, name*) (Vihman and Velleman, 1989).

The two girls also differed in phonological organization. Although Molly gradually increased the number of different consonants she would attempt, she largely restricted herself to stops and nasals throughout this period of early word use. Even in a session in which she used over 20 different words (at 15 months), she still did not attempt any words with sibilants or liquids. Deborah, on the other hand, used a broad array of consonants from the beginning. By the end of this period she had greatly expanded her repertoire by attempting words with interdentals as well as sibilants. In general, Deborah seemed to advance in an exploratory way, whereas Molly's progress was more systematic or constrained.

Finally, the two girls differed in the extent of variability in their productions of different tokens of a single word. Molly's word production was highly repetitive (i.e., she produced many tokens of a single word type), with remarkably little variation across the different tokens or productions of a single word. In contrast, Deborah produced a different shape for almost every token of a given word. This appeared to result, in part, from her inclusion of extra syllables at the beginning of a word, perhaps as a tentative effort to reproduce the sound of the English articles *a* and *the* and the possessive pronoun *my* (*a baby, my baby, the glasses*: cf. Peters, 2001, on "filler syllables"). Here again, Molly's highly stable word production seems to reflect a systematic approach to the learning of phonology, whereas Deborah appears to be exploring new forms before she has a good grasp of their function. The difference between the two girls illustrates Ferguson's (1979) distinction between a cautious, analytic (systematic) style and an unanalytic, risk-taking (exploratory) style.

In summary, these two children differed widely in the phonetic preferences they displayed during babbling although they were matched for sex, socioeconomic status, amount of vocalization, and relative rate of lexical development. These same individual phonetic preferences appeared to carry over to the children's choices of early words. We see the beginnings of phonological structure as each child gradually expanded her range of phonetic segments and attempted increasingly complex syllable shapes.

Systematization and Reorganization: From Word to Segment

The earliest units the child targets for production are whole-word patterns rather than segments or even syllables (Menn, 1983). At least three different kinds of evidence were advanced to support this view: (1) The child's production of a given sound may vary, depending on the particular word attempted. Some words may be produced in a stable (though not necessarily accurate) form, while others are highly variable (Ferguson and Farwell, 1975). Such data suggest that the child has knowledge of particular words but has not yet developed abstract categories of sounds for production. (2) A child's word shapes may have a clear *holistic* relationship to adult models, based on a frequently produced pattern or "template." At the same time, the relationship of particular segments in the adult word to the child's production remains idiosyncratic (Waterson, 1971). This strongly suggests that the child is targeting a whole gestalt, not a sequence of individual segments. Similarly, (3) the child's own word forms may be clearly interrelated at a given time, again providing evidence of a favorite pattern or template which may distort adult models (Macken, 1979). In 30 years of diary-based or small-scale longitudinal studies of infant first word production, a good deal of evidence for this "holistic start" to phonology has accumulated (Vihman and Velleman, 1989; Vihman et al., 1994; Beckman and Edwards, 2000; Velleman and Vihman, 2002).

As the child begins to acquire new vocabulary at an accelerated pace, typically after accumulating 50 words or more, there is pressure to "systematize" the phonological representations and production routines to allow smoother functioning of word production (cf. Chiat, 1979; Menn, 1983). The changes that occur at this time reflect a process of internal reorganization, like that shown to occur in other domains of language acquisition, such as syntax and semantics (cf., e.g., Slobin, 1973; Bowerman, 1982; Karmiloff-Smith, 1992). The classic examples come from English morphology. Although the child at first produces apparently correct (irregular as well as regular) plural and past tense forms (*shoes, feet, walked, broke*), at a later point, he or she will begin to apply the regular inflectional endings to words that happen to have irregular plural or past tense forms in English (*foots, breaked*). This is generally taken as evidence that the child has "analyzed out" or "discovered" the productive inflectional suffixes marking regular plural and past tense forms. The "overregularized" forms thus reflect new knowledge and reorganization. Only much later will the child again begin to use the correct irregular forms, which, at that point, have a new status as known exceptions to the general morphological rule.

Evidence for phonological reorganization is indirect and thus difficult to trace in terms of specific stages. Nevertheless, there are data from a range of children learning difficult languages that suggest that such reorganization, based on internal analysis and systematization, does occur (see Vihman et al., 1994). This reorganization will affect the basic unit of the child's phonological system. Although the primary unit at the earliest stage appears to be the word, reanalysis will allow the child to operate with a more efficient, segment-based system (see Macken, 1979, who traces a single child's development from whole words to segments).

Summary

We have suggested that differences in approach to learning can be discerned among children early in their language acquisition. We provided evidence of individual differences in phonetic preferences, word selection, and stability or variability of word shapes. One child showed a cautious, systematic approach, while the other made bold leaps from one point to another in word selection, with exploration of a wide range of sounds in both babble and first words. In both cases, the child's phonetic preferences were found to influence her choice of early words.

The first units targeted in the earliest period of adult-based word production appear to be whole-word patterns rather than segments. This is suggested by the variation typically found in the treatment of individual segments across different words and by the gestalt-like match of early child forms to adult models. After this early period, experience in production and in the representation of increasing numbers of different words, along with the pressure of finding word forms in a larger lexicon, leads to gradual reorganization. Indirect evidence of this process may be found in the phenomenon of nonlinear progression, in which superficially more advanced forms are later produced in a less adultlike form—but one that fits into the child's repertoire of phonological forms and appears to reflect the operation of regular phonological processes.

Linguistic Perception Beyond the Transition Period: Representing Speech Sounds

We began our account of the origins of phonological development by asking what perceptual abilities or natural biases the infant brings to the task of learning to pronounce. Before reviewing phonological development beyond the transition period, we will consider what is known about perceptual development during the period of rapid phonological advance, from the transition to speech through the mastery of the sound system by age 5–8. Current theories of phonological development differ on the issue of the timing of perceptual development. Some scholars view linguistic perception, or the ability to identify and represent or store the sound pattern of lexical items, as essentially complete even before the child has acquired a lexicon of 50 words or so. From this perspective, the child's production errors may be largely ascribed to difficulties in motor control, phonological organization, or phonological memory. Other scholars believe linguistic perception continues to develop during the preschool period and even beyond, so that some production errors may be due to perception-based differences between the adult word and the sound pattern the child is targeting—that is, to inaccuracies and gaps in the child's perception and consequent internal representation of the adult word.

It is important to note that the term *linguistic perception* refers not only to the auditory perception or identification of contrast between different sounds but also to the *representing* and *accessing for recognition* of the particular sound patterns that constitute words and phrases in the language being acquired. Previously, we dealt with the child's auditory capacities. Here, we are concerned with the child's use of those capacities in constructing a repertoire of word forms and extrapolating from them knowledge of the sound system of his or her language.

In our account of infant perception, we stressed that infants in the first few months of life seem to respond to graduated differences in the acoustic signal in a categorical way and, furthermore, that these categorical responses resemble adult responses, which are based on knowledge of phonemic (meaning-bearing) contrasts in the language. We ascribed the infants' surprising discriminatory ability to natural biases in the auditory structure of humans (and other mammals). Given the wide range of phonemic differences to which infants have been found to be sensitive, it is easy to see why some scholars have concluded that perception of speech patterns can be assumed to be completely accurate by the time children begin to produce lexical items on their own. It is important, however, to bear in mind the distinction between the nonlinguistic *sensory capacity* (the ability to make same-different distinctions) tested in studies of infant perception and the *use* of that discriminatory capacity to distinguish different meaningful lexical items, as well as to store or remember them (**internal representation**). Infant perception tasks used in research investigations involve an essentially **passive response** to change in the signal, which indicates auditory sensitivity to the change. But perception of sound patterns as a basis for language use involves **active attention** to contrasting speech sounds and sequences in order to identify, store, and recognize distinct lexical items (Ferguson, 1975). Furthermore, discrimination between phonemes involves a learned response to a range of different and variable acoustic signals in terms of a single (abstract) linguistic category. With respect to the child who is beginning to speak, we shift our focus from the perception of differences between sounds per se to the perception of phonemic contrasts and the use of that perception to recognize different words (e.g., *pit* vs *bit*) and, thus, to understand language. This shift in focus naturally leads to a shift in the methods used to investigate linguistic perception.

We cannot directly observe a child's perception of speech sounds. Instead, tasks must be devised requiring the child to respond in a way that reveals something about his or her perceptions. As Locke (1980a) has pointed out, this is a formidable challenge since both linguistic perception itself and the required behavioral responses are complex processes involving several steps. First, the salient features of the speech sound stimuli must be *heard* ("go in the ear of the subject") and then *registered* and *interpreted* by the child ("reach and reside briefly in the brain": Locke, 1980a; 433). In other words, the child's perception of a speech sound involves receiving the auditory stimulus and identifying the auditory cues in terms of the phonemic system, or the speech sound categories, of the adult language. Secondly, in order for the observer to judge the "accuracy" of the child's perception, or the extent to which it agrees with that of adults from the child's linguistic community, the perception must be *translated* into an interpretable behavioral response. Considerable ingenuity is required to devise satisfactory tasks since they not only must be within the child's conceptual capacities and repertoire of behavioral responses but also require the child to make a comparison of an adult surface form with his or her own internal representation. Additional ingenuity is needed to determine the critical acoustic cues leading to the child's response.

The difference between two speech sounds may depend on any combination of multiple acoustic cues (cf., e.g., Lisker, 1978). This built-in redundancy helps to make speech intelligible even in noisy or otherwise distracting surroundings. For example, the difference between voiced and voiceless final stops in English is cued by the length of a preceding vowel (which is greater before voiced consonants), by the voicing of the voiced stop, and by differences in the release, if any, of the voiced versus the voiceless stop. The discrimination of contrasting sounds, then, involves *knowledge of a particular phonemic system* as well as discrimination per se. Fluent users of a language disregard some sound-differences that are irrelevant to the phonemic categories of their language (recall the earlier discussion of categorical perception). In the case of children, auditory discrimination is subject to multiple interpretations; we do not necessarily know which cues the child is attending to (for example, vowel lengthening or voicing or release burst in the discrimination of the voicing contrast: Greenlee, 1978).

Research with Young Children

Methodological difficulties are the most acute with younger children. By the age of 10 or 12 months, children are beginning to understand and produce language and, thus, have already internalized a certain number of meaningful sound patterns. It would be of great interest to determine if children's internal representations of words conform more completely with adult models than do the word patterns they are able to produce. At this age, however, the child's cognitive capacities (e.g., attention span) and repertoire of behavioral responses are limited, and it is difficult to obtain on command consistent responses, such as pointing to a named picture or fetching a named object, from a child under the age of 2 or 3. Considerable ingenuity has gone into the development of experiments usable with children under 3, but the results remain disappointingly ambiguous.

Full versus Partial Linguistic Perception

In an effort to test the idea that full perception is achieved very early, Barton (1980) tested 2-year-old children on discrimination of voicing contrasts, among others, using pairs of cards or, for the youngest children, a set of small objects likely to be familiar. The children were trained on words they were found not to know already. On the whole, children were able to discriminate the sounds tested, but failures to discriminate were common when one of the words had to be trained.

The significance of this word familiarity effect should not be overlooked. If children make more errors in discriminating contrasts in *new words*, we cannot assume that they are typically able to draw on accurate internal representations of surface forms when they produce words. Instead, it seems likely that children's internal representations continue to change for some years. When first attempting a word, the child may be operating with an internal representation that is only partially correct. In time, this representation becomes more accurate as the child profits from additional exposure to the adult form. But the child may fail to notice the discrepancy between his or her initial internal representation and the adult surface form and could then persist in the perception-based error for some time.

Examples of such changing internal representations are difficult to obtain in any systematic or experimental way but may be revealed by careful analysis of longitudinal data (Macken, 1980). Specifically, when a child begins to produce a new adult sound (such as /θ/) for which he or she formerly produced a substitute sound (such as /f/), we can look to see if the change seems to occur "across the board" (Smith, 1973), in all and only the words containing the relevant phoneme. If so, we can assume that the words were correctly represented although they were not yet correctly produced. On the other hand, if the child begins to use the new sound /θ/ in words that were formerly correctly produced with the substituting sound (*wife, frosty* as /waiθ/, /θrɔsti/), we conclude that /θ/ words had formerly been mistakenly represented with /f/, and the child is now faced with the problem of sorting out which are actually /θ/ words and which are /f/ words. This process may take a matter of months or even years (cf. Vihman, 1982, for a fuller account of just such an error).

Interaction of Perception and Production

To resolve the question of whether or not internal representations may be assumed to reflect adult surface forms accurately from the earliest stages of lexical acquisition, data are needed on both production and perception from the same subjects. Several studies of this kind have been reported for normal children.

Eilers and Oller (1976) were able to show that some production errors in 2-year-olds may derive from perceptual difficulties although others (e.g., the contrast in voicing or aspiration) are more likely to relate to motor constraints. Strange and Broen (1980) conducted a careful test of both the production and the perception of word-initial /w/, /r/, and /l/ by 3-year-old children. Identification accuracy was clearly related to /r/ and /l/ production ability. Strange and Broen tentatively concluded that both perception and production of phoneme contrasts develop gradually and that perception of a contrast normally precedes its production. However, they emphasized that their test situation was highly constrained; it involved only two response alternatives and a long series of tests using the same stimuli, which could serve as training on the contrast. Thus, the study does not reflect "intentional, coordinated perception," such as ordinary life requires, in which the child-listener is actively involved in extracting the relevant phonetic cues from a complex set of stimuli in order to determine which words were intended by the speaker.

Locke (1980b) has argued that evaluation of a child's perception of speech sounds should be based on the child's patterns of sound substitutions, with attention paid to the **particular phonetic contexts** that give rise to the child's production errors. He developed a *speech production-perception task* in which the perceptual stimuli used are based on a preliminary test of the child's productions. The child is tested on the sounds he or she misarticulated (the *stimulus phoneme*), on the substituting sound (the *response phoneme*), and on a perceptually similar control sound. The different stimulus types are presented six times each in a live-voice object or picture identification task ("Is this X?"), with the tester seated beside the child. For more detail and a copy of the test form, see Chapter 5.

Locke reported that of 131 children tested, ranging in age from 3 to 9 (mean age 5;3), most had speech substitutions, but they did not necessarily have speech disorders. About one third of the contrasts misproduced were also misperceived. However, misperception was not equally likely to be involved in all production errors. Specifically, only 49 percent of those errors consisted of the substitution of one voiceless fricative for another, yet this type of substitution accounted for fully 89 percent of the misperceived contrasts. The pair that accounted for the largest number of perception errors was /f/-/θ/ (67 percent incidence of misperception). Of 52 children who substituted /f/ for /θ/ in production, the 26 younger subjects (mean age 3;7) were much more likely also to misperceive the contrast than were the older subjects (mean age 6;2).

Finally, Velleman (1988) designed a study to test the hypothesis that some English phonemes typically involved in production errors (e.g., /s/) are easy to perceive, so late acquisition is likely to be due to articulatory difficulty. She predicted that in the case of /s/, poor production would occur in the *absence* of poor perception. For other phonemes, the production problem might be related to a perceptual problem; specifically, the articulation of /θ/ and /f/ yields signals that are relatively weak and can be confused with one another. Velleman predicted that in this case, production would be dependent on perception. Velleman's results confirmed her hypotheses. Perception and production of /s/ showed no correlation. Some children with poor /s/ production had good perception of contrasts involving /s/, and in general, perception errors with /s/ were rare. In contrast, perception and production of /θ/ were highly correlated. More errors were made in both perception and production in the case of /θ/ than in the case of /s/.

In summary, the results of the few studies examining production and perception in the same children all point to an identical conclusion: Some phonemic contrasts remain difficult to discriminate perceptually as late as age 3 or older (e.g., /θ/-/f/, /r/-/w/), and production errors involving these pairs typically continue to occur in the later preschool period. It should be mentioned that the /f/-/θ/ contrast in particular is notoriously difficult for adults as well. Other production errors show no evident relation to perception (voicing in stops at age 2, /s/ at age 3 to 5).

Internal Representations

We can now reconsider the question raised earlier regarding internal representations. Note, first of all, that linguistic perception has not yet been successfully tested in the earliest period of lexical production (age 12 to 18 months). Stager and Werker (1997) have provided evidence that minimal pairs cannot be discriminated at 14 months in an experimental setting, although 8-month-olds are able to make the discrimination. They interpret the difference as reflecting a shift from analytic attention to sound patterns in the early period to a more holistic attention to words in the period in which sound patterns have begun to hold meaning for the infants.

Based on production data from this period, a bias toward perception and/or storage in terms of the favored shapes of the babbling period (e.g., CV syllables) seems likely (Locke, 1983; Vihman, 1991). By about age 2, when the child has a sizable lexicon but many production errors, we can assume that the child is perceiving words in a shape that closely resembles the adult surface forms. For some elements (e.g., fricatives, clusters, and /r/), however, nonadultlike perception may still be the rule, and it is precisely those sound classes that continue to give rise to production difficulties for many children into the later preschool and early school years. It is possible, then, that some children persist in misproducing a few sounds because they are inaccurately storing the adult form. Such errors may arise in an early period, when the child is unable to either produce the relevant articulatory gestures or *represent* (store) the relevant distinction. The production error may persist long after the child's motoric or articulatory difficulty has been resolved, due to the child's lack of self-monitoring or lack of attention to the difference between his or her inaccurately stored form and the adult form.

Summary

Infants have been found to respond differentially to a wide range of contrasting speech sounds. Linguistic perception, however, requires active attention to speech sound contrasts, in order to identify, represent, and access distinct lexical items. Given a variety of potential acoustic cues to speech sound contrasts, the child must be able to select and integrate the relevant cues while disregarding those that play no contrastive role in the phonemic system of the language in question.

The question of whether or not a child's perception of lexical items is fully accurate from the beginning of speech production has long been of theoretical interest. Attempts to test children younger than age 2 have been limited and not entirely successful. In such attempts, the role of word familiarity has proven to be significant. This suggests that some production errors may derive from perceptual misinterpretations, that is, internal representations that fail to match the adult model, since initial attempts at a new word inevitably reflect an internal representation based on perception of a relatively unfamiliar word. The results of studies of production and perception in the same children support the idea that imperfect perception is involved in production errors with respect to certain contrasts, such as /f/ versus /θ/ and /w/ versus /r/. The production errors that appear to be related to perceptual difficulties are errors that typically persist into the later preschool or even early school-age years.

QUESTIONS FOR CHAPTER 2

1. Describe how the following models of phonological acquisition add to our overall picture of how children acquire the sounds of language: generative model, cognitive model, non-linear model and biological model.

2. Delineate the stages of infant vocal production from birth to age 1.

3. Describe the characteristics and accomplishments of the transition stage of phonological acquisition.

4. How do perception and production develop and interact in infants?

REFERENCES

Allen, G. D., and S. Hawkins, "Phonological rhythm: Definition and development." In G. H. Yeni-Komshian, J. F. Kavanagh, and C. A. Ferguson (Eds.), *Child Phonology, Vol. 1, Production*. New York: Academic Press, 1980.

Archibald, J., "The acquisition of stress." In J. Archibald (Ed.), *Phonological Acquisition and Phonological Theory*. Hillsdale, N.J.: Lawrence Erlbaum Associates, 1995.

Barton, D., "Phonemic perception in children." In G. Yeni-Komshian, J. Kavanagh, and C. A. Ferguson (Eds.), *Child Phonology, Vol. 2, Perception*. New York: Academic Press, 1980.

Beckman, M. E., and J. Edwards, "The ontogeny of phonological categories and the primacy of lexical learning in linguistic development." *Child Development*, *41* (2000): 240–249.

Bernhardt, B., "The prosodic tier and phonological disorders." In M. Yavas (Ed.), *First and Second Language Pathology*. San Diego: Singular Publishing Group, 1994.

Bernhardt, B., and J. P. Stemberger, *Handbook of Phonological Development: From the Perspective of Constraint-Based Nonlinear Phonology*. San Diego: Academic Press, 1998.

Bernhardt, B., and C. Stoel-Gammon, "Nonlinear phonology: Introduction and clinical application." *Journal of Speech and Hearing Research*, *37* (1994): 123–143.

Bleile, K. M., R. E. Stark, and J. S. McGowan, "Speech development in a child after decannulation: Further evidence that babbling facilitates later speech development." *Clinical Linguistics & Phonetics*, *7* (1993): 319–337.

Bowerman, M., "Reorganizational processes in lexical and syntactic development." In E. Wanner and L. R. Gleitman (Eds.), *Language Acquisition: The State of the Art*. Cambridge (UK): Cambridge University Press, 1982.

Boysson-Bardies, B. de, P. Hallé, L. Sagart, and C. Durand, "A crosslinguistic investigation of vowel formants in babbling." *Journal of Child Language*, *16* (1989): 1–17.

Boysson-Bardies, B. de, L. Sagart, and C. Durand, "Discernible differences in the babbling of infants according to target language." *Journal of Child Language*, *11* (1984): 1–15.

Boysson-Bardies, B. de, and M. M. Vihman, "Adaptation to language." *Language*, *61* (1991): 297–319.

Braine, M. D. S., "Review of N. V. Smith, The Acquisition of Phonology: A Case Study." *Language*, *52* (1976): 489–498.

Chiat, S., "The role of the word in phonological development." *Linguistics*, *17* (1979): 591–610.

Chomsky, N., "A review of B. F. Skinner's *Verbal Behavior*" (New York: Appleton-Century-Crofts, 1957). *Language*, *35* (1959): 26–58.

Chomsky, N., *Lectures on Government and Binding*. New York: Foris Publications, 1981.

Davis, B. L., and P. F. MacNeilage, "Acquisition of correct vowel production: A quantitative case study." *Journal of Speech and Hearing Research*, *33* (1990): 16–27.

Davis, B. L., and P. F. MacNeilage, "The articulatory basis of babbling." *Journal of Speech and Hearing Research*, *38* (1995): 1199–1211.

Davis, B. L., and P. F. MacNeilage, "An embodiment perspective on the acquisition of speech perception." *Phonetica*, *57* (2000): 229–241.

Demuth, K., "The prosodic structure of early words." In J. L. Morgan and K. Demuth (Eds.), *Signal to Syntax: Bootstrapping from Speech to Grammar in Early Acquisition*. Mahwah, N.J.: Lawrence Erlbaum Associates, 1996.

Deville, G., "Notes sur le développement de l'enfant." *Revue de Linguistique*, *23* (1890): 330–343; 24 (1891): 10–42, 128–143, 242–257, 300–320.

Donahue, M. H., "Early phonological and lexical development and otitis media: A diary study." *Journal of Child Language*, *20* (1993): 489–501.

Donegan, P., and D. Stampe. "The study of natural phonology." In D. Dinnsen (Ed.), *Current Approaches to Phonological Theory*. Bloomington, Ind.: Indiana University Press, 1979.

Echols, K., "A perceptually-based model of children's earliest productions." *Cognition*, *46* (1993): 245–296.

Edwards, M. L., and L. D. Shriberg, *Phonology: Applications in Communicative Disorders*. San Diego, Calif.: College-Hill, 1983.

Eilers, R. E., "Context-sensitive perception of naturally produced stop and fricative consonants by infants." *Journal of the Acoustical Society of America*, *61* (1977): 1321–1336.

Eilers, R. E., and F. D. Minifie, "Fricative discrimination in early infancy." *Journal of Speech and Hearing Research*, *18* (1975): 158–167.

Eilers, R. E., and D. K. Oller, "The role of speech discrimination in developmental sound substitutions." *Journal of Child Language*, *3* (1976): 319–329.

Eimas, P., E. Siqueland, P. Jusczyk, and J. Vigorito, "Speech perception in infants." *Science*, *171* (1971): 303–306.

Elbers, L., "Operating principles in repetitive babbling: A cognitive continuity approach." *Cognition*, *12* (1982): 45–63.

Ferguson, C. A., "Sound patterns in language acquisition." In D.P. Dato (Ed.), *Developmental Psycholinguistics:*

Theory and Application. Georgetown University Roundtable, 1–16. Washington, D.C.: Georgetown University Press, 1975.

Ferguson, C. A., "Learning to pronounce: The earliest stages of phonological development in the child." In F. D. Minifie and L. L. Lloyd (Eds.), *Communicative and Cognitive Abilities—Early Behavioral Assessment.* Baltimore, Md.: University Park Press, 1978.

Ferguson, C. A., "Phonology as an individual access system: Some data from language acquisition." In C. J. Fillmore, D. Kempler, and W. S.-Y. Wang (Eds.), *Individual Differences in Language Ability and Language Behavior.* New York: Academic Press, 1979.

Ferguson, C. A., "Discovering sound units and constructing sound systems: It's child's play." In J. S. Perkell and D. H. Klatt (Eds.), *Invariance and Variability of Speech Processes.* Hillsdale, N.J.: Lawrence Erlbaum, 1986.

Ferguson, C. A., and C. B. Farwell, "Words and sounds in early language acquisition." *Language, 51* (1975): 419-439.

Ferguson, C. A., and M. A. Macken, "The role of play in phonological development." In K. E. Nelson (Ed.), *Children's Language,* Vol. 4. Hillsdale, N.J.: Lawrence Erlbaum, 1983.

Ferguson, C. A., L. Menn, and C. Stoel-Gammon, *Phonological Development: Models, Research, Implications.* Parkton, Md.: York Press, 1992.

Ferguson, C. A., D. B. Peizer, and T. A. Weeks, "Model-and-replica phonological grammar of a child's first words." *Lingua, 3* (1973): 35–65.

Fernald, A., and T. Simon, "Expanded intonation contours in mothers' speech to newborns." *Developmental Psychology, 20* (1984): 104–113.

Fikkert, P., *On the Acquisition of Prosodic Structure.* Dordrecht: Holland Institute of Generative Linguistics, 1994.

Francescato, G., "On the role of the word in first language acquisition." *Lingua, 21* (1968): 144–153.

Fry, D. B., "The development of the phonological system in the normal and the deaf child." In F. Smith and G. Miller (Eds.), *The Genesis of Language: A Psycholinguistic Approach.* Cambridge, Mass.: M.I.T. Press, 1966.

Gerken, K., "A metrical template account of children's weak syllable omissions from multisyllabic words." *Journal of Child Language,* 21(1994): 565–584.

Goldsmith, J. A., *Autosegmental and Metrical Phonology.* Oxford: Blackwell, 1990.

Greenlee, M., "Learning the phonetic cues to the voiced-voiceless distinction: An exploration of parallel processes in phonological change." Ph.D. thesis, University of California, Berkeley, 1978.

Grunwell, P., "The development of phonology." *First Language, 2* (1981): 161–191.

Hallé, P., and B. de Boysson-Bardies, "Emergence of an early lexicon: Infants' recognition of words. *IBAD, 17* (1994): 119–129.

Hallé, P., and B. de Boysson-Bardies, "The format of representation of recognized words in infants' early receptive lexicon. *IBAD, 19* (1996): 435–451.

Hauser, M., *The Evolution of Communication.* Cambridge, Mass.: M.I.T. Press, 1996.

Householder, F. W., "Unreleased PTK in American English." In M. Halle (Ed.), *For Roman Jakobson.* The Hague: Mouton, 1956.

Ingram, D., *Phonological Disability in Children.* London: Edward Arnold, 1976.

Jakobson, R., *Child Language, Aphasia and Phonological Universals, A. R. Keiler (Tr.).* The Hague: Mouton, 1968. [Original title *Kindersprache, Aphasie und allgemeine Lautgesetze.* Uppsala: Almqvist and Wiksell, 1941.]

James, W., *The Principles of Psychology.* New York: Dover Publications, 1890.

Jusczyk, P. W., *The Discovery of Spoken Language.* Cambridge, Mass.: M.I.T. Press, 1997.

Jusczyk, P. W., and D. G. Kemler Nelson, "Syntactic units, prosody, and psychological reality during infancy." In J. L. Morgan and K. Demuth (Eds.), *Signal to Syntax: Bootstrapping from Speech to Grammar in Early Acquisition.* (pp. 389-408). Hillsdale, N.J.: Lawrence Erlbaum Associates, 1996.

Jusczyk, P. W., J. Murray, and J. Bayly, "Perception of place of articulation in fricatives and stops by infants." Paper presented at Biennial Meeting of Society for Research in Child Development, San Francisco, 1979.

Kager, R., J. Pater, and W. Zonneveld, *Fixing Priorities: Constraints in Phonological Acquisition.* Cambridge: Cambridge University Press, in press.

Karmiloff-Smith, A., "Taking development seriously." *Beyond Modularity* (pp. 1–29). Cambridge, Mass.: M.I.T. Press, 1992.

Karzon, R. B., "Discrimination of polysyllabic sequences by one-to-four-month-old infants." *Perception and Psychophysics, 39* (1985): 105–109.

Kehoe, M., and C. Stoel-Gammon, "The acquisition of prosodic structure: An account of children's prosodic development." *Language, 73* (1997a): 113–144.

Kehoe, M., and C. Stoel-Gammon, "Truncation patterns in English-speaking children's word productions." *Journal of Speech, Language, and Hearing Research, 40* (1997b): 526–541.

Kent, R. D., "The biology of phonological development." In C. A. Ferguson, L. Menn, and C. Stoel-Gammon (Eds.), *Phonological Development: Models, Research, Implications.* Parkton, Md.: York Press, 1992.

Kent, R. D., and G. Miolo, "Phonetic abilities in the first year of life." In P. Fletcher and B. MacWhinney (Eds.),

The Handbook of Child Language. Oxford: Blackwell, 1995.

Kent, R. D., and A. D. Murray, "Acoustic features of infant vocalic utterances at 3, 6, and 9 months." *Journal of the Acoustical Society of America, 72* (1982): 353–365.

Kiparsky, P., and L. Menn, "On the acquisition of phonology." In J. Macnamara (Ed.), *Language Learning and Thought*. New York: Academic Press, 1977.

Kuhl, P. K., "Perception of speech and sound in early infancy." In P. Salapatek and L. Cohen (Eds.), *Handbook of Infant Perception, Vol. 2. From Perception to Cognition*. New York: Academic Press, 1987.

Leopold, W. F., *Speech Development of a Bilingual Child, Vol. 2. Sound-Learning in the First Two Years.* Evanston, Ill.: Northwestern University Press, 1947.

Lewis, M. M., *Infant Speech: A Study of the Beginnings of Language*. New York: Harcourt Brace, 1936.

Lieberman, P., "On the development of vowel production in young children." In G. Yeni-Komshian, J. Kavanagh, and C. A. Ferguson (Eds.), *Child Phonology*, Vol. 1, *Production*. New York: Academic Press, 1980.

Lieven, E., "Variation in a cross-linguistic context." In D. I. Slobin (Ed.), *The Crosslinguistic Study of Language Acquisition*, Vol. 5. Mahwah, N.J.: Lawrence Erlbaum Associates, 1997.

Lindblom, B., "Phonological units as adaptive emergents of lexical development." In C. A. Ferguson, L. Menn, and C. Stoel-Gammon (Eds.), *Phonological Development: Models, Research, Implications*. Parkton, Md.: York Press, 1992.

Lindblom, B., "Developmental origins of adult phonology: The interplay between phonetic emergents and the evolutionary adaptations of sound patterns." *Phonetica, 57* (2000): 297–314.

Lindner, G., *Aus dem Naturgarten der Kindersprache*. Leipzig: Th. Grieben's Verlag, 1898.

Lisker, L., "Rabid vs. rapid: A catalogue of acoustic features that may cue the distinction." Haskins Laboratories Status Report on Speech Research (SR-54). New Haven, Conn., 1978.

Lisker, L., and A. S. Abramson, "A cross-language study of voicing in initial stops: Acoustical measurements." *Word, 20* (1964): 384–422.

Locke, J. L., "The inference of speech perception in the phonologically disordered child. Part I: A rationale, some criteria, the conventional tests." *Journal of Speech and Hearing Disorders, 4* (1980a): 432–444.

Locke, J. L., "The inference of speech perception in the phonologically disordered child. Part II: Some clinically novel procedures, their use, some findings." *Journal of Speech and Hearing Disorders, 4* (1980b): 445–468.

Locke, J. L., *Phonological Acquisition and Change*. New York: Academic Press, 1983.

Locke, J. L., "Variation in human biology and child phonology: A response to Goad and Ingram." *Journal of Child Language, 15* (1988): 663–668.

Locke, J. L., "Structure and stimulation in the ontogeny of spoken language." *Developmental Psychobiology, 23* (1990): 621–643.

Locke, J. L., *The Child's Path to Spoken Language*. Cambridge, Mass.: Harvard University Press, 1993.

Locke, J. L., and D. Pearson, "Vocal learning and the emergence of phonological capacity: A neurobiological approach." In C. A. Ferguson, L. Menn, and C. Stoel-Gammon (Eds.), *Phonological Development: Models, Research, Implications*. Parkton, Md.: York Press, 1992.

MacKain, K. S., "Assessing the role of experience on infants' speech discrimination." *Journal of Child Language, 9* (1982): 527–542.

Macken, M. A., "Developmental reorganization of phonology: A hierarchy of basic units of acquisition." *Lingua, 49* (1979): 11–49.

Macken, M. A., "The child's lexical representation: The 'puzzle-puddle-pickle' evidence." *Journal of Linguistics, 16* (1980): 1–17.

Macken, M. A., and C. A. Ferguson, "Cognitive aspects of phonological development: Model, evidence and issues." In K.E. Nelson (Ed.), *Children's Language*, Vol. 4. Hillsdale, N.J.: Lawrence Erlbaum, 1983.

MacNeilage, P. F., and B.L. Davis, "Deriving speech from nonspeech: A view from ontogeny." *Phonetica, 57* (2000): 284–296.

MacNeilage, P. F., B. L. Davis, A. Kinney, and C. L. Matyear, "The motor core of speech: A comparison of serial organization of patterns in infants and languages." *Child Development, 71* (2000): 153–163.

Maxwell, E. M., "On determining underlying phonological representations of children: A critique of the current theories." In M. Elbert, D. A. Dinnsen, and G. Weismer (Eds.), *Phonological Theory and the Misarticulating Child*. ASHA Monographs, 22. Rockville, Md.: ASHA, 1984.

McCune, L., and M. M. Vihman, "Early phonetic and lexical development: A productivity approach." *Journal of Speech, Language, and Hearing Research, 44* (2001): 670–684.

McCune, L., M. M. Vihman, L. Roug-Hellichius, D. B. Delery, and L. Gogate, "Grunt communication in human infants (Homo sapiens)," *Journal of Comparative Psychology, 110* (1996): 27–37.

Menn, L., "Pattern, control, and contrast in beginning speech: A case study in the development of word form and word function." Ph.D. thesis, University of Illinois, 1976. (Reprinted by the Indiana University Linguistics Club, 1978.)

Menn, L., "Phonological units in beginning speech." In A. Bell and J. B. Hooper (Eds.), *Syllables and Segments.* Amsterdam: North-Holland, 1978.

Menn, L., "Theories of phonological development." In H. Winitz (Ed.), *Native Language and Foreign Language Acquisition.* New York: Academy of Sciences, 1981.

Menn, L., "Development of articulatory, phonetic, and phonological capabilities." In B. Butterworth (Ed.), *Language Production,* Vol. 2. London: Academic Press, 1983.

Menn, L., and C. Stoel-Gammon, "Phonological development." In P. Fletcher and B. MacWhinney (Eds.), *The Handbook of Child Language.* Oxford: Blackwell, 1995.

Menyuk, P., L. Menn, and R. Silber, "Early strategies for the perception and production of words and sounds." In P. Fletcher and M. Garman (Eds.), *Language Acquisition: Studies in First Language Development,* 2nd Edition. Cambridge (UK): Cambridge University Press, 1986.

Mitchell, P. R., and R. D. Kent, "Phonetic variation in multisyllable babbling." *Journal of Child Language, 17* (1990): 247–265.

Mowrer, O., *Learning Theory and Symbolic Processes.* New York: John Wiley, 1960.

Mulford, R., "First words of the blind child." In M. D. Smith and J. L. Locke (Eds.), *The Emergent Lexicon: The Child's Development of a Linguistic Vocabulary.* New York: Academic Press, 1988.

Nespor, M., and I. Vogel. *Prosodic Phonology.* Dordrecht: Foris Publications, 1986.

Oller, D. K., "The emergence of the sounds of speech in infancy." In G. Yeni-Komshian, J. Kavanagh, and C. A. Ferguson (Eds.), *Child Phonology,* Vol.1, *Production.* New York: Academic Press, 1980.

Oller, D. K., and R. E. Eilers, "The role of audition in infant babbling." *Child Development, 59* (1988): 441–449.

Olmsted, D., *Out of the Mouth of Babes.* The Hague: Mouton, 1971.

Paradis, C., "On constraints and repair strategies." *The Linguistic Review, 6* (1988): 71–97.

Peters, A. M., *The Units of Language Acquisition.* Cambridge: Cambridge University Press, 1983.

Peters, A. M., "Filler syllables: What is their status in emerging grammar?" *Journal of Child Language, 28* (2001): 229–242.

Priestly, T. M. S., "One idiosyncratic strategy in the acquisition of phonology." *Journal of Child Language, 4* (1977): 45–65.

Rescorla, L., and N. Bernstein-Ratner, "Phonetic profiles of toddlers with specific expressive language impairment (SLI-E)." *Journal of Speech and Hearing Research, 39* (1996): 153–165.

Saffran, J. R., R. N. Aslin, and E. L. Newport, "Statistical learning by 8-month-old infants." *Science, 274* (1996): 1926–1928.

Saffran, J. R., E. L. Newport, R. N. Aslin, R. A. Tunick, and S. Barrueco, "Incidental language learning: Listening (and learning) out of the corner of your ear." *Psychological Science, 8* (1997): 101–105.

Schwartz, R., and L. B. Leonard, "Do children pick and choose? An examination of phonological selection and avoidance in early lexical acquisition." *Journal of Child Language, 9* (1982): 319–336.

Shibamoto, J. S., and D. L. Olmsted, "Lexical and syllabic patterns in phonological acquisition." *Journal of Child Language, 5* (1978): 417–456.

Slobin, D. I., "Cognitive prerequisites for the development of grammar." In C. A. Ferguson and D. I. Slobin (Eds.), *Studies of Child Language Development.* New York: Holt, Rinehart & Winston, 1973.

Smith, B. L., S. Brown-Sweeney, and C. Stoel-Gammon, "Reduplicated and variegated babbling." *First Language, 9* (1989): 175–189.

Smith, N. V., *The Acquisition of Phonology: A Case Study.* Cambridge (UK): Cambridge University Press, 1973.

Snow, D., "A prominence account of syllable reduction in early speech development: The child's prosodic phonology of tiger and giraffe." *Journal of Speech, Language, and Hearing Research, 41* (1998): 1171–1184.

Stager, C. L., and J. F. Werker, "Infants listen for more phonetic detail in speech perception than in word-learning tasks." *Nature, 388* (1997): 381–382.

Stampe, D., "The acquisition of phonetic representation." Paper presented at the Fifth Regional Meeting of the Chicago Linguistic Society, Chicago, 1969.

Stark, R. E., "Features of infant sounds: The emergence of cooing." *Journal of Child Language, 5* (1978): 379–390.

Stark, R. E., "Stages of speech development in the first year of life." In G. Yeni-Komshian, J. Kavanagh, and C. A. Ferguson (Eds.), *Child Phonology,* Vol. 1. *Production.* New York: Academic Press, 1980.

Stark, R. E., "The coupling of early social interaction and infant vocalization." Paper presented at Biennial Meeting of Society for Research in Child Development, New Orleans, 1993.

Stark, R. E., L. E. Bernstein, and M. E. Demorest, "Vocal communication in the first 18 months of life." *Journal of Speech and Hearing Research, 36* (1993): 548–558.

Stoel-Gammon, C., and J. A. Cooper, "Patterns of early lexical and phonological development." *Journal of Child Language, 11* (1984): 247–271.

Stoel-Gammon, C., and K. Otomo, "Babbling development of hearing-impaired and normally hearing subjects."

Journal of Speech and Hearing Disorders, *51* (1986): 33–41.

Strange, W., and P. A. Broen, "Perception and production of approximate consonants by 3-year-olds: A first study." In G. Yeni-Komshian, J. Kavanagh, and C. A. Ferguson (Eds.), *Child Phonology*, Vol. 2. *Perception*. New York: Academic Press, 1980.

Thal, D. J., M. Oroz, and V. McCaw, "Phonological and lexical development in normal and late-talking toddlers." *Applied Psycholinguistics*, *16* (1995): 407–424.

Thevenin, D. M., R. E. Eilers, D. K. Oller, and L. La Voie, "Where's the drift in babbling drift? A cross-linguistic study." *Applied Psycholinguistics*, *6* (1985): 3–15.

Trehub, S. E., "Auditory-linguistic sensitivity in infants." Ph.D. thesis, McGill University, Montreal, 1973.

Trehub, S. E., "The discrimination of foreign speech contrasts by infants and adults." *Child Development*, *44* (1976): 466–472.

Trevarthan, C., and P. Hubley, "Secondary intersubjectivity: Confidence, confiding and acts of meaning in the first year." In A. Lock (Ed.), *Action, Gesture and Symbol: The Emergence of Language*. New York: Academic Press, 1978.

Tyler, A. A., and T. E. Langsdale, "Consonant-vowel interactions in early phonological development." *First Language*, *16* (1996): 159–191.

Velleman, S. L., "The role of linguistic perception in later phonological development." *Applied Psycholinguistics*, *9* (1988): 221–236.

Velleman, S. L., and M. M. Vihman, "Whole-word phonology and templates: Trap, bootstrap, or some of each?" *Language, Speech and Hearing Services in Schools*, *33* (2002): 9–23.

Vihman, M. M., "Phonology and the development of the lexicon: Evidence from children's errors." *Journal of Child Language*, *8* (1981): 239–264.

Vihman, M. M., "A note on children's lexical representations." *Journal of Child Language*, *9* (1982): 249–253.

Vihman, M. M., "Ontogeny of phonetic gestures: Speech production." In I. G. Mattingly and M. Studdert-Kennedy (Eds.), *Modularity and the Motor Theory of Speech Perception*. Hillsdale, N.J.: Lawrence Erlbaum, 1991.

Vihman, M. M., "Variable paths to early word production." *Journal of Phonetics*, *21* (1993): 61–82.

Vihman, M. M., *Phonological Development: The Origins of Language in the Child*. Oxford: Blackwell, 1996.

Vihman, M. M., and B. de Boysson-Bardies, "The nature and origins of ambient language influence on infant vocal production and early words." *Phonetica*, *51* (1994): 159–169.

Vihman, M. M., R. A. DePaolis, and B. L. Davis, "Is there a 'trochaic bias' in early word learning? Evidence from

English and French." *Child Development*, *69* (1998): 933–947.

Vihman, M. M., S. Nakai, and R. A. DePaolis, "The role of accentual pattern in early lexical representation." Poster presented at 12th International Conference on Infant Studies, Brighton, UK, 2000.

Vihman, M. M., C. A. Ferguson, and M. Elbert, "Phonological development from babbling to speech: Common tendencies and individual differences." *Applied Psycholinguistics*, *7* (1986): 3–40.

Vihman, M. M., and M. Greenlee, "Individual differences in phonological development: Ages one and three years." *Journal of Speech and Hearing Research*, *30* (1987): 503–521.

Vihman, M. M., E. Kay, B. de Boysson-Bardies, C. Durand, and U. Sundberg, "External sources of individual differences: A cross-linguistic analysis of the phonetics of mother's speech to one-year-old children." *Developmental Psychology*, *30* (1994): 652–663.

Vihman, M. M., M. A. Macken, R. Miller, H. Simmons, and J. Miller, "From babbling to speech: A reassessment of the continuity issue." *Language*, *61* (1985): 395–443.

Vihman, M. M., and R. Miller, "Words and babble at the threshold of lexical acquisition." In M. D. Smith and J. L. Locke (Eds.), *The Emergent Lexicon: The Child's Development of a Linguistic Vocabulary*. New York: Academic Press, 1988.

Vihman, M. M., and S. Velleman, "Phonological reorganization: A case study." *Language and Speech*, *32* (1989): 149–170.

Vihman, M. M., and S. L. Velleman, "Phonetics and the origins of phonology." In N. Burton-Roberts, P. Carr, and G. Docherty (Eds.), *Phonological Knowledge: Its Nature and Status* (pp. 305-339). Oxford: Oxford University Press, 2000.

Vihman, M. M., S. Velleman, and L. McCune, "How abstract is child phonology? Towards an integration of linguistic and psychological approaches." In M. Yavas (Ed.), *First and Second Language Phonology*. San Diego, Calif: Singular Publishing Group, 1994.

Waterson, N., "Child phonology: A prosodic view." *Journal of Linguistics*, *7* (1971): 179–211.

Werker, J. F., "Ontogeny of speech perception." In I. G. Mattingly and M. Studdert-Kennedy (Eds.), *Modularity and the Motor Theory of Speech Perception*. Hillsdale, N.J.: Lawrence Erlbaum, 1991.

Werker, J. F., J. H. V. Gilbert, K. Humphrey, and R. C. Tees, "Developmental aspects of cross-language speech perception." *Child Development*, *52* (1981): 349–353.

Werker, J. F., and J. E. Pegg, "Infant speech perception and phonological acquisition." In C. A. Ferguson, L. Menn, and C. Stoel-Gammon (Eds.), *Phonological Develop-*

ment: Models, Research, Implications. Parkton, Md.: York Press, 1992.

Werker, J. F., and R. C. Tees, "Developmental changes across childhood in the perception of non-native speech sounds." *Canadian Journal of Psychology, 37* (1983): 278–286.

Werker, J. F., and R. C. Tees, "Cross-language speech perception: Evidence for perceptual reorganization during the first year of life." *Infant Behavior and Development, 7* (1984): 49–63.

Wijnen, F., E. Krikhaar, and E. den Os, "The (non)realization of unstressed elements in children's utterances: Evidence for a rhythmic constraint." *Journal of Child Language, 21* (1994): 59–83.

3

Later Phonological Development

MARILYN MAY VIHMAN

University of Wales—Bangor

In Chapter 2 we discussed the earliest stages of phonological development, emphasizing the biological roots of language, the influence of the language to which the child is exposed (ambient language), and the interaction of perceptual and motor development as they relate to segmental and prosodic aspects of phonology. In this chapter we consider advances in phonological learning from the point at which children have developed an active vocabulary of approximately 50 to 100 words, have begun to combine words productively (the beginnings of productive grammar), and are beginning to use some sounds contrastively (by age 2 or somewhat later). We trace children's advances from this early stage to the point of mastery of adult phonology. Usually this is accomplished by age 8, though refinements in phonology occur into adolescence and subtle phonological changes may occur at any point in adulthood, along with the learning of new vocabulary and exposure to new communicative partners or even to new dialects or languages.

Two research strategies commonly used in the study of later phonological development lead to somewhat different pictures of that process. In **longitudinal** studies of individual children, extensive data are collected from different points in a particular child's development. This strategy, typically used by linguists, highlights the variability in any one child's productions at one point and over time, and across different children. Close analysis of individual differences can provide insight into the learning process. But such intensive data analyses are available for only a relatively small number of children, and therefore the validity of any generalizations about the time-course for acquisition of specific speech sounds is uncertain. Child development specialists and speech-language pathologists interested in the study of normal phonological development for the purpose of comparison with disordered speakers most often use a different strategy—a **cross-sectional** research design. In this approach, no single child is followed over time; rather, different children are tested on their ability to produce speech sounds at different age levels, at a single point in time, and a composite profile is extrapolated from the data.

We will begin our discussion of later phonological development by reviewing some of the best-known large-scale studies. This will set the stage for a closer look at the particular paths followed by a smaller number of individual children. We will also consider issues relating to the perception of running speech by older children in comparison with adults. Finally, we will review ways in which phonetic and phonological variation and change continue beyond the early childhood years.

Establishing Group Norms: Large-Scale Studies

Long before the field of child language acquisition began to burgeon in the 1960s, there was considerable interest in determining the age at which most children are able to correctly produce each of the phonemes of their language; that is, there was a need to establish developmental norms. Such an enterprise has inherent methodological and theoretical problems. In order to establish production norms, one must test large numbers of children, but fully adequate evaluation of any one child's ability to produce contrasts between speech sounds requires both time and patience. Use of imitation may yield different results than spontaneous speech, and speech sound production in single words may differ from that in running conversation, as it does in adults. Many intensive studies of small groups (e.g., Ingram, Christensen, Veach, and Webster, 1980) have confirmed what a careful reading of earlier diary data suggested: Individual differences across children are so great in some areas—in the acquisition of fricatives, for example—that it may be impossible to establish meaningful age norms. Nevertheless, the need for such normative information is undeniable. Furthermore, developmental norm studies are based on the testing of children covering a broad age range (2 to 10 years) and can thus provide a useful overview of development beyond the earliest period of lexical acquisition.

Table 3.1 lists salient characteristics of the major cross-sectional studies undertaken in the United States in this century. These large-sample studies generally follow the same model, which may be described as follows.

TABLE 3.1   Major Cross-Sectional Speech Sound Production Studies in the United States. (I = initial, M = medial, F = final, Sp = spontaneous, Im = imitated).

Date	Author(s)	No.ss	Age Range	Word Position	SP/IM	Criterion
1931	Wellman et al.	204	2;0–4;0	I, M, F	Sp, Im	75%
1934	Poole	140	2;5–8;5	I, M, F	Sp	100%
1957	Templin	480	3;0–8;0	I, M, F	Sp, Im	75%
1963	Snow	438	6;5–8;7	I, M, F		
1967	Bricker	90	3;0–5;0	I	Im	
1971	Olmsted	100	1;3–4;6	I, M, F	Sp	
1972	Sax	535	5;0–10;0	I, M, F	Sp	93%
1975	Prather et al.	147	2;0–4;0	I, F	Sp, Im	75%
1976	Arlt and Goodban	240	3;0–5;6	I, M, F	Im	75%
1990	Smit et al.	997	3;0–9;0	I, F	Sp, Im	75%

Subject Selection

Typically an effort is made to ensure that the sample reflects the socioeconomic distribution of the population as a whole. Templin (1957) conducted an early and widely cited normative study of speech sound development with a weighted sample toward the lower end of the scale (70 percent of the children, based on father's occupation) and included only urban children. In most studies, audiometric screening and parental reports are used to exclude children with hearing losses or delayed language development.

Obtaining the Sample

Children are asked to name a picture representing a target word, usually only once; if the child does not produce the word spontaneously, an imitation is typically elicited. Consonants and clusters are tested in initial, medial, and final position, or a subset of those; vowels and diphthongs are also tested in some studies.

Analysis

A criterion is set to determine "age of acquisition" *for the group as a whole.* For Templin, this criterion was correct production in each of three word positions by 75 percent of the children. For Prather, Hedrick, and Kern (1975), it was correct production in two positions, again by 75 percent of the children, and scores were averaged over the two positions. Vowels and diphthongs were generally found to be acquired by age 3, and will not be further considered here.

In these studies, only group data are used. No results are given regarding individual responses, so there is no information regarding either individual differences between children of the same age or actual errors made for a given sound. The goal is to establish the age at which parents, teachers, and clinicians may reasonably expect a child's production of a given sound to match the adult standard.

Sander (1972) pointed out that the widely quoted ages of acquisition for speech sounds, based on the earlier studies cited in Table 3.1, are misleading if taken to reflect "average" performance. Instead, they must be understood to represent upper age limits for acquisition. In an effort to derive a more representative profile, Sander reanalyzed the Wellman, Case, Mengert and Bradbury (1931) data and the Templin data. He established a range between "customary production" (correct production in two out of three word positions by 50 percent of the children) and "mastery" (correct production in all three word positions by 90 percent of the children). Prather et al. (1975) also utilized this strategy; they presented their normative data in a similar manner, and then compared it with Sander's reanalysis (see Chapter 5, Figure 5.3).

Figure 5.3 vividly illustrates the difference between customary production and mastery, given data based on group behavior. Acquisition of /k/, for example, ranges from customary production (i.e., correct use in two of three word positions by half the children sampled) at age 2 to correct production by virtually all the children at nearly age 4. The data regarding correct production of /t/ are strikingly discrepant in the two studies. Whereas Prather and colleagues report a range from under 24 months to 32 months, Sander's reanalysis of the data from Wellman and colleagues and from Templin shows a range from 24 months to over 48 months. However, Sander points out that the late age of acquisition cited for /t/ in Templin (age 6) is entirely due to the younger children's failure to produce a voiceless [t] in medial position. In fact, in American English /t/ is normally produced as a (voiced) flap in medial position following a stressed vowel (as in *skating*). The coding of an error context likely reflects an unrealistic, idealized standard based on British rather than American usage, since the British do use a true medial [t].

Relatively small differences in methodology may greatly affect the age of acquisition reported. Smit (1986) analyzed the differences between Templin's study, which appears to be the one most frequently consulted by clinicians, and the more recent studies by Prather et al. (1975) and Arlt and Goodban (1976). The latter studies reported younger ages of acquisition for most sounds, as is evident for Prather and colleagues. Arlt and Goodban suggested that children were learning speech sounds at younger ages at the time of their study than 20 years earlier. Use of this more recent standard, then, would entail concern about children at an earlier age if their production of some sounds (most likely fricatives or liquids) failed to meet expectations based on the reported data.

Smit noted several methodological reasons for the discrepancy, particularly differences in analysis, like the decision to use two positions instead of three and to *average* scores across word-positions rather than require that 75 percent of the children produce a sound correctly in *each* position. Furthermore, Templin reported data only for children who attempted all sounds, whereas Prather and colleagues reported *partial* data, especially at the younger ages. Since missing data likely reflect an unwillingness to make errors in producing a difficult sound, this difference alone can have a significant effect on the results.

Given their cursory sampling (one production per segment in each word-position) and the differences in methods of analysis of these large-scale studies, it would clearly be a mistake to place a great deal of faith in an exact age at which a given phoneme can be expected to be produced correctly. Nevertheless, the results of the studies do agree sufficiently to provide a general picture of the order of acquisition of English consonants up to the point of mastery of the system as a whole. Nasals, stops, and glides are acquired relatively early; fricatives and affricates are mastered relatively late. Consonant clusters are also acquired late, with two-consonant clusters (for example, /kl/ and /st/) preceding the three-consonant clusters (for example, /str/ and /spl/). Most single consonants and consonant clusters are apparently mastered by age 7 or 8. As Locke (1983) has pointed out, the consonants acquired early are, generally speaking, those which occur most frequently in the languages of the world.

Three other large-scale studies carried out in the United States provided more qualitative data than those described so far. Snow (1963) tested 438 first-grade children, using two test words per consonant for each of three word-positions. Unlike Templin, Snow reported in some detail the particular errors made on each sound. Bricker (1967) tested imitation of word-initial consonants in nonsense syllables by 90 children aged 3 to 5, and reported substitutions for the 10 consonants, which elicited the most errors. Finally, Olmsted (1971) collected spontaneous speech samples of varying lengths from 100 children aged 1;3 to 4;6. He, too, reported substitutions for the 10 consonants most "prone to error."

Noting that these three studies are "more sophisticated in methodology and interpretation" than the earlier large-scale studies, Ferguson (1975) provided a thorough review and comparison of their data on fricatives, which account for the largest proportion of errors in all three. Despite differences in testing procedure, analysis, and the reporting of results, Ferguson found that the order of acquisition of the eight English fricatives across all three studies could be summarized in terms of three (internally unordered) groups: first /f, s, ʃ/, then /v, z/, and finally /θ, ð, ʒ/—an ordering which is largely consistent with the predictions of Jakobson (1941/68). On the other hand, the specific substitutions reported for these fricatives are not typically stops, as Jakobson predicted, except for /v/ (> /b/) and sometimes /ð/ (> /d/). Instead, /s/ substitutes for several other fricatives, /f/ substitutes for /θ/, and the affricative /dʒ/ is the most common substitute for /ʒ/, which has marginal status in English and is often replaced by /dʒ/ word-finally, even by adults. Linguists have yet to provide a plausible or widely accepted explanation for the occurring pattern of fricative to stop and fricative to fricative substitutions, whether based on the physiology of the speech tract, the nature of mental processes, the structure of English phonology, or the phonological usage of different members of society in the English-speaking world.

Smit, Hand, Freilinger, Bernthal, and Bird (1990) reported on a study conducted in Iowa and Nebraska which was larger in scale than anything undertaken previously. The study excluded data from 2-year-olds because of the large number who either failed to complete the test or refused to produce some of the test words. For the remaining children, Smit et al. reported a significant gender difference for children at ages 4;0, 4;6, and 6;0. Comparing their overall results with Templin's, they reported a plateau in the *boys'* developmental speech sound curve, between ages 3;6 and 4;0. A comparable plateau appears in the Templin data for boys beginning 6 months later. Close analysis of the various speech sounds tested reveals that the gender difference can be traced back to consonant cluster development, with either a plateau or a drop in performance for most clusters for boys, beginning at age 3;6. No explanation for this developmental difference is apparent at this time.

Summary

Despite methodological difficulties, investigators have attempted to establish age norms based on the testing of large numbers of children at different age levels. Several cross-sectional studies of 100 or more English-speaking children have been conducted. Most report group data in terms of a set criterion, such as the age at which three quarters of the children correctly produce each consonant in three word-positions. It is important to bear in mind that there is often a long temporal gap between average age of customary production of a sound (correct use by 51 percent of the children in two out of three positions), and mastery of the sound (correct use in all positions by 90 percent of the children). Analysis in terms of customary production yields lower ages of acquisition. Other methodological variables-such as inclusion versus exclusion of data from subjects who fail to attempt some of the target sounds-also strongly affect the resultant chronology.

Large-scale studies do agree on certain general points. Nasals, stops, and glides are acquired early; fricatives, affricates, and consonant clusters are acquired later. Reporting of qualitative results (e.g., specification of the errors made for each sound) greatly enhances the value of a cross-sectional study. Developmental norm studies are designed to provide information about a large number of children and thus afford an overview of phonological development. Their limitation in principle is their inability to reveal the particular course of development of any one child. In providing a broad range of data, such studies can serve as a useful complement to the more narrowly based diaries and longitudinal studies of small groups of children.

Phonological Processes: Systematicity in Production Errors

One fact about phonological development on which linguists agree is the **systematic** nature of the child's simplifications and restructuring of adult words (Macken and Ferguson, 1981). As Oller (1975) explicitly puts it, "the sorts of substitutions, deletions and additions which occur in child language are not merely random errors on the child's part, but are rather the result of a set of systematic tendencies" (299). It is the systematic relationship between the adult target and the child's reproduction of that target that is expressed by the linguist's "rewrite" or "realization rule":

$$X \rightarrow Y/Z$$

or "X 'goes to' [is substituted by or realized as] Y in the environment Z." For example, when a 3-year-old produces a series of words like [tænt] for *can't*, [tɔz] for *'cause*, [taᵘ] for *cow*, and [oᵘt'eⁱ] for *okay*, the linguist formulates a rule to express the observed regularity: [k] → [t]; in this case no "conditioning environment" or context is given since the substitution appears to occur in a wide range of contexts. In fact, when we notice that the child also says [dɛt] for *get*, [doᵘ] for *go*, ['doᵘfɚ·s] for *gophers*, and [di:n] for *green*, we can express the rule more generally as "a velar stop is realized as a dental (or alveolar) stop."

Phonological substitutions typically show great regularity in the language of children past the earliest stage of lexical acquisition. Linguists express such regularity with phonological rules, or what have come to be known in the child language literature as "phonological processes" or phonological patterns. The theoretical status—and the psychological reality—of these processes remains highly controversial. If perception of phonological contrasts continues to develop over the preschool years, the phonological processes that the child appears to operate with may not be strictly production rules; rather, they may be perception or "interpretation" rules, meaning that the error underlying the mismatch between child form and adult form is actually present in the child's internal representation of the target word. Most likely, distortions of different kinds occur in both perception and production and may be due to a variety of factors including such idiosyncrasies as affective peculiarities of certain words and interrelationships between lexical items which the child is exposed to and uses. Our understanding of phonological development has undoubtedly benefited from the extensive cataloging of common processes used by different children learning different languages. At our present stage of knowledge regarding the child's actual processing of language, references to phonological processes or phonological patterns are generally a descriptive convenience rather than an attempt to directly reflect the child's mental activity. (See discussion in Chapter 5.)

Let us now take a closer look at the most common phonological processes that children have been found to apply to adult words. In general, these processes appear to be used regardless of the particular language the child is learning, although the structure of the adult language may affect the frequency with which a given process is used (Ingram, 1986; Vihman, 1978, 1980; Vihman and Velleman, 2000). The processes are used to some extent by virtually all children in the earlier stages of word acquisition, but a given child will quickly master certain difficulties (e.g., the production of velars or fricatives or closed syllables, depending on his or her phonetic preferences and the words he or she has been attempting) and thereby obviate the need for the corresponding processes (velar fronting, stopping, final consonant deletion) while continuing to make use of other processes. Finally, more than one process may be implicated in a child's production of a single word (e.g., cluster simplification as well as velar fronting must be posited to account for the realization of *green* as [di:n], cited above).

Phonological processes may be grouped into two functionally distinct categories: **whole-word processes**, which simplify word or syllable structure and segmental contrast within a word (generally through reduction or assimilation), and **segment change processes**, which involve (context-free) changes in specific segments or segment types, regardless of syllable- or word-position. We will briefly characterize a few of the most common processes representing each of these types; further discussion, using examples taken from the extensive literature on normal phonological acquisition, follows. For a fuller list of common phonological processes, see Chapter 5.

Whole-Word Processes

Unstressed syllable deletion: omission of an unstressed syllable of the target word

> *Ramon* → [mən] (Si: Macken, 1979)

Final consonant deletion: omission of a final consonant of the target word

> *because* → [pi'kʌ]
>
> *thought* → [fɔ] (Vihman and Greenlee, 1987)

Reduplication: production of two identical syllables, based on one or more of the syllables of the target word

> *Sesame Street* → [si:si] (Deborah: Vihman, Ferguson, and Elbert, 1986)
>
> *hello* → [jojo] (Hildegard: Leopold, 1947)

Consonant harmony: one of the contrasting consonants of the target word takes on features of another consonant in the same word

> *duck* → [gʌk]
>
> *tub* → [bʌb] (Daniel: Menn, 1971)

Consonant cluster simplification: a consonant cluster is simplified in some manner

cracker → [kæk] (Molly: Vihman et al., 1986)

Assimilatory processes (like consonant harmony) take the whole word as their domain, whereas reduction processes (involving consonant or syllable deletion) alter the phonotactic or syntagmatic structure of the adult model, reducing the number of syllables or simplifying the shape of syllables. The two types of reduction processes are often treated together and have variously been referred to as "phonotactic rules" (Ingram, 1974), "syllable structure processes" (Ingram, 1986: see also Ch. 5), "structural simplifying processes" (Grunwell, 1981), "syntagmatic processes" (Nettelbladt, 1983), or "processes affecting sequential structure" (Magnusson, 1983). Following the order of processes given above, we will first consider two of the most common reduction processes, syllable deletion and consonant deletion, and then two assimilatory processes, reduplication and consonant harmony; finally, we will illustrate consonant cluster simplification, which is closely related to the segment change processes.

Reduction Processes

Vihman (1980) examined "long word reduction" in 11 children (aged 1;0 to 2;9) acquiring five languages. She restricted analysis to words of three syllables or more in the adult model. She found a language-based order for the proportion of long words attempted in a given child's corpus of utterances. Frequencies ranged from about 25 percent for two Spanish-speaking children to about 3 percent for three English-speaking children (see Savinainen-Makkonen, 2000). Use of syllable deletion or "truncation" to handle the long words varied independently of the particular language spoken, and ranged from 90 percent of all long words attempted by Hildegard Leopold (German- and English-speaking) to 26 percent for Jiri, a Czech-speaking child.

Syllable deletion most often affects an unstressed syllable. Even a stressed syllable may be omitted, especially if it is the first of three or more syllables. There is a strong tendency for children to preserve a final syllable, whether it is stressed or not, presumably because final position is perceptually salient. Klein (1981) provides a great many examples of syllable deletion. The following instances were produced by Jason, a child who made moderate use of the process of deletion.

alligator → ['ægejʌ]
banana → ['nænæ)]
butterfly → ['bʌfaɪ]
watermelon → ['mõmĩn] (omitting the stressed initial syllable)

One of the 3-year-olds included in the study reported in Vihman and Greenlee (1987) was continuing to apply syllable deletion to many words:

animals → ['æmlz]
ambulance → ['æmʌns]
dessert → [ʒrt]

Consonant deletion most often affects final consonants, though initial and medial consonants may also be omitted. Berman (1977) reported that her daughter Shelli (age 18 to 23 months, acquiring both Hebrew and English) frequently used consonant deletion, particularly to avoid producing word-forms with both initial and final consonants. Difficulty with individual segments appears to have dictated the choice of segment to omit: Stops and nasals were retained, with preference for stops; fricatives and liquids were omitted. The chief mark of phonological advance in the period under study was the production of formerly omitted consonants and the admission of new CVC words without reduction. Some examples of consonant deletion (from Berman, 1977):

1. Word-initial
   /ˈruti/ → [ˈuti] "Ruthie" (mother's name)
   /ʃaˈlom/ → [ˈalom] "hello"
   /xam/ → [am] "hot"
2. Word-final
   peach → [pi]
   spoon → [pu]
   /tov/ → [to] "good"

Deletion of a medial consonant is cited for one 3-year-old in Vihman and Greenlee (1987):

   mommy → [mãi]

Assimilatory Processes

Although some writers view use of *reduplication* as the mark of a developmental stage that all children pass through at a very young age (Moskowitz, 1973; Fee and Ingram, 1982), others maintain that reduplication, like other phonological processes, represents an individual strategy characterizing the speech of some but not all children at the same developmental point (Schwartz, Leonard, Wilcox, and Folger, 1980; cf. also Schwartz and Leonard, 1983). The function of reduplication is also a subject of controversy. It may serve as a strategy for producing multisyllabic adult words—retaining the syllable count while reducing the number of contrasting elements.

Schwartz and colleagues collected spontaneous speech data from 12 (English-speaking) children aged 1;3 to 2;0, half of whom proved to be "reduplicators," using full or partial reduplication in 20 percent or more of their recorded lexicon. Fee and Ingram drew on 24 heterogeneous data sets (mostly parental diaries) for children aged 1;1 to 2;6. Some examples of reduplication provided by Schwartz and colleagues (1980):

   Christmas → [dzɪdzɪ]
   kitten → [kɪkɪ]
   water → [wɔwɔ]

Whereas Schwartz and colleagues found no correlation between age or linguistic stage and relative use of reduplication for their narrower age range, Fee and Ingram found that the reduplicators in their sample were younger than the non-reduplicators (they did not assess stage of linguistic development). Both studies found that reduplication is primarily used to reduce the complexity of multisyllabic words. (Application of the process to monosyllables— e.g., *ball* → [bʌbə]—proved rare.) The relation between reduplication and final consonants remains unclear.

Ferguson (1983) pointed out that reduplication has also been found to serve a "play" or "practice" function, not only in babbling but also in the sound-play of 2- to 5-year-olds (cf. Ferguson and Macken, 1983). Furthermore, reduplication may help the child to identify and learn to produce phonologically distinctive syllables and segments. For example, production of a reduplicative pattern reflecting the shape of one of the syllables of the adult model seems to provide the child with a strategy to move from a whole-word to a segment-based phonology (cf. Macken, 1978; Lleó, 1990).

Consonant harmony, or the assimilation of non-contiguous consonants, is essentially the same as "partial reduplication" (vowel harmony is a parallel process but is less frequently noted in child language data). Unfortunately, neither Schwartz et al. nor Fee and Ingram specified the proportion of full versus partial reduplication (i.e., assimilation) in their data. In a study of relatively large data sets from 13 children (aged 1;0 to 2;9) acquiring six languages, Vihman (1978) found a range from 1 percent to 32 percent in the use of consonant harmony (for words containing different consonants in the adult model); mean use was 14 percent. Differences in frequency of harmony use did not appear to be tied to differences across languages.

Smith suggested that consonant harmony is "part of a universal template which the child has to escape from in order to learn his language" (1973; 206). In some children, however, harmony is rare, and when used, enters the child's lexicon as a simplification of words produced earlier in a form closer to the adult model. The use of consonant harmony can be taken to reflect the child's effort to systematize his or her word production. More specifically, consonant harmony often provides a way of avoiding difficult segments (such as liquids and fricatives) or of allowing the child to produce new segments or longer words by reducing overall complexity. For a study of patterns of consonant harmony in a large sample of children acquiring English, see Stoel-Gammon and Stemberger, 1994.

Consonant harmony may also be described as "full" or "partial," depending on the form in the child's production. In full harmony, the consonants of a word that contrasted in the adult model, are identical in the child form; in partial harmony, the consonants of the child form are more similar than in the adult model but are not identical. Some examples (from Vihman, 1978; the examples below from her daughter Virve are in Estonian):

1. Full
   Amahl Smith   *tiger* → [gaigə]
   Virve Vihman   *tuppa* → [pup:a] "into the room"
2. Partial
   Virve Vihman   *suppi* → [fup:i] "some soup"

Notice that the differences reflected here between adult and child forms could all be described in terms of a single distinctive feature: alveolar to velar (plus automatic word-initial voicing) for *tiger*, alveolar to labial or labiodental for *tuppa* and *suppi*. Full versus partial harmony describes only the child's form, not the difference between adult and child form.

Grunwell's chronology (1981) showed that neither reduplication nor consonant harmony is normally used by age 3. Full reduplication did not occur in the 3-year-old samples in Vihman and Greenlee (1987), and consonant harmony occurred only sporadically (a few instances in a three-hour sample) and only for a few of the children.

1. Full
   yellow —> [ˈlɛlou]
   mailboxes —> [ˈmeɪlmaksɪz]
2. Partial
   slimy —> [ˈsnaɪmi]

Consonant Cluster Simplification

Like the reduction processes, cluster simplification alters syllable structure, but it is also closely related to the segment change processes in that the specific consonants omitted or changed are typically those difficult to produce as singleton consonants. Cluster simplification is virtually always present in the first year of language use, and it is one of the longest lasting processes. At age 3, cluster simplification still accounted for a substantial proportion of the phonological errors made by the 10 children followed in Vihman and Greenlee (1987), and it still accounts for over 10 percent of the errors of 5-year-olds responding to standardized test items (Haelsig and Madison, 1986; Roberts, Burchinal, and Footo, 1990).

Among the 11 younger subjects (12–33 months) of Vihman (1980), cluster simplification affected from 52 percent to 100 percent (mean 80 percent) of all target words with clusters (which themselves made up nearly a third of the children's words). Several general relationships emerged in this study. In clusters made up of liquid plus another consonant, the liquid was typically omitted, and when stop and fricative were combined, the stop was the more likely to be preserved. Nasal plus stop clusters were more likely to be maintained as clusters, but when such a cluster was reduced, the nasal was likely to be retained before a voiced stop and omitted before a voiceless stop. Perceptual rather than articulatory factors may be at work here (Braine, 1976) since nasals, like vowels, are longer before voiced obstruents and, thus, may be more easily perceived in that context.

In a study of the **acquisition of stop-plus-liquid clusters**, Greenlee (1974) found the course of development to be very similar in all six of the languages investigated. She identified three stages: (1) omission of the liquid, (2) substitution for the liquid (usually by a glide), and (3) correct production. Some examples (from Greenlee, 1974):

Amahl Smith: *bread* → [bɛd], [blɛd]

Edmond Grégoire (a Belgian child acquiring French):

bras → [bwa] "arm"
croute → [tut] "crust"
grillé → [dije] "toasted"
tram → [kam], [tʃam] "streetcar"

From English-speaking 3-year-olds (Vihman and Greenlee, 1987):

flower → [ˈfawr]
monster → [ˈmãtr]
stinker → [ˈsɪŋkr]
thread → [sɛd]

Segment Change Processes

Velar fronting: a velar is replaced by an alveolar or a dental

/kikeriki:/ → [titi:] (Virve: Vihman, 1976)

Stopping: a fricative is replaced by a stop

sea → [ti:]
say → [tʰei] (Amahl: Smith, 1973)

Gliding: a liquid is replaced by a glide

lie → [jaɪ] (Hildegard: Leopold, 1947)

Of the commonly found changes, **velar fronting** is the only one to affect stops, and it is, no doubt, the first common change process to be outgrown (Preisser, Hodson, and Paden, 1988). A case study by Berg (1995) provides an unusually detailed account of the loss of velar fronting—or, more accurately, the acquisition of velar stops (both as single-tons and in clusters)—as his daughter acquired her first language, German, between the ages of 3 and 4 years. The study, based on daily recording, begins with the first successful production of a word-initial velar and ends with virtual mastery of velar production; the process took a full 15 months. Of the ten 3-year-olds described in Vihman and Greenlee, only one exhibited consistent velar fronting. Regular use of velar fronting contributed significantly to the relative unintelligibility of the speech of that child, who was very advanced syntactically and thus often produced long, complex sentences. For example:

called → [tald]
cow → [taʊ]
gophers → [ˈdoᵘfɚs]

The process of **gliding**, which also plays a role in the acquisition of stop + liquid clusters, persists considerably longer. Examples can be found in many languages, but Ingram (1986) claimed that this process does not appear in French acquisition data. Examples of gliding from English-speaking 3-year-olds (Vihman and Greenlee, 1987):

love → [jʌv]

red → [wɛd]

Mastering Fricatives

The most common process affecting fricatives is **stopping**, but replacement by a stop is not the only error type found. In particular, the interdentals—the most difficult segments for English-speaking children to acquire (comparable to r-trills in languages which have them)—are frequently substituted by other fricatives (/f/ or /s/ for /θ/, somewhat less commonly /v/, /z/, or even /l/ for /ð/). As mentioned earlier, perceptual difficulties have been implicated in production errors involving both fricatives and liquids, although the low incidence of fricatives in babbling suggests that these sounds present articulatory problems for many children. Some examples of stopping from English-speaking 3-year-olds (Vihman and Greenlee, 1987):

move → [mu:b]

shoes → [ʃu:t]

some → [tʌm]

Perhaps the most important lesson to be learned from the rather extensive literature on the acquisition of fricatives (e.g., Moskowitz, 1975; Edwards, 1979; Ingram et al., 1980) is that each fricative is acquired by its own individual path of development. There is no rapid spread of a feature of "frication" or "continuancy" to relevant segments (Ferguson, 1975). Other points of particular interest raised by Ferguson include the following: (1) fricatives may be acquired first in postvocalic, final position or intervocalically before initial position (although the first consonants acquired word-finally are usually stops: Kehoe and Stoel-Gammon, 2001), and (2) language-specific constraints on the frequency and freedom of occurrence of particular fricatives may affect the order of acquisition (e.g., English /ʒ/ is rare and largely limited to word-medial position, and it consequently tends to be a late acquisition).

Summary

The regularity found in phonological substitutions after the earliest stage of lexical acquisition can be conveniently formulated in terms of phonological rules or processes. Two types of processes are usually distinguished. *Whole-word processes* simplify word or syllable structure and segmental contrast within a word, and *segment change processes* account for errors involving difficulty with specific segments. Whole-word processes are generally typical of the earlier stages of phonological development. They include assimilatory processes (reduplication and consonant harmony) and consonant cluster simplification. Clusters of obstruent plus liquid have been found to be produced in stages, first as obstruent only and then as obstruent + glide, before being produced correctly. The most common segment changes include velar fronting—the most common phonological process affecting stops, gliding of liquids, and various substitutions affecting fricatives. Fricatives are sometimes substituted by stops, but may also substitute for one another, e.g. the earlier learned /f/ or /s/ replacing interdental /θ/. Fricatives tend to be acquired first in word-final position.

Profiling the Preschool Child: Individual Differences Revisited

We have reviewed both the findings of large-scale studies aimed at establishing norms for the acquisition of particular phonemes of the adult language and the phonological processes found to apply most often in intensive studies of small groups of children (or even just one child). In both cases, the analyses involved may be termed relational; that is, they are concerned with the relationship between the child's productions and the adult forms (Stoel-Gammon and Dunn, 1985). "Independent" analyses, on the other hand, describe the sounds and syllable structures of the child's productions in their own right, without reference to the adult forms. In order to form an idea of the kind of phonological production that we can expect to characterize a normally developing 2- or 3-year-old child, we will consider the results of two studies reporting phonological analyses of data drawn from naturally occurring conversation. The first is a study of 2-year-olds and makes use of both relational and independent analyses; the second is an intensive examination of the kinds of errors made by a smaller group of 3-year-olds. In addition, we will consider the results of two longitudinal studies, one comparing the phonological status at age 3 of the two 1-year-old girls profiled in Chapter 2, the other comparing phonological process use in two boys at ages 2, 3, and 6 years.

Phonetic Tendencies of Two-Year-Olds

Stoel-Gammon (1987) characterized the "phonological skills" of thirty-three 2-year-old children acquiring English. The children's productions were recorded from the age of 9 to 24 months on a trimonthly basis (cf. also Stoel-Gammon, 1985; Kehoe and Stoel-Gammon, 2001). The data were derived from two half-hour play sessions involving conversational interaction between child and observer. Stoel-Gammon pointed out that the "large-scale" studies of Wellman et al. (1931), Templin (1957), and Prather et al. (1975) were, in fact, based on a rather small number of 2-year-old subjects (no more than 10 or 20), since a large number of children failed to produce many of the target words. She argued that a better assessment of a 2-year-old's phonological skills can be attained through the recording of naturally occurring conversational data.

Stoel-Gammon established the use of at least 10 different adult-based words in the course of one hour of recording as a criterion for including a speech sample in the 2-year-old analyses. She then developed a corpus of up to 50 words for each subject, taken from the first fully or partially intelligible utterances in each sample. No one word *type* was represented by more than two variable *tokens* or productions of the same word (e.g., [su] and [du] for *shoe*). The number of words analyzed ranged from 20 to 50 per child (mean 36). Three different analyses were carried out.

Word and Syllable Shapes, Based on the Co-Occurrence of Consonants and Vowels

All the children produced at least two different open monosyllables (CV), and only one child failed to produce two different closed monosyllables (CVC). Disyllabic word shapes (CVCV[C]) occurred in over half the samples, as did word-initial clusters. Word-final clusters were produced by 48 percent of the children but medial clusters by only 30 percent.

Phonetic Inventories

The findings regarding consonant use in this study are presented in Table 3.2, along with age three data from Templin's (1957) large sample normative study. For the 2-year-olds, word-initial consonant inventories typically included stops at all three places of articulation ([t, k, b, d, g] occurred in at least 50 percent of the samples). In addition, nasals ([m, n]), fricatives ([f, s, h]), and a glide ([w]) typically occurred in initial position. In final position, three voiceless stops, one nasal ([n]), one fricative ([s]), and one liquid ([r]) were typically used. There was a strong tendency for children with large inventories in initial position to have a large inventory in final position as well. No one cluster (such as [sp-, pl-]) was used by more than half the children in either initial or final position. Templin's data for 3-year-old children are similar; however, she also included sound usage in the medial position. Direct comparison of data between these studies is difficult because of differences in age levels and sampling procedures.

Accuracy of Consonant Production

The mean percentage of correct consonants, based on a procedure developed by Shriberg and Kwiatkowski (1982), was 70 percent (range 43 percent to 91 percent). There was a tendency for the children with larger inventories to achieve greater accuracy with respect to the adult form than those with smaller inventories. Stoel-Gammon pointed out that the difference in inventory size between adult English and the "typical" 2-year-old in her study is considerable, and thus, the 70 percent accuracy level achieved by the children suggests that 2-year-olds *mainly attempt words with consonants that fall within their productive range*. The relationship between the number of different consonants produced and the use of consonant phones that match adult segments further suggests that phonetic and phonological abilities are developing in parallel.

Phonological Process Use at Age Three

After age 3, the majority of simplifying phonological processes no longer apply regularly in most cases. The data we will describe were derived from three hours of recorded nat-

TABLE 3.2   Acquisition of Consonants

Cs Typically Produced	Age 2 Years (N = 33) Stoel-Gammon, 1987	Age 3 Years (N = 60) Templin, 1957
Initial Position		
stops	t, k, b, d, g	p, b, t, d, k, g
fricatives	f, s, h	f
affricates		
nasals	m, n	m, n
liquids		
glides	w	w, j
clusters		
Medial Position		
stops		p, b, d, k, g
fricatives		f, s, z
affricates		
nasals		m, n, ng
liquids		
glides		w, j
clusters		
Final Position		
stops	p, t, k	p, t
fricatives	s	f
affricates		
nasals	n	m, n, ng
liquids	r	
glides		
clusters		

ural interaction between each of ten 36-month-old children and the child's mother (30 minutes), a familiar peer (30 minutes) and the observer (including phonological, grammatical, and cognitive probes: Vihman and Greenlee, 1987). The children were drawn from a middle-class population in California. Despite the socioeconomic homogeneity of the sample, wide differences were found in intelligibility, specific processes used, and phonological organization.

Intelligibility

All of the children could be clearly understood more than half the time; on average, 73 percent of their utterances were judged intelligible by three raters unfamiliar with the children, but the range was broad: 54 percent to 80 percent. As might be expected, the children judged most intelligible were generally those who made the fewest phonetic or phonological errors. Yet misarticulation and phonological process use were not the only factors contributing to unintelligible speech at this age. The children who used the highest proportion of complex sentences tended to be relatively difficult to understand. Some examples of complex sentences produced by these children:

> It's sort of necklace, but it's a string where you put beads on.

> It hurts when I crash into something.

> I can buckle 'em when people say that's all right, and then when they say that's not all right, I don't do it.

Most of the 3-year-olds were apparently unable to produce complex sentences and still speak clearly enough to be easily understood by unfamiliar adults.

Only the substitution of interdental fricatives by other consonants (stops or other fricatives) was regularly used by all subjects. Two other processes—gliding and palatal fronting—were regularly used by over half the subjects. The remaining processes were used by no more than one to three subjects. Of the processes affecting sequential structure, cluster simplification was regularly used by three subjects, but the phonological processes typical of 1-year-olds were each regularly used by only one or (in the case of consonant and syllable deletion) two of these 3-year-old subjects.

Phonological Organization: Profile of Two Three-Year-Old Girls

Earlier, we described two talkative firstborn girls, Deborah and Molly. Both had developed large vocabularies by the time they were 16 months old, but they showed different phonetic preferences and differences in phonological organization; we characterized Deborah's style as exploratory and Molly's as systematic. To what extent were the differences between the two girls present at age 3?

Both the girls were still quite talkative. Molly ranked first and Deborah fourth in average length of conversational turn at age 3 (based on interaction with their mothers). Both were also still lexically advanced, with Deborah ranking first and Molly second on a scale of lexical diversity (reflecting the number of different words used in the course of interaction with their mothers). And, with respect to phonology, they continued to diverge. Deborah was judged the most intelligible of the 10 children in the study and was found to make the next-to-least use of phonological processes (i.e., had the next-to-fewest phonological errors). Molly was third from last of the 10 children on both the intelligibility ranking and the phonological error score.

Deborah and Molly continued to differ in their respective error patterns. Deborah's errors were fairly evenly balanced between whole-word and segment change processes. She was the only 3-year-old who made relatively high use of **metathesis**, the reordering of segments. She made regular use of the segment change processes typical of the majority of the 3-year-olds (**palatal fronting, interdental fricative substitution**), and she was one of four children who did not replace liquids with glides. All of Molly's whole-word errors were sporadic or rare, as was true of the group as a whole, but she had a great many more cluster and segment errors than Deborah had. She was one of the three children who often, although inconsistently, reduced Cl-clusters.

What kind of comparison can be made with the specific phonetic preferences exhibited by these children at age 1 (see Chapter 2)? Several of the phonetic preferences seen at age 1 are no longer present at age 3. For example, place of articulation errors were rare at this age and were not made by Deborah or Molly. At age 1, Deborah made unusually extensive use of fricatives, yet at age 3, it was Molly, not Deborah, who showed relatively high accuracy in fricative use. On the other hand, Molly was exceptional at age 1 in her high use of final consonants, yet it was Deborah, not Molly, who showed no tendency to delete final consonants at age 3. In general, the specific phonetic tendencies found at age 1 seemed to be unrelated to the phonological errors made at age 3 (Vihman and Greenlee, 1987).

Turning to the question of phonological organization, the chief difference between Deborah and Molly at age 3 was Deborah's willingness to abbreviate words and to slur or scramble segments (e.g., ['dalfoz]~[du'ralfoz] for *Ruldolfo's*, the name of a local pizza place), despite her relatively accurate production of individual consonants. Molly made relatively few errors affecting the structure of the word as a whole, yet she was unintelligible some of the time because of her difficulty with a number of individual consonants (especially /l/, /r/, and /ʃ/). Recall that Molly's systematic approach to phonological learning was expressed in (1) her highly constrained choice of words - rarely attempting fricatives (whereas Deborah attempted a wider range of sound patterns), and (2) the unusually low degree of variability across different tokens of the same word. In general, the children who, like Molly, were relatively more constrained in their word selection patterns at age 1 were very likely to make little use of whole-word processes at age 3, and those who, like Deborah, explored a wide range of sounds at age 1 were also more likely to delete consonants and syllables, assimilate consonants, and change the order of segments in a word at age 3. Furthermore, there was a tendency for children whose word shapes were more variable at age 1 to make more *inconsistent* use of phonological processes at age 3 (Vihman and Greenlee, 1987). In summary, Deborah's phonological style at both ages was typical of more *exploratory* children, those with a high "tolerance for variability" (Kamhi, Catts, and Davis, 1984), and Molly's was typical of children with a lower tolerance for variability and hence, a more systematic approach.

Profile of Two Boys Recorded at Ages Two, Three, and Six Years

Klein (1985) reported the results of a longitudinal study of the phonological process usage of two boys, Jason and Joshua. The boys were first recorded at ages 1;8 and 2;0, during a four-hour naturalistic play session with the investigator (see also Klein, 1981). Analyses focused on a comparison of monosyllabic versus polysyllabic productions. The boys proved similar in many ways, each attempting polysyllabic words in a little over half of their single-word productions (Jason 60 percent, Joshua 51 percent), and each matching the syllable count of the adult model in the majority of their productions. However, they differed in their more specific production strategies. Joshua tended to use consonant harmony and reduplication, while Jason typically replaced the consonants in unstressed syllables with either glottals or glides. In addition, Jason made greater use of syllable deletion than Joshua, and was thus more variable in his approach to the production of polysyllabic words. These are some examples of words produced by both boys in the course of the first recording:

Adult model	Joshua	Jason
bunny	[babi]	[bʌɪ]
tiger	[tada]	[daɪja]
pocketbook	[bababuk]	[paʔəwu]
motorcycle	[mumulalak]	[modaɪʔu]

At ages 3 and 6 the boys were recorded for about one hour each, including both **continuous speech**, produced during play with the same materials provided at age 2, and **single words**, produced in response to the *Photo Articulation Test* (Pendergast, Dickey, Selmar, and Soder, 1969). Analysis of these data focused on comparison of phonological process use (instances of use relative to opportunities for use in the child's productions) in single-word versus continuous speech. A "whole word accuracy" score was derived by comparing the number of error-free words with the total number of intelligible productions. Based on norms reported by Schmitt, Howard, and Schmitt (1983), Joshua was found to fall one standard deviation above the mean for his age at both ages 3 and 6, while Jason fell slightly more than one standard deviation below the mean for his age. At both ages the boys made many more errors in continuous speech than on single-word productions; in fact, at age 6 Joshua failed to make any errors on the articulation test, while Jason evidenced **stopping** and **deaffrication**. In continuous speech both children sometimes deleted final consonants, stopped /ð/, and simplified consonant clusters.

The relationship between use of supraglottal consonants at age 2 and relative accuracy in phonological production at ages 3 and 6 is striking. Klein (1985) suggested that an **articulatory timing factor** may explain Jason's difficulty with the production of both affricates (or consonant clusters which function as **single units** in English) and consonant clusters in general, particularly in the flow of running speech (see Gilbert and Purves, 1977, discussed below). As Klein pointed out, the same difficulty with articulatory timing may account for Jason's earlier overuse of glottals and glides, which require less precise articulatory control than other consonants. Interestingly, Vihman and Greenlee (1987) found low use of "true consonants" (or overuse of glottals and glides) to be the best phonetic indicator at age 1 of slower phonological acquisition at age 3.

Summary

Analysis of the naturally occurring conversation of 2-year-old English-speaking children revealed that open monosyllables were still the dominant word shapes at this time, followed by closed monosyllables, and open or closed disyllables. Word-initial consonant clusters were used frequently as well. Stops and nasals continued to be the most common consonants; word-initial inventories were richer than word-final inventories in every consonant category except liquids. The children were more accurate in consonant production than might be expected, given their relatively incomplete inventories.

Analysis of ten 3-year-old English-speaking children engaged in natural conversation revealed that over half their speech was intelligible to outsiders. Both specific phonological errors and high use of complex sentences appeared to contribute to unintelligibility. All the children made errors involving interdental fricatives; gliding and palatal fronting were also common.

Comparison of the phonological error patterns of two 3-year-old children whose phonological development at age 1 was described earlier showed that the specific phonetic strengths they had exhibited at age 1 bore no relationship to the errors made at age 3. On the other hand, their differing approaches to phonological learning—systematic versus exploratory—manifested themselves at both ages.

Comparison of two boys across three time points, ages 2, 3, and 6 years, suggested that difficulty with articulatory timing may underlie relatively slow phonological development, and may be identifiable as early as age 1 or 2 years in the use of glottals and glides, or relatively slow mastery of supraglottal articulation.

Development of Perception Beyond Early Childhood: Understanding Running Speech

Perceptual issues relevant to the time when the child must both develop a store of knowledge about the sound system of the language and construct a repertoire of lexical or word forms were discussed previously. As the child becomes a more fluent speaker and enters the world of oral communication with unfamiliar adults as well as peers, one challenge is to master the complex task of understanding continuous or running speech, speech that is not simplified by the baby talk or "infant-directed speech" that characterizes much of the input in the first two years. What factors enter into that task? Do children process spoken language differently than adults?

Under ordinary circumstances, listeners do not identify isolated words but rather retrieve a message from the flow of speech. In the 1980s, investigators began to study the factors affecting the perception of continuous speech, by children as well as adults. A variety of research methods were designed to investigate the complex process by which listeners interpret speech "on-line," without taking the time to make sure of what was heard, consult a lexicon of possible words, and compare the plausibility of one word or interpretation against another.

Recognizing spoken words is thought to involve integrating two different sources of information (Elman and McClelland, 1986; Tyler and Frauenfelder, 1987): (1) **sensory input**, or "bottom-up" (phonetic) information, deriving from the speech signal itself; and (2) **contextual constraints**, or "top-down" information, deriving from the speaker's knowledge of what has already been said, what might plausibly follow, what semantic and syntactic structures the language allows, and what words the language makes available, given the unfolding message.

Experimental evidence suggests that words are typically (though not always) identified *before* sufficient acoustic-phonetic information has become available to allow a listener to be certain of a word on the basis of the sound pattern alone (Marslen-Wilson, 1987). Such "early selection" means that word recognition is based on informed guessing as well as perception. That is, the listener is continually engaged in constructing an interpretation of the incoming message, so that the more predictable a particular word is, given the conversation up to that point, the preceding sentence, or the phrase in which the word is located, the more rapidly a listener can guess or "recognize" it from a brief phonetic clue—such as the first sound or the first syllable.

In addition to the important role of context in word recognition, word frequency must also be taken into account: Experimental manipulations have shown that high-frequency words are recognized more rapidly than low-frequency words, when both provide equally good matches to the initial phonetic shape of the input and each is plausible in context.

To what extent do children resemble adults in the recognition of words in running speech? Each of the factors that enter into adult word recognition—ongoing analysis of the acoustic-phonetic signal, expectations based on the semantic, syntactic, and pragmatic context, and relative lexical familiarity—may potentially reflect a long period of development. Both increasing *experience with language* and possible changes in *processing abilities* may affect the child's capacity to carry out the complex task of interpreting running speech.

Adult-Child Differences in Word Recognition

Analysis of the Phonetic Signal

Elliott, Hammer, and Evan (1987) tested children, teenagers, and adults aged 70 to 85 on their recognition of highly familiar spoken monosyllabic nouns under conditions of **limited acoustic information**. The teenagers recognized more words and did so more rapidly than either the children or adults. Their guesses were usually real words which were phonetically compatible with the sounds heard, whereas the children's responses sometimes failed to match the phonetic stimuli. These results are consistent with the hypothesis, advanced by Walley (1984), that children require more acoustic information to identify stimuli than do teenagers or adults.

Cole and his colleagues (Cole and Jakimik, 1980; Cole and Perfetti, 1980) compared the processing of continuous speech by children and adults. Cole's work supports three major theoretical assumptions regarding the process of decoding or recognizing words in running speech.

1. Words are recognized through the *interaction* of sound perception and linguistic and pragmatic knowledge.
2. Words are typically recognized *in order*. As each word is recognized, it allows the listener to establish word boundaries. In addition, each decoded word imposes syntactic and semantic constraints on the following words, which enables the listener to progressively narrow the field of possible interpretations.
3. Words are decoded sequentially, using earlier-occurring sounds to narrow the range of possible candidates.

In three experiments with 4- and 5-year-old children and adults, Cole (1981) investigated the effects of word-position, consonant substituted, and phonotactic structure, or permissible versus impermissible consonant clusters, on the detection of mispronunciations in running speech. The children were tested on familiar songs and nursery rhymes. The main results were:

1. The children, like the adults, paid most attention to initial position and least to final position.
2. In word-initial position, children were most sensitive to changes in place of articulation of stops and to changes of stop to nasal and of voiced to voiceless stop. Interchanges among nasals, fricatives, or liquids were less often detected. Most easily detected were common articulatory substitutions of a stop for a fricative. In a follow-up study, Bernthal, Greenlee, Eblen, and Marking (1987) also found that developmental substitutions were more easily detected than nondevelopmental substitutions by normally developing and misarticulating 4- to 6-year-old children as well as by adults.

Contextual Effects

Tyler and Marslen-Wilson (1981) investigated the role of discourse and of syntactic context alone on the comprehension of running speech of children aged 5, 7, and 10 years. Children were tested on two tasks, **identical monitoring**, in which the occurrence of a particular word is to be noted as soon as it is spoken, and **category monitoring**, in which a word belonging to a particular category (body part, fruit, furniture) is to be identified when heard. The target words fell toward the end of the second of a pair of sentences of one of three kinds: normal prose, in which the first sentence provides a normal discourse context for the second; syntactic prose, in which the sentences are anomalous in meaning but syntactically correct; and random word order, which violates both semantic and syntactic structure and thus provides no contextual support for word recognition. Examples (with the target word in boldface):

> John had to go back home. He had fallen out of the swing and had hurt his hand on the ground. (normal)
>
> John had to sit on the shop. He had lived out of the kitchen and had enjoyed his **hand** in the mud. (syntactic)
>
> The on sit shop to had John. He lived had and kitchen the out his of had enjoyed **hand** mud in the. (random)

The results suggested that children as young as age 5 are able to make good use of discourse and even of syntactic context. Mean reaction times decreased significantly with age, but all three groups showed a marked facilitatory effect from the normal discourse and a lesser effect from normal syntax only. The category monitoring task was considerably more difficult for the children than the identical monitoring task. The normal discourse context again aided recognition, but the semantically anomalous "syntactic" sentence sequences gave no significant advantage in this case.

Another study suggested that children's ability to make use of semantic knowledge continues to improve up to as late as age 15. Elliott (1979) tested 24 children at each of four age levels (11, 13, 15, and 17 years) on their understanding of sentences against a background of multitalker babble. The test sentences were designed to fall into two groups: **high predictability** and **low predictability**—a function of the presence or absence of two or three semantically related "pointer" words that could help cue the listener as to the identity of the final (target) word, always a monosyllabic noun. The test consisted of 25 sentences of each type; none was longer than 8 syllables. The subject's task was to repeat back the last word of the sentence.

Under just one set of conditions, when the target sentence was presented at the same intensity as the noise, a significant age trend was found, with the 11- and 13-year-olds performing less well on high-predictability sentences than the 15- and 17-year-olds, who did about as well as young adults tested earlier with written responses. No age differences were found in quiet or in comprehension of the low-predictability sentences. A later test of 9-year-old children showed significantly poorer performance than that of the 11-year-olds. The age-related differences are not a direct auditory effect since only the high-predictability sentences proved easier for older subjects. Rather, the difference appears to reflect the extent to which children of different ages were able to use the semantic information in the pointer syllables to guess at the final, difficult-to-hear, target noun.

Lexical Familiarity

Cole and Perfetti (1980) reported a significant difference between children and adults in the detection of mispronunciations in a simple, clearly articulated story: On average, preschool children (ages 4 to 5) detected about 50 percent of the mispronounced words, children kindergarten through fifth grade about 60 percent, and adults 95 percent. Cole and Perfetti suggested that children probably treat mispronunciations as unfamiliar words: "It seems likely that children learn to tolerate (or actively ignore) unfamiliar words, so that each occurrence of an unfamiliar word does not result in a breakdown of the comprehension process" (313).

It is important to note that the children detected mispronunciations in isolated words (95 percent) far more readily than in fluent speech. The high detection rate for isolated words is due in part to their slower articulation, and also to the cues provided by pictures that accompanied the test words. This procedure is commonly used in clinical tests of phonetic discrimination, and therefore, the tests may overestimate children's ability to perceive phonetic differences in the course of conversational speech (Cole, 1981).

The issue of word familiarity itself has also received attention. Walley and Metsala (1990) used mispronunciation tasks to test children aged 5 and 8. Subjective age-of-acquisition ratings were used to categorize test words as "early," "current," and "late." The familiarity factor proved to be important: Young children were more likely to detect mispronunciations in early and current words. Furthermore, the children were biased toward identifying late (or for age 5, both late and current) words as mispronounced—including words which were correctly pronounced ("intact" words). Thus, whereas the subjects in Cole and Perfetti (1980) were found to treat mispronounced words as unfamiliar, Walley and Metsala showed through analysis of "false alarms" that their subjects were reluctant to treat unfamiliar words as intact, and preferred to label them mispronounced. These results call to mind the biasing role of familiarity in early tests of linguistic perception, mentioned in Chapter 2 (Barton, 1976; Clumeck, 1982). They are reminiscent also of several anecdotes reported in Vihman (1981: 248), in which preschool children misperceived unfamiliar words as relatively more familiar ones, disregarding the fact that their interpretation was at odds with the ongoing discourse context.

Summary

Word recognition is a complex process, involving the integration of the sensory input (acoustic-phonetic signal), contextual information (including both pragmatic and general knowledge-based inferences regarding the gist of the incoming message) and specific structural effects relating to the phonotactic, syntactic, and semantic restrictions characteristic of the language code. The listener's lexical expectations are also influenced by word frequency.

On the whole, school-age children process continuous speech in an adultlike way, making use of context to aid in the interpretation of the acoustic signal. Also, developmental mispronunciations are more salient than other consonant substitutions to children as young as age 4 as well as to adults. In several respects children are different from adults, however. They appear to need more acoustic information before they commit themselves to a decision as to word identity, perhaps because so many words continue to be unfamiliar, at least up to the teens. Furthermore, their use of semantic knowledge as a clue to the unfolding message is not fully developed until the teen years. Finally, school-age children, like younger children, perceive familiar words more accurately than unfamiliar words, and take a cautious approach to apparent mispronunciations in running speech.

Production in the School-Age Child: Continuing Change

In characterizing the phonological production of 3-year-olds, we noted that the majority of simplifying phonological processes no longer apply at that age although consonant clusters are still frequently reduced and certain segment types (especially fricatives and liquids) continue to be substituted by other segments. According to the normative articulation data presented in Figure 5.3, half of the children tested had succeeded in using all of the relevant sounds correctly by age 4. However, for fricatives and liquids correct production by 90 percent of the children was achieved only later.

It is reasonable, then, to ask whether phonetic and phonological acquisition can be said to be complete for most normally developing children by the time they reach school age. With respect to basic articulatory mastery and intelligibility outside the family, the answer is yes. It is important to note, however, that both phonetic and phonological variation and change continue in a number of respects, not only beyond early childhood but also throughout a person's life span. We will illustrate this point by briefly discussing three areas of continuing change: (1) temporal coordination of speech production, (2) phonological reorganization under the influence of literacy, and (3) phonetic and phonological influence from the peer group.

Temporal Coordination of Speech Production

Smith (1978) inferred from durational measurements that segment and word production by 2- and 4-year-old children was consistently slower than adult productions of the same forms. However, the proportional relationships between segments were much like those of adults. For example, final syllables and stressed syllables tended to be longer than non-final and unstressed syllables; voiceless stops were longer than voiced stops while vowels were shorter before the (longer) voiceless stops. Smith concluded that children possess quite sophisticated timing-control systems, despite their still immature neuromuscular control capacities (as reported for other aspects of motor performance, such as reaction time in general, maximum rate of syllable repetition, and maximum finger-tapping rate).

A gradual increase in rate of articulation with age was reported by Hulme, Thomson, Muir, and Lawrence (1984). They tested children aged 3 to 4, 7 to 8, and 10 to 11 as well as adults on their maximum rate of repetition of one-, two-, and three- or four-syllable words. They found an increase in speech rate with age, as well as a tendency for subjects to repeat short words more quickly than long ones, but with less difference in rate for different word lengths in the younger subjects. Hulme and colleagues were not primarily interested in speech rate per se, however, but in the possible relationship between speech rate—and, hence, maximum potential rate for *verbal rehearsal*—and short-term memory. Their results showed a close connection between increases in verbal short-term memory and speech rate. They viewed this finding as strong support for the hypothesis that verbal short-term memory "is a time-based system limited by the amount of speech which it can store" (251): see Baddeley, Thomson, and Buchanan (1975); Baddeley (1986).

A number of studies of children's speech production have addressed the question of the timing of individual segments embedded in clusters, syllables, and words. There is evidence that word-initial clusters may first be represented as single consonants combining features of both the consonants in the cluster (cf., e.g., Menyuk, 1972). Only later is the cluster "unpacked" into its separate component segments. Gilbert and Purves (1977) pointed out that the level at which the child represents the cluster as a single segment—in perception, in the production plan, or only in the execution of the plan—is not clear. If, for example, the child perceives the cluster but cannot produce the segments sequentially, the problem could be purely articulatory (difficulty with the timing and/or motor control of the separate articulatory gestures), or it could reflect difficulty in applying the appropriate "segmentalization rules," that is, in sorting out the overlapping articulatory gestures (at the planning level) to achieve the proper sequential output. It has been hypothesized that the child may be constrained at first by a **timing-dominant system**, in which a rigid time schedule governs the execution of articulatory gestures (cf. Ohala, 1970; Hawkins, 1973). As the timing-dominant system is gradually replaced by an **articulation-dominant system**, the limited time constraints are relaxed, leading to slower but more accurate speech production.

Results from detailed analyses of children's productions tend to support such a developmental sequence. Hawkins (1973) measured consonant durations based on production by seven children aged 4 to 7. Comparing her findings with results reported for adults, Hawkins found that in clusters, /l/ tended to be longer in the children's speech. There was, however, no apparent age trend in her data. Hawkins suggested that once the child is able to produce "acceptable but not necessarily mature forms" of particular sounds or sequences of sounds, speech production may remain essentially unchanged for several years (perhaps until puberty) (204).

Gilbert and Purves (1977) tested four groups of five children, one group each at age 5, 7, 9, and 11, and five adults on the production of closed monosyllables, beginning with

/s/, /f/, /l/, /w/, /sl/, /fl/, and /sw/, to determine the relative duration of the fricatives, liquids, and glides as singletons and as part of a cluster. They found greater variation in duration values in the younger children's productions. Like Hawkins (1973), they also found that the only significant timing differences across age groups involved clusters with /l/. In adult production, consonants are shorter when combined in a cluster. Five-year-olds failed to shorten /l/ appropriately; they produced a longer /l/ after fricatives. For the remaining age groups, there was a progressive decrease in the duration of /l/ in clusters, as compared with single-ton /l/, up to age 11, when the relative durations were about the same as those for adults. The positional differences in duration, however, were not significant.

In the view of Gilbert and Purves, these results reflected a late stage in the acquisi-tion of consonant clusters. At first, /l/ is likely to be omitted. Later, some children "split" the cluster, producing *blue* (/blu/) as [bəlu]. This may reflect the child's attempt to circum-vent the constraints of a timing-dominant system. Since the child lacks the articulatory con-trol needed to produce the cluster within a single syllabic unit, an additional syllable is produced. Gilbert and Purves' data suggest that the elongation of the /l/ may represent a fur-ther stage in the splitting process. As the child's timing control improves, the lengthening of /l/ is no longer needed.

In summary, studies of timing problems posed by the production of consonants in clusters and in long words have shown that school-age children, although able to produce acceptably adultlike speech, are continuing to develop fluency in the planning and produc-tion of complex sequences of sounds.

Phonological Reorganization: The Influence of Literacy

Linguistic theory in this century has strongly emphasized the primacy of oral as opposed to written language. As a corollary, it is typically assumed that the unconscious systemic knowledge which underlies productive language use derives solely from the learning of oral language in early childhood. Yet in a literate society, individuals spend many of their for-mative years learning to read, to write, to spell, and to alphabetize. Indeed, as Ferguson (1968) has pointed out, spoken language changes in subtle ways as a society becomes lit-erate, as indicated, for example, by the sporadic occurrence of spelling pronunciations (such as /'fɔr`hɛd/ in lieu of /'fɔrɪd/ for *forehead*; /'ɔftən/ in lieu of /'ɔfən/ for *often*). It is likely that what children are taught in school "reshapes the psychological structures . . . built up previously, so that what is psychologically real for literate speakers includes at least some of what they have been taught about their language" (Jaeger, 1984; 22). Three types of studies have investigated the role of literacy in forcing a restructuring of phonological knowledge. These studies have focused on (1) knowledge of the vowel alternations par-tially reflected in the English spelling system, (2) the influence of spelling on perception and production, and (3) differences in lexical organization between children and adults.

Knowledge of Vowel Alternations

In their highly influential work *The Sound Pattern of English*, Chomsky and Hallé (1968) posited a set of phonological rules to capture the systematic relationship between different vowels that is reflected in such word-pairs as *divine–divinity* (/ai:ɪ/), *serene–serenity* (/i:ɛ/), *profane–profanity* (/ey:æ/), *cone–conical* (/ow:a/), *lose–lost* (/u:ɔ,a/), *profound–profundity* (/aw:ʌ/). These and other phonological rules in Chomsky and Hallé's account have been said to reflect psychologically real patterns of alternation; that is, it is assumed that speakers will unconsciously apply these rules to new words fitting into the same pattern. But this particular set of rules, which reflects a historical sound change known as the Great English Vowel Shift (fourteenth to seventeenth century), is no longer productive or evident in present-day English, since many words entered the lexicon *after* the shift took place and now participate in other alternations (e.g., *retain–retention* (/e:ɛ/), *genteel–gentility* (/iː:ɪ/). Jaeger (1984) reviewed a series of psycholinguistic tests carried out on adults and children in an effort to probe the psychological reality of the vowel shift rule for English speakers.

Moskowitz (1973) obtained positive results on a concept formation task used in testing children aged 9 to 12 on knowledge of the vowel shift alternations. She concluded, however, that these results were based on the children's knowledge of *spelling rules* rather than of the phonological rules underlying derived words that were still largely unfamiliar to them. Jaeger (1984) followed up on Moskowitz's suggestion with a concept formation task carefully designed to distinguish between responses based on the vowel shift alternations and responses based on spelling rules. The crucial patterns involved the pair /aw/–/ʌ/, in which the alternations are not spelled with the same letter, and /u/–/ʌ/, in which the alternations are spelled with *u* (as in *reduce–reduction*) but are not part of the vowel shift rule. Jaeger trained 15 adults to respond positively to English words reflecting the vowel shift alternations and negatively to other derivationally related word-pairs exhibiting other phonological relationships, such as tense–lax (*retain–retention*, *peace–pacify*), or the same vowel (*promise–promissory*). She then tested subjects with new word-pairs exhibiting these two types of relationships as well as pairs belonging to the two critical categories (/aw/–/ʌ/ or /u/–/ʌ/). The results were clear. Pairs containing the critical spelling-based pair /u/–/ʌ/ were generally accepted, while pairs containing the irregular vowel shift pair /aw/–/ʌ/ were generally rejected. Later interviews with the subjects further confirmed a tendency to rely on the spelling rule, as when the training category was described by one subject as "a long and a short version of the same vowel." Jaeger (1984) concluded that "certain entities can be psychologically real either because they have been brought to speakers' conscious attention as part of their education or because they have been intuited from the orthographic system of their language" (34).

Influence of Spelling on Perception and Production

Ehri (1984) reviewed the various ways in which learning to read and spell have been found to affect children's competence in the production and perception of speech. In Ehri's view, "the full representational system offered by printed language is acquired and stored in memory during acquisition" (123), including both the whole-word ("lexical") gestalt and the segmental ("phonetic") letter-sound correspondences that characterize each word. Specifically, Ehri maintains that in the course of learning to read, the "alphabetic" or "orthographic" image of a word is *added* to the store of information associated with each item in the mental lexicon. The orthographic image is integrated with other information about a word as printed words are read and understood in context. Gradually, orthographic representations come to stand for a word's meaning as well as its form and to be as intimately associated with the word as are the phonological, semantic, and syntactic aspects of its identity. (For words acquired later, through reading, the orthographic image may even be established *before* the actual oral pronunciation is known.)

Ehri's experimental investigations on the effect of orthography on perception and production have led to a number of interesting results. She found that knowledge of spelling helps children to detect and accurately segment out the sounds embedded in words. For example, through spelling children become aware of extra syllabic segments (e.g., in words like *different, comfortable, decimal*). On the other hand, knowledge of spelling may also misleadingly influence perception, as in the case of the English alveolar flap /D/ (as in *latter* or *ladder*), which children typically hear as /d/ until they learn that many words containing the flap are spelled with *t*. Surprisingly, knowledge of related words in which the flap is realized as /t/ or /d/ (*sit–sitting, ride–riding*) was not found to affect perception.

In a series of studies of older children, Templeton (1979, 1983; Templeton and Scarborough-Franks, 1985) established that knowledge of the complex phonological alternations between derivationally related English words, such as those investigated by Moskowitz and Jaeger, continues to increase at least through grade 10 and is typically acquired through *prior* learning of the more transparent orthographic relationship between these words. Templeton and Scarborough-Franks pointed out that it is easier to relate complex derived English words through spelling than through verbal production for two reasons: The derivational stem is more stable in orthography than in surface phonetics, and the processes which must be applied to relate the base and derived forms of the word are also less complex (compare the spelling and pronunciation shifts needed to relate *incline* and *inclination*, for example). These authors concluded that the subjects in their study (both "good" and "poor" spellers, in grades 6 and 10) had abstracted the orthographic patterns associated with such words by the end of elementary school, but in grade 10 they were still in the process of abstracting the patterns in pronunciation (so that they could be automatically applied to the production of novel forms, for example: see also Jaeger, 1986).

Differences in Lexical Organization

The study of malapropisms (e.g., *ornaments* or *monuments* in lieu of *condiments*), or the mistaken production of one word in lieu of another, can shed light on the organization of the mental lexicon. Aitchison and Straf (1981) analyzed 680 malapropisms, almost a third of which were produced by children (aged 12 or under). Separate analysis of the adult and child malapropisms in comparison with their target words was carried out with respect to number of syllables, stress pattern, initial and final consonant, and identity of the stressed vowel. The results for adults and children were then compared. The child malapropisms were found to be as close to the targets as those produced by adults. For both adults and children, the number of syllables, initial consonant, and stressed vowel all were likely to match the target. Where all three were not retained, adults were most likely to produce the same initial consonant (e.g., *Acapulco* in place of *acupuncture*: 77 percent), whereas children were more likely to retain the number of syllables (e.g., *naughty story* in place of *multistory* [carpark]: 84 percent, vs. 68 percent for adults) and least likely to retain the initial consonant (57 percent). Stress pattern largely correlated with number of syllables for both adults and children. Although final consonants were retained more or less equally often by adults (e.g., *jungle* for *conjugal*: 72 percent) and children (e.g., *faint* for *fête*: 68 percent), the initial consonant was more often retained than the final consonant in the adult data; children retained the final consonant (marginally) more often than the initial consonant. In longer words, the final consonant was especially likely to be preserved by both children and adults, perhaps because of the derivational suffixes in which target and malapropism often matched (especially in the adult data where about 50 percent of the malapropisms included a suffix: Recall the errors for *condiments*).

Aitchison and Straf (1981) suggested five interacting factors to account for the differences between adult and child lexical retrieval and storage:

1. Children may pay more attention to perceptually salient aspects of words, such as rhythm (i.e., *giggle* for *wriggle*, *fascination* for *vaccination*).
2. Children appear to pay more attention to word endings (cf. Slobin, 1973) and, perhaps consequently, less attention to initial consonants.
3. Consonant harmony, a preference for open syllables, and a tendency to alter unstressed syllables appear to affect older children's memory for unfamiliar words, just as they affect word production in younger children and perhaps for the same reasons (cf. Aitchison and Chiat, 1981, who implicate "faulty perception," or incomplete representation, together with memory overload to account for the role of phonological processes in both younger and older children).
4. Literacy and experience with dictionaries may enhance the importance of initial consonants for adults.
5. Growth in importance of word beginnings may accompany growth in vocabulary since the high frequency of derivational affixes in more sophisticated English vocabulary renders attention to word endings relatively inefficient as a way of differentiating between words.

In summary, the analysis of adult and child malapropisms reveals some of the salient features that must characterize words in the mental lexicon since these features influence word retrieval. Rhythmic structure and word endings are salient from early childhood (cf. Vihman, 1981); with schooling, experience with dictionary and library work, and the growth of a more abstract, derived lexicon, the importance of the initial consonant increases. An experimental study of ninety 5- to 9-year-olds showed that, at those ages, the consonants of the stressed syllable were still more likely to be recalled than the initial consonant (Aitchison and Chiat, 1981). It is not clear at what age the shift to a preferential reliance on initial consonants begins to affect lexical retrieval.

Influence from the Peer Group

In the introduction to Chapter 2 we mentioned that by the time children are speaking clearly enough to be understood outside the family, their speech patterns will have been stamped with the phonetically distinguishing features of the language of their home community. Yet phonetic and phonological development do not come to an end at this point. An extensive sociolinguistic study by Payne (1975, 1980) demonstrated the influence of the peer group on both the phonetic and the phonological levels after the period of early childhood.

In order to investigate ongoing linguistic change, Payne designed a study to observe the speech patterns of a large number of children who had moved from one dialect area to another. By noting the age at which the children moved to the new community as well as their length of stay there, she was able to roughly distinguish between parental and peer influence.

Payne carried out her investigation in King of Prussia, a small middle-class community on the outskirts of Philadelphia that had become a thriving industrial center attracting a large number of recent arrivals. She interviewed some 200 families, making contact through children playing on the block and through church leaders, and finally, extended her investigation to the school where some 50 groups of children were interviewed, including 10 of the children originally approached in the family context. Payne (1975) presented in detail the acquisition of the Philadelphia dialect by one family of four children that had moved to the area from New York five years earlier; the children were aged 8, 10, 11, and 13 at the time of the study.

Payne concentrated her analysis on seven specific vowel patterns that characterize the "stable, central core" of the Philadelphia dialect. These patterns include three phonological differences from other dialects of English (splitting or merger of classes of phonemically distinct vowels; for example, the stressed vowels of *merry–Murray* and *ferry–furry* are merged) and four phonetic differences, in which the phonemic structure is not affected (e.g., the nucleus of /oy/ is raised to [u]).

Payne found that the phonetic variables had all been acquired by all of the children, whereas the phonological variables were only incompletely acquired. Furthermore, she found a correlation for the three older children between degree of acquisition of the Philadelphia dialect and number of years spent under the influence of the King of Prussia peer group. The youngest child, Mike, aged 3 on arrival in the new area, showed about the same degree of influence as the oldest child, Richard (aged 8 on arrival). Liz (aged 6 on arrival) showed more influence and Dan (aged 5 on arrival) showed full acquisition of the phonological and phonetic variables. Payne explained this pattern of dialect change in terms of the proportion of a child's peer-influence years (from about 4 to 14) spent in the new dialect area (see Figure 3.1). Liz and Dan had spent a larger proportion of their peer-influence years in King of Prussia than had Richard, and they showed it by sounding more like Philadelphians; Mike was presumably too young to be influenced by peers for two of the five years he had spent in the area at the time of the study.

Although Payne (1975) reported results for only a single family, she noted that observation of the community as a whole supports the generality and consistency of the pattern of findings reported. Payne's study suggests that the dialect a child learns from his or her parents can change almost completely in later years under the influence of peers (but see Deser, 1991).

Summary

Phonetic and phonological variation and change continue at least into the school-age years. Difficulties with the precise timing of sequential articulatory gestures continue to be smoothed out over a period of several years. The learning of a written language supplies a visual-spatial model for speech that is internalized as a representational system in memory

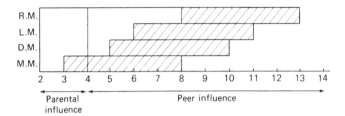

FIGURE 3.1   Peer group influence. Number of years the Morgan children have spent under King of Prussia peer-group influence versus New York City and parental influence.
Source: From A. Payne, "The Reorganization of Linguistic Rules: A Preliminary Report." *Pennsylvania Working Papers on Linguistic Change and Variation*, 2, 1975. Used with permission.

(Ehri, 1984). Once children begin learning to read and spell, they acquire an important added dimension of language that subtly affects many aspects of language processing and use. Lexical organization, as revealed by lexical selection errors, is also influenced by literacy skills and by the growth, associated with advancing education, of the derived-word vocabulary. Finally, language in the school-age years comes under strong peer influence. Where parental and peer dialects differ in this period the peer norm is likely to triumph.

QUESTIONS FOR CHAPTER 3

1. Review the large scale normative data and identify early, mid, and late developing sounds.

2. Differentiate customary production and sound mastery. How is each of these a useful concept?

3. Describe young children's use of phonological processes. What are phonological processes? How is the concept used clinically?

4. How are children similar and different in phonological acquisition?

5. What is the influence of literacy on phonological development in school-age children?

REFERENCES

Aitchison, J., and S. Chiat, "Natural phonology or natural memory? The interaction between phonological processes and recall mechanisms." *Language and Speech*, 24 (1981): 311–326.

Aitchison, J., and M. Straf, "Lexical storage and retrieval: A developing skill?" In A. Cutler (Ed.), *Slips of the Tongue and Language Production*. Amsterdam: Mouton, 1981.

Arlt, P. B., and M. J. Goodban, "A comparative study of articulation acquisition as based on a study of 240 normals, aged three to six." *Language, Speech, and Hearing Services in Schools*, 7 (1976): 173–180.

Baddeley, A., *Working Memory*. Oxford: Clarendon Press, 1986.

Baddeley, A. D., N. Thomson, and M. Buchanan, "Word length and the structure of short-term memory." *Journal of Verbal Learning and Verbal Behavior*, 14 (1975): 575–589.

Barton, D., "The role of perception in the acquisition of phonology." Ph.D. thesis, University of London, 1976.

(Reprinted by the Indiana University Linguistics Club, 1978).

Berg, T., "Sound change in child language: A study of inter-word variation." *Language and Speech, 38* (1995): 331–363.

Berman, R. A., "Natural phonological processes at the one-word stage." *Lingua, 43* (1977): 1–21.

Bernthal, J. E., M. Greenlee, R. Eblen, and K. Marking, "Detection of mispronunciations: A comparison of adults, normal speaking children and children with articulation errors." *Applied Psycholinguistics, 8* (1987): 209–222.

Braine, M. D. S., "Review of N. V. Smith, The Acquisition of Phonology: A Case Study." *Language, 52* (1976): 489–498.

Bricker, W. A., "Errors in the echoic behavior of preschool children." *Journal of Speech and Hearing Research, 10* (1967): 67–76.

Chomsky, N., and M. Hallé, *The Sound Pattern of English.* New York: Harper & Row, 1968.

Clumeck, H., "The effects of word-familiarity on phonemic recognition in children aged 3 to 5 years." In C. E. Johnson and C. L. Thew (Eds.), *Proceedings of the Second International Congress for the Study of Child Language,* Vol. 1. Lanham, Md.: University Press of America, 1982.

Cole, R. A., "Perception of fluent speech by children and adults." In H.B. Winitz (Ed.), *Native Language and Foreign Language Acquisition.* New York: New York Academy of Sciences, 1981.

Cole, R. A., and J. Jakimik, "A model of speech perception." In R. A. Cole (Ed.), *Perception and Production of Fluent Speech.* Hillsdale, N. J.: Lawrence Erlbaum, 1980.

Cole, R. A., and C. A. Perfetti, "Listening for mispronunciations in a children's story: The use of context by children and adults." *Journal of Verbal Learning and Verbal Behavior, 19* (1980): 297–315.

Deser, T., "Dialect transmission and variation: An acoustic analysis of vowels in six urban Detroit families." Ph.D. thesis, Boston University, 1990. (Reprinted by the Indiana University Linguistics Club, 1991).

Edwards, M. L., "Patterns and processes in fricative acquisition: Longitudinal evidence from six English-learning children." Ph.D. thesis, Stanford University, 1979.

Ehri, L. C., "How orthography alters spoken language competencies in children learning to read and spell." In J. Downing and R. Valtin (Eds.), *Language Awareness and Learning to Read.* New York: Springer-Verlag, 1984.

Elliott, L. L., "Performance of children aged 9–17 years on a test of speech intelligibility in noise using sentence material with controlled word predictability." *Journal of the Acoustic Society of America, 66* (1979): 651–653.

Elliott, L. L., M. A. Hammer, and K. E. Evan, "Perception of gated, highly familiar spoken monosyllabic nouns by children, teenagers, and older adults." *Perception and Psychophysics, 42* (1987): 150–157.

Elman, J., and J. L. McClelland, "The TRACE model of speech perception." In D. E. Rumelhart, J. L. McClelland, and the PDP Research Group (Eds.), *Parallel Distributed Processing: Explorations in the Microstructure of Cognition.* Cambridge, Mass.: MIT Press, 1986.

Fee, J., and D. Ingram, "Reduplication as a strategy of phonological development." *Journal of Child Language, 9* (1982): 41–54.

Ferguson, C. A., "Language development." In J. A. Fishman, J. Das Gupta, and C. A. Ferguson (Eds.), *Language Problems of Developing Nations.* New York: John Wiley, 1968.

Ferguson, C. A., "Fricatives in child language acquisition." In L. Hellman (Ed.), *Proceedings of the Eleventh International Congress of Linguists.* Bologna: Mulino, 1975. (Also in V. Honsa and M. H. Hardman-Bautista (Eds.), *Papers on Linguistics and Child Language.* The Hague: Mouton, 1978.)

Ferguson, C. A., "Reduplication in child phonology." *Journal of Child Language, 10* (1983): 239–243.

Ferguson, C. A., and M. A. Macken, "The role of play in phonological development." In K. E. Nelson (Ed.), *Children's Language,* Vol. 4. Hillsdale, N.J.: Lawrence Erlbaum, 1983.

Gilbert, J. H. V., and B. A. Purves, "Temporal constraints on consonant clusters in child speech production." *Journal of Child Language, 4* (1977): 417–432.

Greenlee, M., "Interacting processes in the child's acquisition of stop-liquid clusters." *Papers and Reports on Child Language Development, 7* (1974): 85–100.

Grunwell, P., "The development of phonology." *First Language, 2* (1981): 161–191.

Haelsig, P. C., and C. L. Madison, "A study of phonological processes exhibited by 3-, 4-, and 5-year-old children." *Language, Speech, and Hearing Services in Schools, 17* (1986): 107–114.

Hawkins, S., "Temporal coordination of consonants in the speech of children: Preliminary data." *Journal of Phonetics, 1* (1973): 181–217.

Hulme, C., N. Thomson, C. Muir, and A. Lawrence, "Speech rate and the development of short-term memory span." *Journal of Experimental Child Psychology, 38* (1984): 241–253.

Ingram, D., "Phonological rules in young children." *Journal of Child Language, 1* (1974): 49–64.

Ingram, D., "Phonological development: Production." In P. Fletcher and M. Garman (Eds.), *Language Acquisition: Studies in First Language Development* 2nd ed. Cambridge (UK): The University Press, 1986.

Ingram, D., L. Christensen, S. Veach, and B. Webster, "The acquisition of word-initial fricatives and affricatives in English by children between 2 and 6 years." In G. Yeni-Komshian, J. Kavanagh, and C. A. Ferguson (Eds.), *Child Phonology*, Vol. 1, *Production*. New York: Academic Press, 1980.

Jakobson, R., *Child Language, Aphasia and Phonological Universals*, A. R. Keiler (Tr.). The Hague: Mouton, 1968. [Original title Kindersprache, Aphasie und Allgemeine Lautgesetze. Uppsala: Almqvist and Wiksell, 1941.]

Jaeger, J. J., "Assessing the psychological status of the vowel shift rule." *Journal of Psycholinguistic Research, 13* (1984): 13–36.

Jaeger, J. J., "On the acquisition of abstract representations for English vowels." *Phonology Yearbook, 3* (1986): 71–97.

Kamhi, A. G., H. W. Catts, and M. K. Davis, "Management of sentence production demands." *Journal of Speech and Hearing Research, 27* (1984): 329–338.

Kehoe, J., and C. Stoel-Gammon, "Development of syllable structure in English-speaking children with particular reference to rhymes." *Journal of Child Language, 28* (2001): 393–432.

Klein, H., "Productive strategies for the pronunciation of early polysyllabic lexical items." *Journal of Speech and Hearing Research, 24* (1981): 389–405.

Klein, H., "Relationship between early pronunciation processes and later pronunciation skill." *Journal of Speech and Hearing Disorders, 50* (1985): 156–165.

Leopold, W. F., *Speech Development of a Bilingual Child*, Vol. 2. *Sound-Learning in the First Two Years*. Evanston, Ill.: Northwestern University Press, 1947.

Lleó, C., "Homonymy and reduplication: On the extended availability of two strategies in phonological acquisition." *Journal of Child Language, 17* (1990): 267–278.

Locke, J. L., *Phonological Acquisition and Change*. New York: Academic Press, 1983.

Macken, M. A., "Permitted complexity in phonological development: One child's acquisition of Spanish consonants." *Lingua, 44* (1978): 219–253.

Macken, M. A., "Developmental reorganization of phonology: A hierarchy of basic units of acquisition." *Lingua, 49* (1979): 11–49.

Macken, M. A., and C. A. Ferguson, "Phonological universals of language acquisition." In H. B. Winitz (Ed.), *Native Language and Foreign Language Acquisition*. New York: New York Academy of Sciences, 1981.

Magnusson, E., *The Phonology of Language Disordered Children: Production, Perception, and Awareness*. Travaux de l'Institut de Linguistique de Lund, 17. Lund: CWK Gleerup, 1983.

Marslen-Wilson, W. D., "Functional parallelism in spoken word-recognition." In U. H. Frauenfelder and L. K. Tyler (Eds.), *Spoken Word Recognition*. Amsterdam: Elsevier-Science Publishers, 1987.

Menn, L., "Phonotactic rules in beginning speech." *Lingua, 26* (1971): 225–251.

Menyuk, P., "Clusters as single underlying consonants: Evidence from children's production." *Proceedings of the Seventh International Congress of Phonetic Science, Montreal, 1971*. The Hague: Mouton, 1972.

Moskowitz, A. I., "The acquisition of phonology and syntax: A preliminary study." In K. J. J. Hintikka, J. M. E. Moravcsik, and P. Suppes (Eds.), *Approaches to Natural Language*. Dordrecht: Reidel, 1973.

Moskowitz, A. I., "The acquisition of fricatives: A study in phonetics and phonology." *Journal of Phonetics, 3* (1975): 141–150.

Nettelbladt, U., *Development Studies of Dysphonology in Children*. Travaux de l'Institut de Linguistique de Lund, 19. Lund: CWK Gleerup, 1983.

Ohala, J. J., "Aspects of the control and production of speech." *U.C.L.A. Working Papers in Phonetics, 15* (1970).

Oller, D. K., "Simplification as the goal of phonological processes in child speech." *Language Learning, 24* (1975): 299–303.

Olmsted, D., *Out of the Mouth of Babes*. The Hague: Mouton, 1971.

Payne, A., "The reorganization of linguistic rules: A preliminary report." *Pennsylvania Working Papers on Linguistic Change and Variation, 2* (1975).

Payne, A. C., "Factors controlling the acquisition of the Philadelphia dialect by out-of-state children." In W. Labov (Ed.), *Locating Language in Time and Space*. New York: Academic Press, 1980.

Pendergast, K., S. Dickey, J. Selmar, and A. L. Soder, *Photo Articulation Test*. Danville, Ill.: Interstate, 1969.

Prather, E., D. Hedrick, and C. Kern, "Articulation development in children aged two to four years." *Journal of Speech and Hearing Disorders, 40* (1975): 179–191.

Preisser, D. A., B. W. Hodson, and E. P. Paden, "Developmental phonology: 18–29 months." *Journal of Speech and Hearing Disorders, 53* (1988): 125–130.

Roberts, J. E., M. Burchinal, and M. M. Footo, "Phonological process decline from $2\frac{1}{2}$ to 8 years." *Journal of Communication Disorders, 23* (1990): 205–217.

Sander, E., "When are speech sounds learned?" *Journal of Speech and Hearing Disorders, 37* (1972): 55–63.

Savinainen-Makkonen, T., "Learning long words—a typological perspective." *Language and Speech, 43* (2000): 205–225.

Schmitt, L. S., B. H. Howard, and J. F. Schmitt, "Conversational speech sampling in the assessment of articulatory proficiency." *Language, Speech, and Hearing Services in Schools, 14* (1983): 210–222.

Schwartz, R., and L. B. Leonard, "Some further comments on reduplication in child phonology." *Journal of Child Language, 10* (1983): 441–448.

Schwartz, R., L. B. Leonard, M. J. Wilcox, and K. Folger, "Again and again: Reduplication in child phonology." *Journal of Child Language, 7* (1980): 75–88.

Shriberg, L., and J. Kwiatkowski, "Phonological disorders III: A procedure for assessing severity of involvement." *Journal of Speech and Hearing Disorders, 47* (1982): 256–270.

Slobin, D. I., "Cognitive prerequisites for the development of grammar." In C. A. Ferguson and D. I. Slobin (Eds.), *Studies of Child Language Development.* New York: Holt, Rinehart & Winston, 1973.

Smit, A. B., "Ages of speech sound acquisition: Comparisons of several normative studies." *Language, Speech, and Hearing Services in Schools, 17* (1986): 175–186.

Smit, A. B., L. Hand, J. J. Freilinger, J. E. Bernthal, and A. Bird, "The Iowa articulation norms project and its Nebraska replication." *Journal of Speech and Hearing Disorders, 55* (1990): 779–798.

Smith, B. L., "Temporal aspects of English speech production: A developmental perspective." *Journal of Phonetics, 6* (1978): 37–67.

Smith, N. V., *The Acquisition of Phonology: A Case Study.* Cambridge (UK): Cambridge University Press, 1973.

Snow, K., "A detailed analysis of articulation responses of 'normal' first grade children." *Journal of Speech and Hearing Research, 6* (1963): 277–290.

Stoel-Gammon, C., "Phonetic inventories, 15–24 months: A longitudinal study." *Journal of Speech and Hearing Research, 28* (1985): 505–512.

Stoel-Gammon, C., "The phonological skills of two-year-olds." *Language, Speech, and Hearing Services in Schools, 18* (1987): 323–329.

Stoel-Gammon, C., and C. Dunn, *Normal and Disordered Phonology in Children.* Baltimore: University Park Press, 1985.

Stoel-Gammon, C., and J. P. Stemberger, "Consonant harmony and phonological underspecification in child speech." In M. Yavas (Ed.), *First and Second Language Phonology.* San Diego: Singular Publishing Group, 1994.

Templeton, S., "Spelling first, sound later: The relationship between orthography and higher order phonological knowledge in older students." *Research in the Teaching of English, 13* (1979): 255–264.

Templeton, S., "The spelling-meaning connection and the development of word knowledge in older students." *Journal of Reading, 27* (1983): 8–14.

Templeton, S., and L. Scarborough-Franks, "The spelling's the thing: Knowledge of derivational morphology in orthography and phonology among older students." *Applied Psycholinguistics, 6* (1985): 371–390.

Templin, M. C., *Certain Language Skills in Children.* Minneapolis: University of Minnesota Press, 1957.

Tyler, L. K., and U. H. Frauenfelder, "The process of spoken word recognition: An introduction." In U. H. Frauenfelder and L. K. Tyler (Eds.), *Spoken Word Recognition.* Amsterdam: Elsevier-Science Publishers, 1987.

Tyler, L. K., and W. D. Marslen-Wilson, "Children's processing of spoken language." *Journal of Verbal Learning and Verbal Behavior, 20* (1981): 400–416.

Vihman, M. M., "From pre-speech to speech: On early phonology." *Papers and Reports on Child Language Development, 3* (1976): 51–94.

Vihman, M. M., "Consonant harmony: Its scope and function in child language." In J. H. Greenberg (Ed.), *Universals of Human Language*, Vol. 2. *Phonology.* Stanford, Calif.: Stanford University Press, 1978.

Vihman, M. M. "Sound change and child language." In E. C. Traugott, R. Labrum, and S. Shepherd (Eds.), *Papers from the Fourth International Conference on Historical Linguistics.* Amsterdam: John Benjamins B.V., 1980.

Vihman, M. M., "Phonology and the development of the lexicon: Evidence from children's errors." *Journal of Child Language, 8* (1981): 239–264.

Vihman, M. M., C. A. Ferguson, and M. Elbert, "Phonological development from babbling to speech: Common tendencies and individual differences." *Applied Psycholinguistics, 7* (1986): 3–40.

Vihman, M. M., and M. Greenlee, "Individual differences in phonological development: Ages one and three years." *Journal of Speech and Hearing Research, 30* (1987): 503–521.

Vihman, M. M., and S. L. Velleman, "Phonetics and the origins of phonology." In N. Burton-Roberts, P. Carr, and G. Docherty (Eds.), *Phonological Knowledge: Its Nature and Status* (pp. 305–339). Oxford: Oxford University Press, 2000.

Walley, A. C., "Developmental differences in spoken word identification." Ph.D. thesis, Indiana University, 1984.

Walley, A. C., and J. L. Metsala, "The growth of lexical constraints on spoken word recognition." *Perception and Psychophysics, 47* (1990): 267–280.

Wellman, B. L., I. M. Case, E. G. Mengert, and D. E. Bradbury, *Speech Sounds of Young Children.* University of Iowa Studies in Child Welfare, 5. Iowa City: University of Iowa Press, 1931.

4

Etiology/Factors Related To Phonologic Disorders

NICHOLAS W. BANKSON
James Madison University

JOHN E. BERNTHAL
University of Nebraska-Lincoln

Introduction

In the study of phonologic disorders, an abiding concern is the identification of variables that may relate to the presence of speech sound disorders. Various factors, including (1) speech/hearing mechanism, (2) cognitive linguistic, and (3) psychosocial, as they relate to speech sound production have been studied. Investigators continue to be interested in the influence that physiological, cognitive, and environmental factors may have on phonologic development and phonologic disorders. Since clients, family, and clinicians are all interested in etiological variables that might be related to phonologic disorders, it is important that a book on phonologic disorders include a discussion of current understandings of causality and correlational factors related to the presence of phonologic impairment.

As discussed in later sections of this chapter, certain **causal factors** may precipitate, accompany, and/or maintain the presence of phonologic/articulatory disorders. In general, the most established causal factors are related to impairments and/or interference with the structure and function of the speech and hearing mechanism. Since the percentage of clients in whom causal factors can be easily identified is relatively small, researchers have been interested in variables, called **causal correlates**, that may coexist with phonologic impairments. From 1930 to around 1970 an extensive body of literature related to causal correlates was developed. An interest in etiological research again emerged in the late 1980s that focused on familial history in individuals with phonologic disorders, as well as the impact of otitis media on phonological disorders. A knowledge of related factors is helpful in our understanding of phonologic impairments.

Correlational studies have been a primary method used to explore whether phonologic proficiency and selected variables covary or coexist within individuals. Stated more simply, such studies seek to determine whether one variable (such as status of articulation) is related to another variable (such as intelligence). A *high* correlation between two variables implies that such variables are related to each other. For example, a high correlation between a measure of intelligence and the acquisition of speech sounds would indicate that a high number of correct articulatory responses co-occur with a high score on a measure of intelligence, and a low number of correct articulatory responses co-occur with a low score on a measure of intelligence. A *low* correlation, on the other hand, would indicate that the score obtained on an articulatory measure and the score on an intelligence measure do not covary and are not systematically related to each other. When a correlation is high, the status of one variable can sometimes be predicted from knowledge of the status of the second variable. This does not mean, however, that a causal relationship exists between the two; it simply means that they are related to each other. The frequently cited warning, "Correlation does not imply causation," speaks to precisely this issue. Correlational studies are useful for purposes of identifying topics worthy of further study, as selected factors may precipitate, accompany, or maintain phonologic performance.

In correlational studies, investigators typically have looked at a single variable (for example, speech sound discrimination) as it relates to articulatory status. Several investigators have used **multivariate analysis** techniques to look at the relationship between articulation status and several variables simultaneously within individuals. Winitz (1969) suggested it is "quite possible that substantial relationships between articulation and other independent variables would be forthcoming if the independent variables were examined collectively rather than singularly" (216).

A procedure used to examine factors potentially related to phonologic impairment involves comparisons between normal children and children who are phonologically delayed on a variable of interest, for example, reading performance. When reviewing studies of this type, several points should be kept in mind. First, a statistically significant difference between a group of normal persons and a group of phonologically impaired persons on a particular variable (for example, language comprehension) does not imply a causal relationship between that variable and phonology. Other variables may account for the differences found between the phonologically impaired and normal-speaking groups. For example, if children with phonological disorders were found to have poorer reading skills than a normal control group, differences in reading performance may be related to something other than poor articulation (e.g., phonological awareness). Such studies, however, may point to areas that are worthy of further exploration in terms of how they relate to phonological performance. Second, statistical significance does not imply clinical/practical significance for two reasons: (1) group trends frequently do not reflect individual performance, and (2) relatively small quantitative differences resulting in statistically significant differences may have limited clinical utility. In a study reported by Dubois and Bernthal (1978), a small but statistically significant difference was found between two types of articulation measures (spontaneous picture naming and a delayed imitation sentence production), and yet the numerical difference in average performance, based on a 20-item task, was less than 2 items. Because of the small numerical difference, the clinical or practical significance of such group findings might be questioned.

A fourth procedure used to examine causal-correlates is to present descriptive profiles of children who evidence developmental phonologic disorders and trace their history in therapy. A comprehensive investigation of speech-language prosody and voice characteristics of children with developmental phonologic disorders was reported by Shriberg and Kwiatkowski (1994). None of the factors studied were good predictors for short- or long-term normalization of phonology. Williams and McReynolds (1975) reported that improvement in articulation covaried with improved performance in speech sound discrimination. Correlational studies demonstrating that improvement in one or more variables results in improvement in articulation may have potential for predicting clinical outcomes.

Winitz (1969) has suggested that some variables that have been studied in relation to articulation disorders may best be viewed as **macrovariables** (variables formed from several other variables). The variable of age, for example, may be comprised of such components as physical maturation, motor coordination, cognition, and linguistic maturity. As Winitz pointed out, although a macrovariable may be found to correlate with articulation, the individual components accounting for the correlation may be difficult to identify.

At the present time, most of the identified causal factors are in the area of structure and function of the speech and hearing mechanism. Other factors that have been studied offer potential for variables worthy of further study as they relate not only to the presence of a phonological disorder, but may also have implications for predicting treatment outcomes and/or impacting the nature of instruction. Such treatment may be a critical part of the speech remediation plan. In the next section of this chapter, defects in structure and function of the speech and hearing mechanism that might interfere with the individual's phonologic productions are reviewed, including hearing loss, structural anomalies, and neuromotor pathologies. After this we will discuss cognitive-linguistic factors associated with phonological impairments, and in the final section we will discuss psychosocial factors.

Structure and Function of the Speech and Hearing Mechanisms

An obvious consideration when evaluating an individual's phonologic status relates to the potential for problems that may be manifested in the structure and function of the speech and hearing mechanisms. Medically related interventions, for example, surgical management for a cleft palate, are often a critical part of helping a client achieve maximal phonologic proficiency.

Hearing Loss

Among the variables influencing articulation, perhaps none is as important as the ability to hear. Lundeen (1991) reported that the prevalence of school-age children with pure tone averages greater than 25 dB HL was 2.63 percent. Through hearing, an individual is able to receive incoming messages as a listener and monitor his or her own productions as a speaker.

One of the most important elements underlying the production and comprehension of speech is an intact auditory system that is sensitive to the frequency range where most speech sounds occur (500 to 4000 Hz). Individuals with more severe hearing loss will have difficulty decoding the incoming sound signal and will perceive words differently than individuals with normal hearing mechanisms.

The child who is hard of hearing or deaf faces the challenging task of learning how to produce speech by watching how sounds look on the face, how they feel through vibrations, and what he or she can perceive from a distorted auditory signal. A certain level of hearing is required to learn and maintain normal speech production. Ling (1989) summarized this relationship by noting that the more normal a person's hearing, the more natural his or her speech is likely to be.

Several aspects of hearing loss have been shown to affect speech perception and production; these include the level of hearing sensitivity, speech recognition ability, and configuration of the hearing loss. Individual hearing losses range from mild to severe or profound (greater than 70 dB HL). Labels such as *hard of hearing* and *deaf* are frequently applied to persons with varying degrees of hearing impairment.

Hearing sensitivity typically varies somewhat from one frequency to another, with speech and language differentially influenced by the frequency configuration and severity of the hearing loss. Although information recorded on an audiogram is a useful prognostic indicator of speech reception ability, predictions based on pure-tone measurements are not always accurate. Two children with similar audiograms may not perceive speech sounds in the same way. A pure-tone audiogram cannot measure a person's ability to distinguish one frequency from another or to track formant transitions (a skill critical to speech perception). For these and other reasons (e.g., age of fitting and full-time use of amplification, concomitant factors, quality of early intervention programs), individuals with similar pure-tone audiograms can differ greatly in their understanding of speech.

A second hearing-related factor important to phonologic acquisition and maintenance is the age of onset and the age of detection of the hearing loss. If a severe loss has been present since birth, even in children with cochlear implants, acquisition of language including phonology, syntax, and semantics is difficult, and specialized instruction is necessary to develop speech and language. Such instruction may rely on visual, tactile, and kinesthetic cues, and signing as well as whatever residual auditory sensation the person possesses or has been afforded via technology. For a discussion of the influence of hearing loss on infants and toddlers phonologic development, see Stoel-Gammon and Kehoe (1994). Children and adults who suffer a serious loss of hearing after language has been acquired usually retain their articulation patterns for a time, but frequently their articulatory skills deteriorate. Even those assisted with amplification may find it difficult to maintain their previous level of articulatory performance.

Influence on Speech

Investigators have explored the influence of hearing loss on speech sound productions. Levitt and Stromberg (1983) observed the following vowel characteristics in individuals with hearing loss: (1) a number of vowel substitutions (e.g., tense-lax substitutions [i for ɪ], substitution of the intended vowel by a neighboring vowel in the vowel quadrilateral); (2) substitution of diphthongs for vowels (diphthongization) and vowels for diphthongs; (3) some omissions of the intended vowel or diphthong; and (4) schwa or schwa-like vowel substitutions (neutralization). Tye-Murray (1991) reported that some deaf speakers used excessive jaw movement to establish different vowel shapes instead of appropriate tongue movement. The less flexible tongue movement reduces the formation of the acoustic vowel formants (particularly the second formant) necessary to discriminate vowels.

There seems to be general agreement that consonant errors reflect difficulties with voiced-voiceless distinction, substitutions (voice-voiceless, nasal-oral, fricative-stop) omission of initial and final consonants, distortions, inappropriate nasalization of consonants, and final consonant deletions (Paterson, 1994).

In addition to segmental difficulties, the suprasegmental patterns of persons who are deaf or persons with moderate to severe hearing loss differ from those seen in normal-hearing speakers. Such speakers generally speak at a slower rate than normal-hearing speakers because of longer duration of both consonants and vowels, and they also use more frequent pauses and slower articulatory transitions. Stress patterns may also differ from those of normal-hearing speakers as many persons who are deaf or hearing impaired do not distinguish duration associated with stressed and unstressed syllables. Finally, persons who are deaf or hearing impaired sometimes use too high or too low a pitch, use nonstandard inflectional patterns, use harsh or breathy voice quality, and are hypo- or hypernasal (Dunn and Newton, 1986).

There is a great deal of variation in the speech patterns of individuals with hearing impairments. There is still no definitive description of the speech and language of persons who are hearing impaired because of the complexity involved in analyzing their speech. Less information is available for individuals with mild to moderate hearing losses than for those with more severe losses.

Calvert (1982) reported that errors of articulation common to deaf children are not confined to productions of individual phonemes; errors also occur because of the phonetic context in which the phones are embedded. Calvert delineated the following common errors of articulation in the speech of persons who are deaf (defined as those with hearing threshold levels for speech of greater than 92 dB) for whom everyday auditory communication is impossible or nearly so.

1. Errors of Omission
   a. Omission of final consonants
   b. Omission of /s/ in all contexts
   c. Omission of initial consonants
2. Errors of Substitution
   a. Voiced for voiceless consonants
   b. Nasal for oral consonants
   c. Low feedback substitutions (substitution of sounds with easily perceived tactile and kinesthetic feedback for those with less; for example, /w/ for /r/ substitution)
   d. Substitution of one vowel for another
3. Errors of Distortion
   a. Degree of force (stop and fricative consonants are frequently made with either too much or too little force)
   b. Hypernasality associated with vowel productions
   c. Imprecision and indefiniteness in vowel articulation
   d. Duration of vowels (deaf speakers tend to produce vowels with undifferentiated duration, usually in the direction of excess duration)

      e. Temporal values in diphthongs (deaf speakers may not produce the first or the second vowel in a diphthong for the appropriate duration of time)

   4. Errors of Addition

      a. Insertion of a superfluous vowel between consonants (e.g., /sʌnoʊ/ for /snoʊ/)

      b. Unnecessary release of final stop consonants (e.g., [stopʰ])

      c. Diphthongization of vowels (e.g., *mit* → [mɪʌt])

      d. Superfluous breath before vowels

Calvert further reported that in those who become deaf after acquiring speech and language, distortions and omissions occur for speech sounds characterized by low intensity and high frequency, such as /s/, /ʃ/, /tʃ/, /f/, and /θ/. In addition, such individuals may produce consonants in the final position of words with so little force that they are not heard by the listener.

There is no one-to-one correspondence between level and type of hearing loss and patterns of misarticulations. In general, however, the less severe the loss, the less speech and language are affected. Since consonants, especially those with high-frequency energy (e.g., sibilants), have less inherent intensity in their production than vowels, consonants tend to be most frequently misarticulated.

Even relatively mild fluctuating hearing losses seen in children with recurrent middle-ear problems may affect those children's speech and language acquisition. Investigators have reported that children who are experiencing otitis media with effusion usually score more poorly on articulation tests than those free of this condition. Researchers have reported that a delay in speech and language development at 3 years and older often follows otitis media, with effusion and its accompanying fluctuating hearing loss. It has been reported that many children seen for phonologic and articulation deficiencies have a history of middle-ear involvement, and children with a history of middle-ear involvement can be differentiated from those without such a history by the phonologic patterns in their speech (Shriberg and Smith, 1983; Shriberg and Kwiatkowski, 1982). Shriberg and Kwiatkowski (1982) reported that up to one third of the children with moderate to severe phonologic delays may have histories of middle-ear involvement. For a complete review of the literature on the relationship of otitis media to speech perception and phonology, see Roberts and Clarke-Klein (1994).

Shriberg and Smith (1983) reported that children with positive histories of middle-ear involvement made sound changes (errors) in nasals and word-initial consonants more frequently than phonologically delayed children without such histories. Initial consonants were deleted (e.g., *got* → [ot]), or replaced by [h] (e.g., *tie* → [haɪ]) or glottal stop replacements (e.g., *to* → [ʔu]). The other changes noted were that nasal sounds were (1) replaced by another nasal or stop (e.g., *not* → [ma] or *my* → [baɪ]; (2) replaced by denasalization (e.g., *knee* → [ni:]); or (3) preceded or followed by an epenthetic stop (e.g., *no* → [ᵈnoʊ]). Shriberg and Smith (1983) suggested that it may be possible to differentiate children who have a positive history of middle-ear involvement from those who do not on the basis of the phonologic patterns in their speech. Churchill, Hodson, Jones, and Novak (1985) reported that deletion of the stridency feature was the distinguishing characteristic of children with middle-ear involvement.

Paden, Novak, and Beiter (1987) attempted to identify differences between children with frequent or persistent middle-ear problems who later required phonologic intervention from those who did not. They reported no distinguishing phonological patterns in their subjects with a history of middle-ear involvement. They concluded that children with similar hearing thresholds and length of time the middle-ear involvement persisted differed widely in their mastery of phonological skills. They also suggested that guidelines based on a number of variables—for example, the percentage of deviancy from age norms on velars, deletions of postvocalic obstruents, liquid durations, age of initial diagnosis of middle-ear problems, length of time the middle-ear problem persisted, and severity of the hearing impairment—could be developed to aid in the identification of 18- to 36-month-old children with a history of middle-ear involvement who are at risk phonologically. In a subsequent study, Paden, Matthies, and Novak (1989) attempted to identify which young children, 19 to 35 months, who were delayed in phonologic development and had otitis media with effusion were at risk for continued phonologic delay even when pressure equalization tubes were inserted. They reported that of the original group they studied, 24 percent, even with aggressive medical treatment, did not attain normal phonologic development by age 4. It can be inferred from this finding that with aggressive medical treatment most children who are prone to have middle-ear problems will catch up with their peers without intervention but about 25 percent will not. A statistical procedure called *discriminant analysis* indicated that the best predictors between children who would likely achieve normal phonology by age 4 and those who would not were four variables:

1. Presence of velar deviations
2. Presence of cluster reduction
3. Lack of improvement on an articulation retest four months following insertion of tubes
4. A time period of six months or more between initial diagnosis of otitis media and the first significant remission of this condition

Roberts, Burchinal, Koch, Footo, and Henderson (1988) studied 55 children in a longitudinal study and reported no significant relationship between otitis media during the first three years of life and the subsequent use of phonologic processes and/or consonant errors during the preschool years. They concluded that "the magnitude of any adverse speech outcome associated with early childhood middle-ear problems is small and more likely to be evident when children are school age" (431). Although there is disagreement in the literature about the role early middle-ear problems have on phonological acquisition, otitis media may be a contributing factor to later speech difficulties. Because middle-ear involvement has the potential to adversely affect speech development, the speech of children with reoccurring otitis media should be periodically monitored.

Roberts and Clarke-Klein (1994), summarizing the literature on otitis media with effusion and later speech processing and production, concluded that these investigations were characterized by conflicting results and that further studies are needed concerning the relationship between a history of otitis media in childhood and later phonologic development. They suggested that phonologic development in these subjects needs to be followed from early infancy through the elementary school years to determine the effect of ottis media on phonology.

Intelligibility

In evaluating the speech intelligibility of persons with hearing impairment, the listeners, the stimulus material, and the context for evaluation should be taken into account. As a listener becomes familiar with the speech of persons with a hearing impairment, understanding improves; most listeners develop this familiarity in a short time.

Judgments of speech intelligibility have also been shown to vary with the samples on which they are based. For example, one-syllable words do not provide the linguistic redundancy available in sentence productions. Judgments based on utterances produced spontaneously may differ from judgments based on speech samples involving reading or elicited through questions. Judgments based on live speech may differ from those based on tape recordings.

Monson (1983) studied 10 adolescents with severe hearing impairment and reported that:

1. Subjects used simple sentences with few consonant clusters and few polysyllabic words and were more intelligible when using less complicated syntax than when using more complex sentences.
2. Experienced listeners understood more from those who are hearing impaired than did inexperienced listeners.
3. Sentences presented within a verbal context were more intelligible than those presented out of context.
4. Sentences where the speaker was both seen and heard were better understood than those that were only heard.

Wolk and Schildroth (1986), in a study of intelligibility of hearing-impaired speakers, indicated that the greater the degree of hearing loss the less the intelligibility. They further indicated, however, that this relationship did not hold when the student's method of communication was considered (i.e., those who used oral communication were 73 percent intelligible, those who used sign language were 4.8 percent intelligible, and those who used both were 24.7 percent intelligible).

Speech Sound Perception in Individuals with Normal Hearing

Speech-language pathologists have long been interested in a possible relationship between the perception (often referred to as discrimination) and production of speech sounds in individuals with normal auditory acuity. In the early days of the profession, many clinicians assumed that the reason children produced sounds in error was because they didn't properly discriminate one sound from another. Phonemic perception is a form of auditory perception in which the listener and/or speaker distinguishes the sound contrasts used in a language. Linguistic or phonemic perception also includes the storing and accessing of sounds for the recognition of words that are heard. From a clinical perspective, this skill includes the ability to detect differences between sounds in the language and differences between correct and incorrect productions. Clinicians are interested in determining whether or not production errors are related to errors in perception of speech sounds. Numerous investigations have been conducted to ascertain the relationship between production and perception in children with normal phonologic development and children with delayed phonologic development.

As was stated in the discussion of phonologic acquisition (see Chapter 2), some scholars view phonemic perception as essentially completed by the time the normally developing child has acquired the first 50 words. If this assumption is correct, it follows that the child's speech sound production errors can be ascribed primarily to difficulties in motor (articulatory) control and/or phonologic (linguistic) factors, rather than perception. If, however, the acquisition and development of speech sound perception continues into the preschool and even the early school years, or if some children with phonological delays also are delayed in the development of speech sound perception, some production errors may be the result of a mismatch between the adult form of the word and the child's perception and underlying representation (storage) of the word. In other words, some children's production errors may be related to phonemic perception. Finally, many treatment programs include auditory perceptual tasks (e.g., discrimination, auditory bombardment) on the assumption that such tasks help the child to learn the adult sound system.

Before discussing studies concerning the relationship between production and perception, it is useful to recall some of the previously reviewed data on auditory perception in normal infants and young children. In Chapter 2, evidence was presented that infants can perceive many contrasts used in the phonology of their language at the time they begin to speak. Indeed, experiments have shown that infants under 1 year of age are able to discriminate between many speech sounds (Eimas, Siqueland, Jusczyk, and Vigorito, 1971; Butterfield and Cairns, 1974; Jusczyk and Luce, 2002). Apparently, within the first few months of life infants perceive differences in the acoustic signal as categorical differences similar to those serving as phonemic contrasts in adult languages. Speech sound perception experiments also suggest that as children begin to speak words, they do not perceive all of the relevant phonologic contrasts. This finding may be explained in part by the fact that infant perception tasks typically require only that the subject note changes in the acoustic signal, whereas linguistic or phonemic perception involves an active attention to contrasting speech sounds and sequences in order to identify, store, recognize and retrieve distinct lexical items. The skills required for nonlinguistic discrimination (same-different distinctions) tested in investigations of infant perception are very different from those required to distinguish and store lexical items.

Perceptual discrimination experiments with preschoolers, beginning with children at approximately age 2, have shown that young children can make most of the phonologic distinctions in English. Barton (1976) who attempted to determine whether normal 2-year-olds had full or partial linguistic perception (see Chapter 2), reported that his subjects were not able to make all of the perceptions required on the experimental tasks but were able to perceive sounds they were not producing. He concluded that his subjects' perception was more advanced than their production and suggested that they may have had full or nearly full perception at this early age. He also pointed out that word familiarity influenced the children's performance on perceptual tasks: children made more errors on the perception of new or unfamiliar words than on words they knew well.

Perceptual errors may result from a partially correct internal representation that becomes more accurate with increased exposure to the adult speech models. If a child fails to notice the discrepancy between his or her initial internal representation and the adult form, a perceptually based error may exist.

The study of young children's perceptual skills has continued to be of interest to both clinicians and researchers. The extent to which the findings based on children with normal perceptual and production skills are applicable to the phonologically delayed population is unclear since it is not certain that inferences can be drawn from normal to phonologically delayed speakers. Locke (1980) suggested that a difference may exist between the role of perception in the acquisition of phonologic errors and its role in the maintenance of a phonologic disorder.

Clinical research on speech sound perception and its relationship to phonological disorders has sought to determine (1) if a relationship exists, (2) the relationship between general and phoneme-specific measures of discrimination and production as well as that between external and internal discrimination, and (3) the relationship between perceptual training and production.

Relationship between Phonologic Disorders and Speech Sound Discrimination

The possibility of a relationship between articulation disorders and speech sound (auditory) perception was first investigated in the 1930s. This early perceptual research, referred to as speech sound discrimination research, relied primarily on general measures of speech sound discrimination (tests measuring many sound contrasts), which required the subject to judge whether word or nonsense pairs verbally presented by the examiner were the same or different. In such tests, there was generally no attempt to compare the specific phoneme production errors with the specific perception errors the subject might have made.

Travis and Rasmus (1931) found that on a discrimination test of 366 paired nonsense-syllable items, normal subjects performed significantly better than subjects with mild articulation disorders. Other researchers comparing the discrimination skills of normal speakers and speakers with articulation errors (Kronvall and Diehl, 1954; Clark, 1959) reported similar findings; that is, that normal speakers had significantly better skills, and several investigators found a positive correlation between performance on an articulation test and performance on a test of speech sound discrimination (Reid, 1947a; Carrell and Pendergast, 1954).

A number of studies, however, found no relationship between discrimination and speech sound productions. In a study similar to that of Travis and Rasmus, Hall (1938) reported no significant differences in discrimination skill between normal speakers and two groups of speakers with mild and severe articulatory disorders. Hansen (1944), who studied discrimination and articulation in a college-age population, also reported little relationship between the two variables; likewise, Mase (1946), Prins (1962b), Garrett (1969), and Veatch (1970) found no significant differences in speech sound discrimination skills between children with articulation disorders and normal speakers.

Sherman and Geith (1967) suggested that one reason for the equivocal findings may have been that experimental groups were chosen on the basis of articulatory proficiency rather than speech sound discrimination performance, and consequently etiologies associated with articulatory-impaired students may not have been limited to individuals with poor speech sound discrimination skills. To control for perceptual skill, Sherman and Geith administered a 50-item speech sound discrimination test to 529 kindergarten children and then selected from this group 18 children with high discrimination scores and 18 with low scores. These two groups were given a 176-item picture-articulation test. The authors reported that children with high speech sound discrimination scores obtained significantly higher articulation scores than the group with lower discrimination scores. They concluded that poor speech sound discrimination skill may be causally related to poor articulation performance.

Schwartz and Goldman (1974) investigated the possible effects on performance by young children of the type of discrimination task required and found that their subjects consistently made more errors when stimulus words were presented in a paired-comparison context (*goat* and *coat*; *coat* and *boat*) than when target words were included in carrier phrase and sentence contexts (as in, "The man brought a *coat*"). They also found that when background noise was present during stimulus presentation performance was poorer, particularly for the paired-comparison words. The authors urged speech-language pathologists to test discrimination with tasks that are meaningful and familiar to children, and under the kind of listening conditions the child is likely to encounter in his or her environment.

After reviewing the early articulation and discrimination literature, Weiner (1967) attributed variations in findings to the fact that (1) different types of discrimination tasks were used; (2) subjects of different age levels were used; and (3) subjects reflected varying degrees of articulatory defectiveness from one study to another. He further concluded that speech sound discrimination is a developmental skill, which ceilings at about 8 years, and that a positive relationship exists between auditory discrimination problems and more severe articulation difficulties at age levels below 9 years. After reviewing the studies on the relationship between auditory discrimination and articulation performance, Winitz (1984) identified a number of factors that may account for the absence of consistent reports of a positive relationship between articulatory performance and speech sound discrimination measures: (1) a lack of relevance of the discrimination test items, (2) a lack of consideration of the child's specific articulation errors, and (3) a lack of consideration of phonetic context in which the production error occurs.

Relationship between General and Phoneme—Specific Measures; External and Internal Monitoring

In most of the investigations cited above, discrimination was tested through general speech sound discrimination measures—that is, tasks comprised of items sampling a wide variety of sound contrasts (e.g., *s*un-*b*un, *k*ey-*t*ea, *s*hoe-*z*oo) and designed to examine the subject's overall capacity to distinguish among a large number of speech sounds in a variety of phonetic contexts. Locke (1980) pointed out that in testing speech sound perception of articulatory-impaired clients, the critical issue is the clients' ability to discriminate the sound or segments that they misarticulate. Although clients may not have a general problem with speech sound discrimination, they may have phoneme-specific perceptual difficulties on sounds they misarticulate. Perceptual testing should involve stimuli that focus on the children's production errors.

Locke (1980) recommended going a step further, urging that measures of sound perception should not only be phoneme specific, but also context specific. He argued that perceptual tasks should reflect the child's production errors and reflect those phonetic environments (words) in which error productions occur and include both the error productions and the target productions.

Locke studied children's ability to discriminate sounds they produced in error when those sounds were reproduced and contrasted with the correct sound by the adult examiner. Specifically, 131 children were tested on a perceptual task in which the examiner produced imitations of the subject's error productions, and the subjects were then required to judge whether the examiner's productions were correct productions of the target word. Locke reported that 70 percent of the children correctly perceived the correct and incorrect forms of the target words, thus indicating that many children could correctly discriminate sounds made by an adult, that they produced in error. About one-third of the contrasts misproduced were also misperceived, but the misperceptions were not evenly distributed across all misproductions. Although the substitution of one voiceless fricative for another accounted for 49 percent of the production errors, these contrasts accounted for 89 percent of the misperceptions.

In a study of fourteen 2-year-old children, Eilers and Oller (1976) found some perceptual confusions in word and nonsense pairs where production of one segment was substituted for another. Yet other common production errors were discriminated by most of their subjects. They concluded that some production errors may be related to perceptual difficulties and others to motor constraints.

Strange and Broen (1980) compared 21 children between the ages of 2 and 11 on their production and perception of word-initial /w/, /r/, and /l/. They concluded from their data that both perception and production of phonemic contrasts develop gradually and that perception of a contrast usually preceded its production.

Velleman (1983) collected data from children aged 3 to 5 on a production task that included naming of pictures and objects in a play situation and the imitation of nonsense syllables. She then tested the children's perception of /s/ and /θ/—/s/ because it is easy to perceive and /θ/ because it is not "acoustically salient" and is thus relatively difficult to perceive—and computed a correlation between the two tasks. The data confirmed her hypothesis that some frequently occurring production errors in children's speech are easier to perceive than others. Since contrasts involving /s/ were relatively easily perceived, Velleman inferred that the late acquisition of /s/ could be ascribed to motor constraints. In contrast, the /θ/ versus /f/ contrast is a difficult distinction to make and, as she predicted, only children with high perception scores (over 80 percent) obtained high production scores on these phonemes. More errors were made on both perception and production in the case of /s/, and there was no significant correlation between the two measures.

In summary, some speech sound contrasts remain difficult to discriminate as late as 3 years or older, even in normal developing children. There does not, however, appear to be a correlation between many of the production errors seen in children and measures of speech sound perception. This finding suggests that while perception might be a factor in some misarticulations, this factor cannot account for others.

An additional testing variable frequently considered in phoneme-specific discrimination testing is the source of the speech production that the subject is required to judge. When the task involves discrimination of a stimulus presented from an external source, such as speech productions from another person or recorded stimuli, it is termed **external discrimination** or monitoring. External discrimination can also include **external self-discrimination**, of which listening to and making judgments of tape-recorded samples of one's own speech is an example.

When the discrimination or perceptual task involves a judgment of one's own ongoing speech sound productions, it is called **internal discrimination** or internal monitoring. During internal discrimination, the speaker has available both air- and bone-conducted auditory cues.

Studies of speech sound discrimination skills of young children with delayed phonologic development have indicated that subjects frequently were able to make external judgments of sound contrasts involving their error sounds (Locke and Kutz, 1975; Chaney and Menyuk, 1975). In a study employing phoneme-specific discrimination tasks, Aungst and Frick (1964) utilized the *Deep Test of Articulation* (McDonald, 1964), in which the /r/ was tested in 58 productions, to study the relationship between /r/ production and four measures of speech sound discrimination. Three of the discrimination tasks were designed by the investigators to assess subjects' discrimination of their own /r/ productions as they occurred in a set of 30 words. These discrimination tasks required each subject to (1) make an immediate right-wrong judgment of his or her /r/ production after speaking each word, (2) make right-wrong judgments of his or her /r/ productions after such productions had been audio recorded and played back, and (3) make same-different judgments of his or her /r/ productions as they followed the examiner's correct productions presented via audio tape recording. The fourth discrimination task was the *Templin Test of Auditory Discrimination* (Templin, 1957), a general test of external discrimination. The subjects were children, 8 years or older, who made articulation errors only on /r/. The authors reported high correlations for relationships among their three discrimination tasks but low correlations between each of those tests and the Templin general discrimination measure. Moderate correlation coefficients of .69, .66, and .59 were obtained between each of the three phoneme-specific discrimination tasks and scores on the *Deep Test of Articulation* for /f/. In contrast, the Templin discrimination test scores (a general discrimination measure) did not correlate well with the articulation measure. These findings indicate some relationship between performance on the *Deep Test of Articulation* and the phoneme-specific discrimination measures but not between the *Deep Test of Articulation* and the general test of discrimination.

Lapko and Bankson (1975) also compared external and internal monitoring with consistency of articulation, as measured by the *Deep Test of Articulation*, in a group of 25 kindergarten and first-grade children exhibiting misarticulations of /s/. All measures were phoneme-specific to /s/. They reported a significant correlation (r = .55) between the child's ability to discriminate his or her own productions of /s/ and the consistency of misarticulation of /s/. In other words, those subjects with the higher number of correct productions on the *Deep Test of Articulation* also had higher scores on the measure of internal discrimination. A significant correlation was not obtained between external monitoring tasks and articulation consistency as measured on the *Deep Test of Articulation*.

Wolfe and Irwin (1973) and Stelcik (1972) provided further evidence of a positive correlation between articulatory skill and self-monitoring (internal monitoring) of error sounds. But the results of other investigations (Woolf and Pilberg, 1971; Shelton, Johnson, and Arndt, 1977) have indicated that the findings in such studies may be influenced by such factors as the consistency of misarticulation, type of discrimination task used to test internal monitoring, and nature of the stimulus items.

Hoffman, Stager, and Daniloff (1983) suggested that current phoneme-specific, external discrimination tasks may not be sensitive to allophonic variations that might be perceived by misarticulating children. For example, the prevocalic voicing contrast that a misarticulating child perceives and produces may not be within the perceptual boundary of an adult phoneme and, consequently, not perceived by the adult; what the child may perceive as a contrast between adult allophones of /z/ may not be perceived by the adult listener because both allophones are within the adult's perceptual boundary of /z/. Such sound variations may be used by some children to contrast forms that are not used in a contrastive manner by adults. It would follow that an adult examiner would evaluate such contrasts as a mismatch between the child's production and the adult standard. These authors have suggested that "meaningful subgroups of misarticulating children may be found to manipulate subphonemic, that is allophonic, acoustic cues in nonstandard manners and thus lead to their identification as misarticulations" (214).

Discrimination Improvement and Articulatory Productions

The influence of discrimination training on production has also been considered by investigators. Historically, clinicians routinely conducted some type of discrimination training, or "ear training," as a precursor to production training; however, that is no longer the case. Investigators have attempted to determine whether or not a functional relationship exists between articulation and discrimination and more specifically, whether or not discrimination training affects production.

Sonderman (1971) reported an investigation designed to assess (1) the effect of speech sound discrimination training on articulation skills, and (2) the effect of articulation training on speech sound discrimination skill. Holland's speech sound discrimination program (1967) and the *S-Pack* (Mowrer, Baker, and Schutz, 1968) were administered in alternate sequence to two matched groups of 10 children between 6 and 8 years old, all of whom produced frontal lisps. Four measures were administered to obtain pre-training and post-training profiles for each child: (1) the *Wepman Test of Auditory Discrimination* (a general test of external monitoring skills), (2) a /s/ specific discrimination test, (3) an examiner-designed general articulation test, and (4) the criterion test from the *S-Pack* (a deep test of the /s/). Improvement in both discrimination and articulation scores was obtained from both discrimination training and articulation training, regardless of the sequence in which the two types of training were conducted. Articulatory improvement did not necessarily mean that speech sound errors were corrected. Rather, shifts from one type of error to another (e.g., omission to substitution; substitution to distortion) were regarded as evidence of improvement.

Williams and McReynolds (1975) explored the same question that Sonderman did. Two subjects were first given production training followed by a discrimination probe, then discrimination training followed by a production probe. Two additional subjects received the discrimination training first and the production training second. The probe measures, administered to determine if changes occurred in one modality after training in the other, indicated that production training was effective in changing both articulation and discrimination; in contrast to Sonderman (1971), however, Williams and McReynolds (1975) found that discrimination training was effective in changing only discrimination and did not generalize to production.

Shelton and colleagues (1977) explored the influence of articulation training on discrimination performance. One group of subjects received articulation training on the /r/ and a second group on the /s/, and pre- and post-discrimination probes, consisting of 40 items specifically related to the error sound, were administered. Results indicated that both groups of subjects improved in articulation performance, but no improvement was noted in discrimination performance. The authors suggested that the variance between their results and those of other investigators presumably could be accounted for by one or more unidentified subjects or procedural variables.

Rvachew (1994) studied the influence of various types of speech perception training that were administered concurrently with traditional speech sound training. Twenty-seven (27) preschoolers with phonologic impairment who misarticulated /s/ were randomly assigned to three groups each of which received one of the following types of discrimination training: (1) listening to a variety of correctly and incorrectly produced versions of the word *shoe*; (2) listening to the words *shoe* and *moo*; and (3) listening to the words *cat* and *Pete*. Following six weekly treatment sessions, children who received types 1 and 2 training demonstrated superior ability to articulate the target sound in comparison to those who received approach 3. Based on her data, Rvachew (1994) suggested that "speech perception training should probably be provided concurrently with speech production training" (355). A later report of Rvachew, Rafaat, and Martin (1999) further supported this conclusion. Through two complementary studies, these researchers explored the relationship of stimulability, speech perception ability, and phonological learning. In the first study, subjects were treated individually using a cycles approach as prescribed by Hodson (1989). They reported that children who were stimulable for a target sound and who demonstrated good pretreatment perceptual ability for that sound made more progress in therapy than those who were stimulable for the target sound but had poor speech sound perception for that sound. Children who were not stimulable did not make progress regardless of their perceptual skills. A second study included both individual and group instruction for subjects. Lessons involved phonetically based production activities, and a computer based program of perceptual training (SAILS, 1995). Results from the second study indicated that all children, regardless of pre-treatment stimulability and /or speech perception skills made progress in production. The authors concluded that "despite the independence of stimulability and speech perception ability before training, there is reason to believe that speech perception training may facilitate the acquisition of stimulability if both production and perception training are provided concurrently to children who demonstrate unstimulability and poor speech perception for the target sound" (40). The results of the studies cited above suggest that for children with poor speech sound perception of a target sound, including perceptual training along with production training produces positive clinical out terms of sound acquisition.

Other groups of investigators (Koegel, Koegel, and Ingham, 1986; Koegel, Koegel, Van Voy, and Ingham, 1988) have looked at a related topic and examined the relationship between self-monitoring skills and response generalization into the natural environment. School-age children were provided specific training in self-monitoring of the speech productions. These investigators reported that generalization of correct articulatory responses of the target sounds did not occur until a self-monitoring task was initiated in the treatment program. They concluded that such self-monitoring was required for generalization of the target sounds in the natural environment to occur.

An effort was made by Gray and Shelton (1992) to replicate these findings. They employed self-monitoring procedures, which differed slightly from those employed in the studies by Koegel and colleagues (1986, 1988) with eight elementary school subjects. Results of their study did not replicate the positive treatment effects found by found by Koegel and colleagues (1986, 1988). The authors indicated that different subject, treatment, and environmental variables may have accounted for different outcomes.

Summary

A relationship appears to exist between speech sound perception and articulation in some subjects with impaired phonology although the precise nature of the relationship has not been determined. The suggestion of Lof and Synan (1997) that perceptual testing should focus on speech sounds that a child misarticulates is well supported by research data. Self-monitoring of error productions would appear to be an important skill for normal articulation, but instruments to assess such a skill are lacking. Further data are needed to better understand the relationship between discrimination errors and phonological disorders. Although the efficacy of speech sound discrimination training as a predecessor to production training has often been questioned, when perceptual deficiencies are present, perceptual training prior to or concurrent with direct instruction would seem appropriate.

Minor Structural Variations of the Speech Mechanism

Speech clinicians, as part of an oral-mechanism examination, are required to make judgments about the structure and/or function of the lips, teeth, tongue, and palate. These oral structures can vary significantly, even among normal speakers. Investigators have attempted to identify relationships between articulatory status and structural variations of the oral mechanism, which can range from minor deviations to gross structural anomalies. Although a cause-and-effect relationship between articulation deviations and minor variations in oral structures has not been established, individuals with significant deformities of the orofacial region (such as patients who have undergone ablative [tongue reduction] surgery) may experience articulatory difficulties. Articulation deviations associated with major structural variations will be discussed later in this chapter.

Lips

Approximation of the lips is required for the formation of the bilabial phonemes /b/, /p/, and /m/; lip rounding is required for various vowels and the consonants /w/ and /hw/. An impairment that would inhibit lip approximation or rounding might result in misarticulation of these sounds. Fairbanks and Green (1950) examined various dimensions of the lips in 30 adult speakers with superior consonant articulation and 30 with inferior consonant articulation and reported no differences on various lip measurements between the two groups. This finding suggests that only major deviations in lip structure or function are likely to impact articulation.

Teeth

Several English consonants require intact dentition for correct production. Labiodental phonemes (/f/ and /v/) require contact between the teeth and lower lip for their production, and linguadental phonemes require interdental tongue placement for /ð/ and /θ/ productions. The tongue tip alveolars (/s/, /z/) require that the airstream pass over the cutting edge of the incisors.

Researchers investigating the relationship between deviant dentition and consonant production have examined the presence or absence of teeth, position of teeth, and dental occlusion. **Occlusion** refers to the alignment of the teeth when the jaws are closed, and **malocclusion** refers to the imperfect or irregular position of the teeth when jaws are closed. Lay terms to describe different types of occlusion include open bite and overjet. Examples of different types of occlusion may be seen in Figure 4.1.

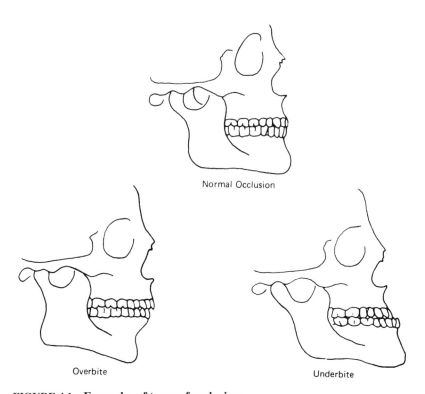

Normal Occlusion

Overbite

Underbite

FIGURE 4.1 Examples of types of occlusions.

Bernstein (1954) identified malocclusions in children with normal and defective speech but did not find a higher incidence of malocclusion in children with articulation problems than in children with normal articulation skills. He found that articulation defects were generally not related to malocclusion, except in the case of the open bite (the teeth do not come together from the first or second molar on one side to the same tooth on the opposite side). Fairbanks and Lintner (1951) examined molar occlusion, occlusion of the anterior teeth, and anterior spaces in 60 adults, 30 of whom were judged to have superior articulation skills and 30 with inferior articulatory skills. They found that neutrocclusion (normal jaw relationship with a slight malocclusion in the anterior segments) tended to predominate in the group of superior speakers, and distocclusion (malocclusion with retrusion of the mandible) and mesiocclusion (malocclusion with protrusion of the mandible) tended to occur more often in the group of speakers with production errors. When data on the subjects were divided according to (1) no marked dental deviation and (2) one or more marked dental deviations, the authors found that marked dental deviations occurred significantly more frequently in the inferior speakers than in the superior ones. Open bite was present in the inferior speaking group but not in the superior speaking group.

Although speakers with normal articulatory skills tend to have a lower incidence of malocclusion than speakers with articulatory errors, malocclusion itself does not preclude normal articulation. Subtelny, Mestre, and Subtelny (1964) found malocclusion to coexist with both normal and defective speech. They also noted that during /s/ production, normal speakers with malocclusion (distocclusion) tended to position the tongue tip slightly to the rear of the lower incisors when compared to normal speakers with normal occlusion.

Starr (1972) reported several clinical observations concerning dental arch relationships and speech production skills. He stated that an articulation problem is highly probable in individuals with a short or narrow maxillary (upper) arch and a normal mandibular (lower) arch. The consonants likely to be affected by such conditions are /s, z, ∫, t∫, f, v, t, and d/. He further noted that rotated teeth and supernumerary (extra) teeth do not generally present significant speech problems.

Another area of interest to investigators has been the influence of *missing teeth* on articulation. Bankson and Byrne (1962) examined the influence of missing teeth in kindergarten and first-grade children on the production of /s/, /∫/, and /f/ in the word-initial, medial, and final positions, and /z/ in the word-medial position. Initially, subjects were identified either as children who had correct articulation with their teeth intact or as children who had incorrect articulation with their teeth intact. After four months, articulation skills were reassessed and the number of missing central or lateral incisors tabulated. A significant relationship was found between presence or absence of teeth and correct production of /s/, but not of /f/, /∫/, or /z/. However, some children maintained correct production of /s/ despite the loss of incisors.

Snow (1961) examined the influence of missing teeth on consonant production in first-grade children. Subjects were divided into two groups: those with normal incisors and those with missing or grossly abnormal incisor teeth. The consonants examined were /f/, /v/, /θ/, /ð/, /s/, and /z/. Although Snow found that a significantly larger proportion of children with dental deviations misarticulated consonants, she also found that three quarters of the children with defective dentition did not misarticulate these sounds. In contrast to Bankson and Byrne, who noted significant differences only for /s/, Snow found significant differences for all phonemes. Snow suggested that although dental status may be a crucial factor in sound productions for some children, it does not appear to be significant for most.

Tongue

The tongue is generally considered the most important articulator for speech production. Tongue movements during speech production include tip elevation, grooving, and protrusion. The tongue is relatively short at birth, growing longer and thinner at the tip with age.

Ankyloglossia, or "tongue-tie," are terms used to describe a restricted lingual frenum. At one time, it was commonly assumed that an infant or child with ankyloglossia should have his or her frenum clipped to allow greater freedom of tongue movement and better articulation of tongue tip sounds, and frenectomies (clipping of the frenum of the tongue) were performed relatively frequently. However, McEnery and Gaines (1941) examined 1,000 patients with speech disorders and identified only 4 individuals with abnormally short frenums. Their most extreme case of a short frenum was a 10-year-old boy, whose only articulation error was a /w/ for /r/ substitution; the error was corrected following speech instruction. The authors recommended against surgery for ankyloglossia because of the possibility of hemorrhages, infections, and scar tissue. It can be inferred from these data that a short frenum is only rarely the cause of an articulation problem.

Fletcher and Meldrum (1968) examined the relationship between length of the lingual frenum and articulation. They compared two groups of sixth-grade students, 20 with limited lingual movement and 20 with greater lingual movement, and reported that subjects with restricted lingual movement scored within normal limits on a measure of articulation but tended to have more articulation errors than the group with greater lingual movement.

Although too large a tongue (**macroglossia**) or too small a tongue (**microglossia**) might be expected to affect articulation skills, there appears to be little relationship between tongue size and articulation although these variables have not been adequately investigated. The tongue is a muscular structure capable of considerable change in length and width and thus, regardless of size, is generally capable of the mobility necessary for correct sound productions.

Hard Palate

The relationship between articulation disorders and variations in hard palate dimensions has received limited attention. Fairbanks and Lintner (1951) measured the hard palates of a group of young adults with superior consonant articulation and a group with inferior consonant articulation. They reported no significant differences in cuspid width, molar width, palatal height, and maximum mouth opening. Removal of any part of the maxilla, if not restored surgically or prosthetically, may create a serious problem for the speaker. Articulation problems related to major structural anomalies of the palate will be discussed in the following section.

Major Structural Variations of the Speech Mechanism

Speech-language clinicians should recognize that significant anomalies of the oral structures are frequently associated with specific speech problems. Oral structural anomalies may be congenital or acquired. Cleft lip and/or palate is perhaps the most common congenital anomaly of the orofacial complex. Acquired structural deficits may result from trauma to the orofacial complex or surgical removal of oral structures secondary to oral cancers. For individuals with orofacial anomalies, the course of habilitation or rehabilitation often includes surgical and/or prosthetic management, and therefore, the speech clinician must work closely with various medical and dental specialists. See Leonard (1994) for more information concerning characteristics of speakers with glossectomy and other oral/oropharyngeal ablation.

Lips

Surgical repair of clefts of the lip can result in a relatively short immobile upper lip. Although this might be expected to adversely affect articulation skills, there is little evidence that this anomaly causes a speech problem for most speakers. Bloomer and Hawk (1973) reported the effects of ablative surgery on production of labial phonemes in a patient who underwent surgical removal of the external and internal nasal structures for treatment of cancer. Although surgery resulted in a relatively immobile and shortened upper lip, the patient maintained good overall speech intelligibility, producing labiodental approximations for all bilabial consonants. The development of compensatory articulatory gestures to achieve acoustically acceptable speech production is very common in many patients with structural anomalies.

Tongue

As we mentioned in addressing minor structural variations, the tongue is a muscular structure capable of considerable changes in length and width. Because the tongue is such an adaptable organ, speakers are frequently able to compensate for extensive amounts of the tongue missing and still maintain intelligible speech. Clinical investigators have repeatedly reported intelligible speech production following partial glossectomies (surgical removal of the tongue). (See Leonard, 1994.) One such case study (Backus, 1940) recorded the speech pattern of a 10-year-old boy with an undersized tongue after excision of the tongue tip and the left half of the tongue. Initially, the child's articulation was characterized by numerous consonant substitutions, but after a period of treatment, he was able to produce all consonants with little identifiable deviation.

For many patients, however, speech production is affected in varying degrees when part of the tongue is excised. Skelly, Spector, Donaldson, Brodeur, and Paletta (1971) reported pre-treatment and post-treatment intelligibility scores for 25 glossectomy (14 total, 11 partial) patients. Intelligibility judgments were based on single-word productions audio tape-recorded and played back to listeners. Intelligibility scores for those who underwent partial glossectomy ranged from 6 to 24 percent on the pre-test and from 24 to 46 percent on the post-test. Intelligibility scores for those who underwent total glossectomy ranged from 0 to 8 percent prior to treatment and from 18 to 24 present after treatment. The investigators noted that the compensatory articulatory patterns of the two groups differed. Partial glossectomy patients utilized the residual tongue stump to modify articulation; total glossectomy patients made mandibular, labial, buccal, and palatal adjustments during speech production.

Massengill, Maxwell, and Picknell (1970) reported that speech intelligibility in three patients decreased as the amount of tongue excised increased. The patients demonstrated minimal difficulty in verbal communication, though speech distortion was present. Skelly and colleagues (1971) reported that unilateral tongue excision required fewer speech adaptations than tongue tip excisions.

Leonard (1994) reported a study where listeners were asked to evaluate consonants produced by 50 speakers with various types of glossectomy. Results indicated that fricatives and plosives were most frequently judged to be inaccurate, while nasals and semi-vowels appeared more resistant to perceptual disruption.

Hard Palate

The removal of any part of the maxilla which includes the hard palate (e.g., necessitated by oral cancer), if not restored surgically or prosthetically, creates a serious problem for the speaker. Most patients receive palatal closure through a prosthetic (dental) appliance. Sullivan, Gaebler, Beukelman, Mahanna, Marshall, Lydiatt and Lydiatt (2002) reported results from 32 cancer patients who had palatal defects because of surgical removal of a portion of the palate as a result of cancer of the maxillar sinus and alveolar ridge. The maxillectomy patients had their defects obturated with a dental appliance. Testing was conducted one month after obturation on measures of speech intelligibility, speaking rate, nasality, and communication effectiveness. With the obturator removed, mean speech intelligibility was 61 percent, speaking rate was 138 words per minutes, and nasality was 5.8 on a 0–7 point scale. With the obturator inserted, mean speech intelligibility was 94 percent, speaking rate was 164 words per minute, and nasality was rated 1.6 The mean self-perception of communication effectiveness by patients was 75 percent of what it was prior to the cancer. The authors concluded that "obturation is an effective intervention for defects of the maxillary sinus and alveolar ridge on speech performance. Variations in effectiveness were noted based on site defect and patient satisfaction with the intervention."

For children born with clefts of the hard palate, the palate is typically repaired within the first 12 to 14 months of life. Scarring associated with the surgery has not been found to interfere with articulatory production.

Soft Palate

The relationship of the soft palate (velum) to articulation has been a topic of considerable research, much of it focusing on the sphincteral closure of the velopharyngeal port and the effect of velopharyngeal competence on articulation. **Velopharyngeal competence** refers to the valving that takes place to separate the nasal cavity from the oral cavity during non-nasal speech production. Inadequate velopharyngeal closure is frequently associated with (1) hypernasal (excessive nasal) resonance of vowels, vocalic consonants, and glides and liquids; (2) reduced or diminished intraoral breath pressure during production of pressure consonants (i.e., fricatives, stops, and affricates); and (3) nasal air emission accompanying production of pressure consonants (e.g., substitutions of glottal stops for stop consonants and pharyngeal fricatives for sibilants). Although velopharyngeal incompetence is often associated with individuals with clefts of the soft palate, some speakers without clefting also demonstrate such incompetence—for example, individuals with dysarthria related to neurogenic paresis or paralysis of the velopharyngeal muscles (Johns and Salyer, 1978).

As stated above, the pharyngeal fricative and the glottal stop are two examples of compensatory articulatory gestures associated with velopharyngeal valving problems. The glottal stop is characterized by interruption of the airstream at the glottis, resulting in a glottal click, or coughlike sound. Glottal stops are generally substituted for stops, particularly velar stops, as well as fricatives and affricates. The pharyngeal fricative is produced with the source of friction in the pharyngeal area and is frequently substituted for fricatives and affricates. The presence of hypernasality, nasal emission of air, weak consonants, glottal stops, and pharyngeal fricatives are all signs of velopharyngeal valving difficulties.

When the oral cavity communicates (is open to) with the nasal cavity, for example, through palatal fistulae (openings), or following ablative surgery or velopharyngeal incompetence, varying degrees of hypernasality will usually result. On the other hand, hyponasality (denasality) may result when the nasopharynx or nasal cavity is obstructed during speech production. Inflammation of the mucous membranes of the nasal cavity or a deviated septum may also cause hyponasality.

Nasopharynx

The nasopharyngeal tonsils (adenoids) are located at the upper or superior pharyngeal area. Hyperthrophied (enlarged) adenoids may compensate for a short or partially immobile velum, by assisting in velopharyngeal closure. Thus, their removal may result in hypernasality. But the adenoids may become sufficiently enlarged as to constitute a major obstruction of the nasopharynx, resulting in hyponasal speech. Enlarged adenoids may also interfere with Eustacian tube function in some individuals. When adenoids constitute an obstruction of the Eustacian tube, they may be removed for medical reasons.

Summary

Although individuals with oral structural deviations frequently experience articulation problems, the relationship between structural deficits and articulation skills is not highly predictable. The literature cites many instances of individuals with structural anomalies who have developed compensatory gestures to produce acoustically acceptable speech. Why some individuals are able to compensate for relatively gross abnormalities and others are unable to compensate for lesser deficits has not been resolved. A speech-language clinician who evaluates or treats individuals with oral structural anomalies must work collaboratively with various medical and dental specialists during speech habilitation or rehabilitation. For an excellent review of the speech characteristics and treatment of individuals with glossectomy and other oral/oropharyngeal ablation, see Leonard (1994).

Oral Sensory Function

Oral sensory and kinesthetic feedback play a role in the development and ongoing monitoring of articulatory gestures, and thus the relationship between oral sensory function and speech sound productions has been of interest. Some treatment approaches include the practice of calling the client's attention to sensory cues. Bordon (1984) indicated the need for awareness of *kinesthesis* (sense of movement and position) during therapy. Almost any phonetic placement technique used to teach speech sounds usually includes a description of articulatory contacts and movements necessary for the production of the target speech sound.

The investigation of *somesthesis* (sense of movement, position, touch, and awareness of muscle tension) has focused on (1) temporary sensory deprivation during oral sensory anesthetization (nerve block anesthesia) to determine the effect of sensory deprivation on speech production, and (2) assessment of oral sensory perception such as two-point discrimination or oral form discrimination to see if such sensory perception was related to articulatory skill. Considerable research into oral sensory functioning was conducted in the 1960s using a variety of methods to assess oral tactile sensitivity in order to understand if a relationship existed between these sensory tasks and articulation performance. Later research examined articulation of individuals during periods of temporary sensory deprivation, sometimes referred to as **oral blockade**.

Netsell (1986) has suggested that it is likely that adults are not consciously aware of specific speech movements during running speech. He also speculated that children may not be aware of articulatory movements during the acquisition period. If Netsell is correct, the clinician who attempts to utilize somesthetic senses in monitoring running speech may be asking the client to respond to information that is not available at a conscious level without instruction.

Oral Tactile Sensitivity

Early investigators of oral sensory function attempted to explore the sensitivity or threshold of awareness of oral structures to various stimuli. Ringel and Ewanowski (1965) studied oral tactile sensitivity utilizing an esthesiometer, a device used in the measurement of two-point discrimination. They examined discrimination sensitivity of various structures in a normal population and found that the maximal to minimal awareness hierarchy for two-point stimulation (awareness of two points rather than one) was tongue tip, finger tip, lip, soft palate, alveolar ridge, and that the midline of structures tended to be more sensitive than the lateral edges.

Fucci and associates (Arnst and Fucci, 1975; Fucci, 1972) measured the threshold of vibrotactile stimulation of structures in the oral cavity in both normal and speech-disordered individuals. These investigators found that subjects with misarticulations tended to have poorer oral sensory abilities than normal speaking subjects.

Oral Form Recognition

Oral sensory function has also been investigated extensively through form recognition tasks. Ringel, Burk, and Scott (1970) speculated that form identification (**oral stereognosis**) may provide information on nervous system integrity since the recognition of forms placed in the mouth was assumed to require integrity of peripheral receptors for touch and kinesthesis as well as central integrating processes. Most form recognition tasks require the subject to match forms placed in the oral cavity with drawings of the forms, or to make same-different judgments. Subjects tend to improve on such tasks until adolescence when they ceiling-out on the task. Stimuli for such testing are typically small, plastic, three-dimensional forms of varying degrees of similarity, such as triangles, rectangles, ovals, and circles.

Investigators who have studied the relationship between oral form recognition and articulation performance have reported inconsistent results. Arndt, Elbert, and Shelton (1970) did not find a significant relationship between oral form recognition and articulation performance in a third-grade population. But Ringel, House, Burk, Dolinsky, and Scott (1970) reported significant differences on an oral form-matching task between normal-speaking elementary school children and children with articulation errors. They noted that children with severe misarticulations made more form-recognition errors than children with mild articulation problems.

Some researchers have investigated the relationship between production of specific phonemes and oral sensory function. McNutt (1977) found that children who misarticulated /r/ did not perform as well as the normal speakers on oral form perception tasks; there were, however, no significant differences between the normal speakers and the children who misarticulated /s/.

Bishop, Ringel, and House (1973) compared oral form-recognition skills of deaf high school students who were orally trained (taught to use speech), and those who were taught to use sign language. The authors noted skill differences that favored the orally trained students and postulated that "while a failure in oroperceptual functioning may lead to disorders of articulation, a failure to use the oral mechanism for speech activities, even in persons with normal orosensory capabilities, may result in poor performance on oroperceptual tasks" (257).

Locke (1968) examined the relationship between articulation skills and oral form-recognition scores from a different perspective. Rather than comparing the performance of normal-speaking children with those of children who demonstrated articulation errors, he compared the performance on an articulation learning task of 10 normal children with high form-recognition scores with that of 10 normal children with low form-recognition scores. Each subject was required to imitate three German sounds heard on a tape recording of a native German speaker. Locke found that the group with high form-perception scores obtained significantly better production scores on two of the three consonant sounds than the group with low form-identification scores.

McDonald and Aungst (1970) pointed out that an individual can have good articulation skills despite poor oral form-recognition scores. They cited the case of a 21-year-old neurologically impaired male who articulated normally yet demonstrated difficulty in oral form identification and in two-point discrimination on the tongue.

Oral Anesthetization

The relationship between speech sound productions and oral sensory functions has also been examined through sensory deprivation. To study the role of oral sensation during speech, researchers have induced temporary states of oral sensory deprivation through the use of oral nerve-block and topical anesthetization (similar to what occurs prior to dental work). Then they have compared speech under normal conditions with speech under anesthetization on a variety of dimensions, such as overall intelligibility, vowel and consonant articulation, rate, phoneme duration, and physiological and acoustic characteristics.

Gammon, Smith, Daniloff, and Kim (1971) examined the articulation skills of eight adult subjects reading 30 sentences under four conditions: (1) normal, (2) with masking noise present, (3) nerve-block anesthesia, and (4) nerve-block anesthesia with masking noise. They noted few vowel distortions under any of the conditions and a 20 percent rate of consonant misarticulation (especially fricatives and affricates) under anesthesia and under anesthesia with noise. Scott and Ringel (1971) studied the articulation of two adult males producing lists of 24 bisyllabic words under normal and anesthetized conditions. They noted that articulatory changes caused by sensory deprivation were largely non-phonemic in nature and included loss of retroflexion and lip-rounding gestures, less tight fricative constrictions, and retracted points of articulation contacts.

Prosek and House (1975) studied four adult speakers reading 20 bisyllabic words in isolation and in sentences under normal and anesthetized conditions. Although intelligibility was maintained in the anesthetized condition, speech rate was slowed and minor imprecisions of articulation were noted. The authors reported that, when anesthetized, speakers produced consonants with slightly greater intraoral air pressure and longer duration than under the normal nonanesthetized condition.

In summary, studies involving anesthetization found that speech remained intelligible although subjects did not speak as accurately under this condition as they did under normal conditions. However, the subjects in these studies were adult speakers with normal articulation skills prior to the sensory deprivation. It is unclear if reduced oral sensory feedback might interfere with the acquisition of speech or affect remediation.

Oral Sensory Function and Articulation Learning

Jordan, Hardy, and Morris (1978) studied the influence of tactile sensation as a feedback mechanism in articulation learning. Their subjects were first-grade boys, nine with good articulation skills and nine with poor articulation skills. Subjects were fitted with palatal plates equipped with touch-sensitive electrodes and taught to replicate four positions of linguapalatal contact, with and without topical anesthesia. Children with poor articulation performed less well on tasks of precise tongue placement than children with good articulation. Subjects with poor articulation were able to improve their initially poor performance when given specific training on the tongue placement tasks.

Wilhelm (1971) and Shelton, Willis, Johnson, and Arndt (1973) used oral form-recognition materials to teach form recognition to misarticulating children and reported inconsistent results. Wilhelm reported articulation improved as oral form recognition improved. Shelton and colleagues reported results that did not support that finding. Ruscello (1972) reported that form-recognition scores improved in children undergoing treatment for articulation.

Summary

The role of normal oral sensory function or somesthetic feedback in the development and maintenance of speech production is complex. Despite efforts to identify the relationship between oral sensory status and articulatory performance, conclusive findings are lacking. A review of the literature, however, has revealed the following:

1. Many methods have been used to measure oral sensory perception: form recognition, touch-pressure threshold, two-point discrimination, oral vibrotactile thresholds, and oral blockade.
2. Oral form recognition improves with age through adolescence.
3. The role of oral sensory feedback in the acquisition of phonology is unclear.
4. Individuals with poor articulation tend to achieve slightly lower scores on form-perception tasks than their normal-speaking peers. However, some individuals with poor form-identification skills have good articulation.
5. Investigators who have anesthetized oral structures reported that intelligibility is generally maintained during sensory deprivation but less accuracy in articulation was noted.
6. Although research has indicated that some individuals with articulation problems may also have oral sensory deficits, the neurological mechanisms underlying the use of sensory information during experimental conditions may differ from those operating in normal running speech.
7. Information concerning oral sensory function has not been shown to have clinical applicability.
8. It is important to distinguish between the effects of sensory deprivation in individuals who have already developed good speech skills and the effects in individuals with defective articulation.
9. The effects of long-term sensory deprivation have yet to be explored.

Motor Abilities

Because speech is a motor act, researchers have explored the relationship between articulation and motor skills, investigating performance on gross motor tasks as well as oral and facial motor tasks.

General Motor Skills

Studies focusing on the relationship between general or gross motor skills and articulatory abilities have yielded inconsistent and inconclusive results. It may be concluded, however, that individuals with articulation problems do not have significant retardation in general motor development.

Oral-Facial Motor Skills

Speech is a dynamic process that requires the precise coordination of the oral musculature. During ongoing speech production, fine muscle movements of the lips, tongue, palate, and jaw constantly alter the dimensions of the oral cavity. An assessment of the client's oral motor skills is typically a part of a speech mechanism examination. Tests of diadochokinetic rate or maximum repetition rate (rapid repetition of syllables) have been used frequently to evaluate oral motor skills. Diadochokinetic rate is established either with a *count by time* procedure, in which the examiner counts the number of syllables spoken in a given interval of time, or a *time by count* measurement, in which the examiner notes the time required to produce a designated number of syllables. The advantage of the time by count measurement is that few operations are required since the examiner need only listen to the syllable count and turn off the timing device when the requisite number of syllables is produced. Performance is then sometimes compared to normative data. The syllables most frequently used to assess diadochokinetic rates are /pʌ/, /tʌ/, and /kʌ/ in isolation, syllable repetition, and the sequence /pʌtʌ/, /tʌkʌ/, /pʌkʌ/, /pʌtʌkʌ/. There is evidence that diadochokinetic rates improve with age. Fletcher (1972) examined diadochokinetic rates in normal children ages 6 to 13 years using a count by time procedure. He reported that children increased the number of syllables produced in a given unit of time at each successive age from 7 to 13 years. Data reported by Canning and Rose (1974) indicated that adult values for maximum repetition rates were reached by 9- to 10-year-olds, whereas Fletcher's data show a convergence after age 15.

McNutt (1977) and Dworkin (1978) examined diadochokinetic rates of children with specific misarticulations and of their normal-speaking peers. McNutt examined the rate of alternating syllable productions (e.g., /dʌgə/) in children with normal articulation, children with /s/ misarticulation, and children with /r/ misarticulation. Both groups of children with misarticulations were noted to be slower than normal speakers in syllable production rates. Dworkin examined lingual diadochokinetic rates for the syllables /tʌ/, /dʌ/, /kʌ/, and /gʌ/, in normal speakers and frontal lisping speakers aged 7 to 12 years. The mean rate of utterances of the syllables tested was significantly lower in subjects in the group with misarticulations.

Some researchers have questioned the usefulness of rapid syllable repetition tasks and their relationship to articulation skills because the movements of articulation are produced by the simultaneous contraction of different groups of muscles rather than the alternating contraction of opposed muscles (McDonald, 1964). Winitz (1969) also pointed out that because normal speakers have a history of success with speech sounds, they may have an advantage over subjects with misarticulations on diadochokinetic tasks. Tiffany (1980) pointed out that little is known about the significance of scores obtained on diadochokinetic tasks and thus "such measures appear to lack a substantial theoretical base" (895). The one exception to this generality relates to those children that might be considered to evidence developmental verbal dyspraxia (discussed elsewhere in this chapter). Poor performance in diadochokinetic tasks is often reflective of syllable sequencing problems evident in this population. Another exception would be clients with a history of unusual or delayed oral-motor development, which may be evidenced in sucking, feeding, and swallowing in addition to delayed speech sound development. These children may evidence problems with muscle tone and movement of the oral structures, including independent movement of the tongue and/or lips from the jaw. It would appear that slow or weak oral-motor development may be a contributing factor to the presence of a speech sound disorder.

Summary

Individuals with articulation problems have not been shown to exhibit significantly depressed motor coordination on tasks of general motor performance. The relationship between oral motor skills and articulation skills in functional articulation disorders remains uncertain. Although individuals with defective articulation have been found to perform more poorly on diadochokinetic tasks than their normal-speaking peers, these results cannot be accurately interpreted until the relationship between diadochokinetic tasks and the ability to articulate sounds in context is clarified. A small percentage of children will evidence abnormal tone, stability, or movement in areas of the oral structure while another subgroup will evidence developmental verbal dyspraxia. These two groups represent subsets of individuals with articulation impairment for whom oral-motor factors may have diagnostic significance.

Oral Myofunctional Disorders/Tongue Thrust

Oral myofunctional disorders (OMD) are observed by speech-language pathologists and include such phenomena as tongue thrusting, unusual oral movements, finger sucking, lip insufficiencies, and dental and oral structure deficiencies. Our concern as speech-language pathologists relates to speech differences and disorders that may be related to such oral variations. Since tongue thrusting is the oral myofunctional disorder most commonly encountered by speech-language pathologists, in this section we will focus on this phenomena.

Tongue thrust has been defined as frontal or lateral tongue thrust or strong contact of the tongue with the teeth during swallowing, as well as inadequate lip closure or incorrect tongue rest posture (Neiva and Wertzner, 1996). Proffit (1986) points out that tongue thrust is something of a misnomer since it implies that the tongue is thrust forward forcefully, when in reality such individuals do not seem to use more tongue force against the teeth than nonthrusters. Rather, *tongue thrust swallow* implies a directionality of tongue activity in swallowing. Other terms sometimes used to describe these behaviors include *reverse swallow*, *deviant swallow*, and *infantile swallow*. These terms should be avoided because of their inherent faulty implications (Mason, 1988). The most salient features of a tongue thrust swallow pattern, according to Mason and Proffit (1974), include one or more of these conditions:

1. During the initiation of a swallow, a forward gesture of the tongue between the anterior teeth so that the tongue tip contacts the lower lip;
2. During speech activities, fronting of the tongue between or against the anterior teeth with the mandible hinged open (in phonetic contexts not intended for such placements); and
3. At rest, the tongue carried forward in the oral cavity with the mandible hinged slightly open and the tongue tip against or between the anterior teeth (116).

Everyone starts out life as a tongue thruster because at birth the tongue fills the oral cavity, making tongue fronting obligatory. Sometime later, prior to about 5 years, most children replace an anterior tongue-gums/teeth seal during swallowing with a superior tongue-palate seal (Hanson, 1988b).

Tongue thrust during swallow and/or tongue fronting at rest can usually be identified by visual inspection. Mason (1988) has pointed out that two types of tongue fronting should be differentiated. The first is described as a **habit** and is seen in the absence of any morphological structural delimiting factors. The second is **obligatory** and may involve factors such as airway obstruction or enlarged tonsils with tongue thrusting being a necessary adaptation to maintain the size of the airway to pass food during swallow. Oral myofunction therapy for obligatory tongue fronting has been questioned by Shelton (1989) because of the poor prognosis for change.

Wadsworth, Maul, and Stevens (1998) indicated that tongue thrust swallow frequently co-occurred with resting forward-tongue posture (63 percent), open bite (86 percent), overjet (57 percent), abnormal palatal contour (60 percent), and open mouth posture (39 percent). Marshall (1992) indicated that some children who tongue thrust are described as having a tongue that is "too big." However, she indicated that low muscle tone (flaccidity) of the tongue is often the real problem. She also attributes tongue thrusting to tongue instability, jaw instability, allergies, and poor sensory awareness.

Hanson (1988a) suggested that a better description for these tongue position and movement behaviors would be "oral muscle pattern disorders." Orthodontists and speech-language pathologists have been interested in tongue thrusting and a forward tongue resting posture because of the perception that tongue function can cause certain types of (1) malocclusion problems, (2) altered patterns of facial development, and (3) articulation problems. The type of articulation disorder associated with tongue thrust and malocclusion is a frontal lisp characterized by anterior tongue placement for /s/ and /z/. The number of lisps is higher in children who evidence tongue thrusting than for children who do not evidence such behavior. Sometimes tongue thrust is also associated with anterior placement of /ʃ/, /tʃ/, /dʒ/, /ʒ/, /t/, /d/, /l/, and /n/.

Impact of Tongue Thrust on Dentition

The current view is that the resting posture of the tongue affects the position of the teeth and jaws more than does the tongue function during swallowing (tongue thrust) or speaking (Proffit, 1986). Tongue thrusting may play a role in maintaining or influencing an abnormal dental pattern when an anterior resting tongue position is present. If the position of the tongue is forward (forward resting position) and between the anterior teeth at rest, this condition can impede normal teeth eruption and can result in an anterior open bite. However, tongue thrusting patients, in the absence of an anterior tongue resting position, are not thought to develop malocclusions. The pressure or force on dentition associated with tongue thrust during speaking and swallowing are of short duration and do not exert enough force on the dentition to cause problems of dental occlusion. Mason (1988) pointed out that individuals who exhibit a tongue thrust pattern and forward tongue posture create morphological conditions that can potentially lead to dental occlusion problems and would be much more likely to develop a malocclusion than when only a tongue thrust is present.

Tongue Thrust and Presence of Articulation Errors

Investigators have reported that articulation errors, primarily sibilant distortions, occur more frequently in children who evidence tongue thrust than in those who do not. Fletcher, Casteel, and Bradley (1961) studied 1,615 school children aged 6 to 18 and found that children who demonstrated a tongue thrust swallow pattern were more likely to have associated sibilant distortions than children who did not. They also reported that subjects with normal swallow patterns demonstrated a significant decrease in sibilant distortion with age, whereas tongue thrusters did not.

Palmer (1962) found that clients referred for marked tongue thrusting nearly always demonstrated a sibilant "difference" but that the difference was perceived as only a slight lisp. He reported that such differences also occurred on /t/, /d/, and /n/.

Jann, Ward, and Jann (1964) examined the relationship among speech defects, tongue thrusting, and malocclusion in children in the early primary grades and reported a high incidence of /s/, /z/, and /l/ variations in children with tongue thrust swallow patterns. Wadsworth and colleagues (1998) reported that of 200 children from grades kindergarten through sixth who were enrolled in speech therapy, 77 percent of children with a defective /s/ evidenced abnormal rest tongue position and 76 percent exhibited a tongue thrust swallow.

Subtelny and colleagues (1964) used radiographic techniques to examine the relationship between normal and abnormal oral morphology and /s/ production. Their subjects, 81 adolescents and adults, were divided into three groups: (1) normal speakers with normal occlusion, (2) normal speakers with severe malocclusion, and (3) abnormal speakers with severe malocclusion. In contrast to earlier investigators, these authors found that the incidence of tongue thrusting and malocclusion in normal speakers was comparable to that in abnormal speakers. This finding is consistent with the reported developmental decrease in the reverse swallow pattern.

Dworkin and Culatta (1980) studied the relationships among protrusive tongue strength, open bite, and articulation in 141 children. They reported no significant difference among their group in tongue strength.

Treatment Issues

Hanson (1994), in a review of the 15 studies that examined the effectiveness of tongue thrust therapy, reported that 14 of the investigators indicated that swallowing and resting patterns were altered successfully. Most studies reviewed patients at least one year following the completion of treatment. Only one study of five subjects (Subtelny, 1970) found therapy to be ineffective in correcting the disorders.

Other support for tongue thrust intervention has often come from clinical reports by clinicians who conduct oral myofunctional therapy. For example, Hilton (1984) stated: "In my experience, many tongue-fronting children who begin speech articulation therapy without having had the early sensorimotor and stretching activities of myotherapy . . . begin with an unnecessary handicap . . . I provide every tongue-fronting speech articulation case these initial oral awareness, control, and flexibility exercises prior to initiation of the place-feature oriented therapy . . ." (51). Umberger and Johnston (1997) agreed that combined articulation therapy and oral myofunctional therapy provides the best opportunity for improved speech accompanying reduced tongue thrusting.

The official statement adopted by the American Speech-Language-Hearing Association (ASHA) Legislative Council (ASHA, 1991) on the role of the speech-language pathologist in assessment and management of oral myofunctional disorders includes the statement:

"Investigation, assessment, and treatment of oral myofunctional disorders are within the purview of speech-language pathology" (7).

1991 Position Statement

It is the position of ASHA that:

1. Oral myofunctional phenomena, including abnormal fronting (tongue thrust) of the tongue at rest and during swallowing, lip incompetency, and sucking habits, can be identified reliably. These conditions co-occur with speech misarticulations in some patients.
2. Tongue fronting may reflect learned behaviors, physical variables, or both.
3. Published research indicates that oral myofunctional therapy is effective in modifying disorders of tongue and lip posture and movement.
4. Investigation, assessment, and treatment of oral myofunctional disorders are within the purview of speech-language pathology.
5. The speech-language pathologist who desires to perform oral myofunctional services must have the required knowledge and skills to provide a high quality of treatment. The provision of oral myofunctional therapy remains an option of individual speech-language pathologists whose interests and training qualify them.
6. Evaluation and treatment should be interdisciplinary and tailored to the individual. The speech-language pathologist performing oral myofunctional therapy should collaborate with an orthodontist, pediatric dentist, or other dentists, and with medical specialists such as an otolaryngologist, pediatrician, or allergist, as needed.
7. Appropriate goals of oral myofunctional therapy should include the retraining of labial and lingual resting and functional patterns (including speech). The speech-language pathologist's statements of treatment goals should avoid predictions of treatment outcome based on tooth position or dental occlusal changes.
8. Basic and applied research is needed on the nature and evaluation of oral myofunctions and the treatment of oral myofunctional disorders (7).

The ad hoc committee report (ASHA, 1989) on the labial-lingual posturing function developed the above statement based on the following concepts relative to oral myofunctional phenomena as they relate to communication disorders:

1. All infants exhibit a tongue thrust swallow as a normal performance.
2. This pattern changes with growth and maturation to the extent that many different swallow patterns can be identified from infancy to adulthood.
3. At some time in development, a tongue protrusion swallow is no longer the norm and can be considered undesirable or as a contributing and maintaining factor in malocclusion, lisping, or both.
4. A related condition that has a stronger link to malocclusion is a forward resting posture of the tongue. . . . This is consistent with orthodontic theory and research that long-acting forces against the teeth result in tooth movement whereas short-acting (intermittent) forces are not as likely to cause tooth movement.

5. There is descriptive evidence that during the course of oral myofunctional therapy some individuals have corrected or controlled a tongue thrust swallow and an anterior resting posture.

6. Diagnostic attention should be directed toward determining whether a tongue thrust swallow and a forward tongue resting posture coexist in a given patient. When these conditions coexist, a greater link to malocclusion would be expected than from a tongue thrust swallow alone. However, there is insufficient evidence to show that a forward tongue posture and tongue thrust swallow are more detrimental than a tongue forward resting posture alone. There is also some evidence that a tongue forward resting posture or tongue thrust swallow and lisping coexist in some persons. Correction of tongue function or posture may facilitate correction of the lisp or the interdentalization of the /t/, /d/, /n/, and /l/ phonemes.

7. In normal development, slight separation of the lips at rest ("lip incompetence") is normal in children. With growth, the lips typically achieve contact at rest in the teenage years. Some individuals, however, persist in a lips-apart posture after development has advanced sufficiently to permit lip closure. Such individuals may be candidates for treatment.

8. There is some evidence that lip exercises can be successful in facilitating a closed-lip posture.

9. Sucking habits (e.g., finger, thumb, tongue, lips) can influence dental development. When tongue thrusting and thumb sucking coexist with dental problems, developmental correction of the tongue thrust would not be expected until the thumb, finger, or sucking habit ceases.

10. Other variables besides learning influence tongue posture. They include posterior airway obstruction, which may involve tonsils, adenoids, nasal blockage, high posterior tongue position with a short mandibular ramus, or a long soft palate. Many morphologic features or combinations of features can reduce oral isthmus size and obligate the tongue to rest forward. Diagnostic procedures should distinguish such patients from those with other forward tongue postures or functions. The obligatory tongue forward posture group would seem unlikely candidates for myofunctional therapy in the absence of medical treatment. Any indicated remedial medical procedures are usually carried out prior to consideration of myofunctional therapy.

Summary

1. Existing data support the idea that abnormal labial-lingual posturing function can be identified, including abnormal fronting (tongue thrust) of the tongue at rest and during swallowing, lip incompetency, and sucking habits.

2. A forward tongue resting posture has the potential, with or without a tongue thrust swallow, to be associated with malocclusions.

3. There is some evidence that an anterior tongue resting posture or a tongue thrust swallow and lisping coexist in some persons.

4. Oral myofunctional therapy can be effective in modifying disorders of tongue and lip posture and movement.

5. Assessment and treatment of oral myofunctional disorders that may include some nonspeech remediation are within the purview of speech-language pathology but should involve interdisciplinary collaboration.

6. Research is needed on the nature and evaluation of oral myofunctions and the treatment of such disorders.

Neuromotor Disorders

Speech production at a motor level requires muscle strength, speed of movement, appropriate range of excursion, accuracy of movement, coordination of multiple movements, motor steadiness, and muscle tone (Darley, Aronson, and Brown, 1975). Damage that impairs one or more of these neuromuscular functions may affect motor speech production, including phonation, respiration, or velopharyngeal function. Neuromotor speech disorders more typically occur in adults than children, since they are often associated with strokes or other forms of brain injury. Cerebral palsy is one example of a condition that results in neuromotor-based speech disorders in children.

Neurologists and speech-language pathologists have sought to understand the possible relationship between the clinical (behavioral) responses associated with neurologically-impaired individuals and the site and extent of the neurological lesions (brain damage). The reason for such inquiry is to identify some potential commonality across patients in the specific brain damage and the concomitant cognitive language impairment.

Although entire books are devoted to motor speech disorders, the following offers a brief introduction to this topic:

Dysarthrias

The **dysarthrias** are neurologic motor speech impairments characterized by slow, weak, imprecise, and/or uncoordinated movements of the speech musculature. Yorkston, Beukelman, Strand, and Bell (1999) state that "dysarthrias form a group of disorders marked by impaired execution of the movements of speech production." Because dysarthrias are caused by different types of lesions, trauma, or disease that cause central or peripheral nervous system damage, dysarthrias cannot be described by a single set of characteristics.

Dysarthrias are characterized by a paralysis, weakness, or incoordination of the speech musculature, which may result from localized injuries to the nervous system, various inflammatory processes, toxic metabolic disorders, vascular lesions or trauma of the brain, and lesion, disease, or trauma to the nervous system. The most significant characteristic of dysarthric speech is reduced intelligibility. Dysarthric speech can involve disturbances in respiration, phonation, articulation, resonance, and prosody. Phonemes misarticulated in spontaneous speech are also likely to be misarticulated in other situations, such as reading and imitation tasks.

Table 4.1 lists the types of dysarthrias and the most prominent speech characteristics associated with each. The most common of these characteristics is the production of imprecise consonants.

TABLE 4.1   Dysarthrias and Associated Speech Deviations

Type	Discrete Neurological Group	Relative Prominence of Speech Deviations
Flaccid dysarthria—(disorders of the lower motor neuron)	bulbar palsy	1. hypernasality 2. imprecise consonants 3. breathiness (continuous)
Spastic dysarthria—(disorders of the upper motor neuron)	pseudobulbar palsy	1. imprecise consonants 2. monopitch 3. reduced stress
Ataxic dysarthria—(disorders of the cerebellar system)	cerebellar lesions	1. imprecise consonants 2. excess and equal stress 3. irregular articulatory breakdown
Hypokinetic dysarthria—(disorders of the extra-pyramidal system)	Parkinsonism	1. monopitch 2. reduced stress 3. monoloudness
Hyperkinetic dysarthria—(disorders of the extra-pyramidal system)	chorea	1. imprecise consonants 2. prolonged intervals 3. variable rate
	dystonia	1. imprecise consonants 2. distorted vowels 3. harsh voice quality
Unilateral upper motor neuron—(disorders on right or left side)	pseudobulbar palsy	1. imprecise articulation 2. hypernasality 3. slow-labored rate
Mixed dysarthrias—	amyotrophic lateral sclerosis with relative prominence in pseudobulbar palsy and bulbar palsy	1. imprecise consonants 2. hypernasality 3. harsh voice quality

Source: Adapted from F. Darley, A. Aronson, and J. Brown, *Motor Speech Disorders* (Philadelphia: W.B. Saunders, 1975).

Apraxia

Apraxia is a motor speech disorder also caused by brain damage, but it is differentiated from the dysarthrias and described as a separate clinical entity. Apraxia of speech is characterized by an impairment of motor speech programming with little or no weakness, paralysis, or incoordination of the speech musculature. Whereas dysarthrias frequently affect all motor speech processes—respiration, phonation, articulation, resonance, and prosody—apraxia primarily affects articulatory abilities with secondary prosodic alterations.

A description of some of the clinical characteristics of this disorder has been provided by Darley and colleagues (1975):

Apraxia of speech is characterized by highly variable articulation errors embedded in a pattern of speech made slow and effortful by trial-and-error gropings for the desired articulatory postures. The off-target productions are usually complications of articulatory performance, that is, substitutions (many of them unrelated to the target phoneme), additions, repetitions, and prolongations. Less frequently, the errors are simplifications, that is, distortions and omissions. Errors are most often on consonants occurring initially in words, predominately on those phonemes and clusters of phonemes requiring more complex muscular adjustment. Errors are exacerbated by increase in length of word and the linguistic and psychologic "weight" of a word in the sentence. They are not significantly influenced by auditory, visual, or instructional set variables. Islands of fluent, error-free speech highlight the marked discrepancy between efficient automatic-reactive productions and inefficient volitional-purposive productions (267).

Some clients who demonstrate apraxia of speech (**verbal apraxia**) also demonstrate similar difficulty in volitional oral nonspeech tasks, a behavior described as **oral apraxia** (De Renzi, Pieczuro, and Vignolo, 1966). For example, an individual may protrude his or her tongue during eating but may be unable to perform this act voluntarily. Although oral apraxia often coexists with verbal apraxia, this is not always the case.

Johns and Darley (1970) compared apraxic and dysarthric speakers on tasks involving spontaneous speaking and reading at a "self-chosen rate" and at a rapid rate. They reported that (1) apraxic speakers were less consistent than dysarthric speakers in their articulatory errors; (2) apraxics made fewer articulation errors and were more intelligible when reading at rapid rates rather than slow rates; (3) apraxics performed better on the spontaneous speaking tasks than on the reading tasks; (4) dysarthrics made fewer errors and were more intelligible when speaking at slow rates rather than fast rates; and (5) distortions accounted for 65 percent of the errors made by dysarthrics but only 10 percent of the errors made by apraxic speakers; substitutions accounted for 50 percent of the errors made by apraxic speakers but only 10 percent of the errors made by dysarthric speakers. Speech sound errors seen in apraxia have usually been identified as sound substitution errors and thereby differentiated from the speech sound distortions seen in dysarthrics. Itoh and Sasanuma (1984) have argued, however, that some of the substitutions seen in apraxia can better be described as distortions, and thus apraxia may be characterized by both substitution and distortion errors. Lapointe and Wertz (1974) described patients who demonstrated a "mixed" articulation disorder consisting of a combination of apraxic and dysarthric speech characteristics.

Developmental Verbal Dyspraxia

A speech sound production disorder, sometimes regarded as neurologically based, is developmental verbal dyspraxia. This disorder is seen in a small percentage of those children who are often labeled as having a "developmental phonological disorder." Such disorders have often been linked to some type of congenital neuromotor impairment in the absence of dysarthria. The labels **developmental verbal dyspraxia** (DVD) and **developmental apraxia of speech** (DAS) are used to identify this subcategory of children. While the literature in this area is almost exclusively focused on children, Haynes, Johns, and May (1978) have suggested that the syndrome of conditions commonly associated with this disorder may persist to adulthood.

Descriptions of this unique subgroup of phonologically impaired children have existed for some time. Morley (1957), and other Europeans, were among the first to call attention to and describe this type of developmental speech disorder. During the 1970s, the diagnostic label **developmental apraxia/dyspraxia** came into prominence in the United States to identify a particular subcategory of children who traditionally were identified as having "functional" articulation disorders (disorders of unknown etiology), but whom clinicians suspected as having a subtle motor or neurological basis to their phonological errors. In more recent years, linguistic variables, including stress and other aspects of language, have been described as an additional characteristic of DVD (Velleman and Strand, 1994; Shriberg, Aram, and Kwiatkowski, 1997).

As stated earlier, apraxia in the adult population is viewed as a motor speech disorder associated with lesions of the nervous system and characterized by an impairment of motor speech programming (i.e., select, plan, organize, and initiate a motor pattern) with no weakness, paralysis, or incoordination of the speech musculature (Darley, 1970; Darley et al., 1975). The term *apraxia* has been borrowed from the adult literature to identify a somewhat behaviorally similar, but etiologically dissimilar phenomenon in children. Thus, the term *developmental verbal dyspraxia* or *developmental apraxia* has come to refer to children with articulation errors who also have difficulty with volitional or imitative production of speech sounds and sequences. These symptoms may or may not be accompanied by symptoms of oral apraxia.

Although DVD is widely discussed and a body of literature has developed that addresses the description, assessment, and treatment of the disorder, some controversy has persisted over the existence of such a disorder. Some have suggested that it is inappropriate to consider DVD as a "diagnostic entity" of phonologically impaired children since the symptoms attributed to the disorder are not consistent enough in occurrence or unique enough to support such a designation. In spite of this concern, however, most clinical phonologists acknowledge the existence of such a diagnostic category.

Characteristics of DVD

Rosenbek and Wertz (1972) and Yoss and Darley (1974) conducted early studies that sought to document the characteristics of DVD. More recently, Velleman and Strand (1994) and Shriberg et al. (1997) summarized the literature and have further described the identifying characteristics of this population. The authors have identified the following features associated with this disorder:

1. Severe and persistent speech difficulty and/or unintelligibility, including vowel misarticulations, poor or reduced production of consonants. Errors tend to increase as length and complexity of utterances increase.
2. Inconsistent errors with some awareness of errors as they occur.
3. Difficulties sequencing phonemes in syllables and words as well as in diadocokinesis tasks.
4. Groping/silent posturing and difficulties in performing volitional oral movements and sequences of movement.
5. Inconsistent timing and control of nasality (and prosody).

6. Inappropriate use of prosody, especially stress.
7. Slow progress in therapy.

In addition, the following exclusionary features are often used to describe children with DVD, although variations and inconsistencies are observed in all of these characteristics:

1. No apparent organic conditions
2. No muscle weakness
3. IQ with normal limits
4. Receptive language within normal limits
5. Normal hearing

In spite of the arguments against the validity of the DVD syndrome, however, the diagnosis is supported by clinicians and researchers. For those clinicians working with children who are perceived to evidence dyspraxic characteristics, several concepts may be useful in guiding professional actions.

1. Jaffe (1986) has pointed out that DVD appears to be a syndrome in which all symptoms and signs need not be present to diagnose the disorder, nor must one typical sign or symptom be present to establish the diagnosis.
2. Velleman and Strand (1994) point out that the controversy about this disorder centers around the characterization of DVD as a purely motoric disorder with some linguistic symptoms versus a linguistic disorder affecting motor speech. They have further stated that "the existence of a subgroup of children with phonological disorders who demonstrate multiple articulation errors, effortful speech and slow progress in remediation is rarely questioned, but the nature, etiology, prognosis, and remediation of this disorder have been the subject of debate for a century" (110).
3. It has been suggested (Crary and Towne, 1984) that clinicians should work to better describe the basic motor properties of the deficits seen in dyspraxic children—in other words, keep better records of children's performance on both speech and non-speech tasks (for both those who are and are not perceived as evidencing motor articulation problems). In this way, we can refine our descriptions and make comparisons among clients.
4. One way to support the presence of a diagnostic category is to demonstrate that particular remediation procedures are effective in ameliorating symptoms. Documenting progress (single subject research designs can be useful in this regard) in response to particular intervention procedures can be helpful in testing the viability of the DAS diagnosis.
5. Love (1992) suggested that "despite the serious questions raised about the etiology, pathology, and validity of the reported signs and symptoms of the DVD syndrome, it remains an appropriate and useful diagnostic category of childhood motor speech disability" (95). He further suggested that DVD "provides substantial assistance in the differential diagnosis of the most prevalent speech disorder encountered by the speech-language pathologist—a developmental phonologic disorder, or so called

'functional articulation disorder.' The appropriate identification of children with phonologic disorders whose etiology is likely neurogenic rather than learned or idiopathic provides added explanatory power to the understanding, assessing, and managing of a select group of children with severe and often unyielding articulation defects that make them special problem cases for the speech-language pathologist" (98).

Chapter 7 presents suggestions for assessment and treatment of DVD.

Cognitive-Linguistic Factors

A second category of variables that have been studied relative to a possible relationship to phonologic productions is that of cognitive-linguistic factors. Historically, the field of communication sciences and disorders has been interested in the relationship between intelligence and the presence of speech sound disorders. In more recent years investigators have sought to describe the relationship between disordered phonology and additional aspects of cognitive-linguistic functioning. This not only is useful in determining the type of instructional/intervention program that may be most efficacious for the child's overall language development, but also helps to provide us with a better understanding of interrelationships of various components of language behavior.

Intelligence

The relationship between intelligence (as measured by IQ tests) and articulation disorders has been a subject of interest for many years, and of several investigations. Reid (1947a, 1947b) in a study of elementary and junior high school students reported that articulation proficiency could not be predicted from intelligence scores when the IQ was 70 or above. Winitz (1959a, 1959b), in his investigation of 150 children, reported similarly low positive correlations between scores obtained on the *Wechsler Intelligence Scale for Children* and the *Templin-Darley Articulation Screening Test*. Thus, in terms of the relationship between intelligence and articulation in children of normal intelligence, data have indicated that one is not a good predictor of the other.

A second perspective on the relationship between intelligence and phonology may be gleaned from studies of the phonological status of developmentally delayed individuals. Prior to 1970, a number of studies were conducted to explore the prevalence of articulation disorders in developmentally delayed individuals. Typical of these studies are those of Wilson (1966), Schlanger (1953), and Schlanger and Gottsleben (1957). Wilson used the *Hejina Articulation Test* in his study of 777 mentally retarded children whose chronological ages ranged from 6 to 16 years. He reported that 53.4 percent of the children evidenced articulation disorders. Errors of substitution, omission, and distortion tended to decrease as the mental ages of the children increased. Wilson (1966) concluded that "there is a high incidence of articulatory deviation in an educable mentally retarded population, and the incidence and degree of severity is closely related to mental-age levels" (432). Wilson's findings also indicated that articulatory skills, which continue to improve until approximately age 8 in the normal population, continue to show improvement well beyond that age in the retarded population.

Schlanger (1953) and Schlanger and Gottsleben (1957) reported similar findings to Wilson in their studies of articulation in the mentally retarded. Schlanger investigated 74 children in a residential school; the children's mean chronological age (C.A.) was 12;1, and their mean mental age (M.A.), 6;8. Of the 74 children, 56.7 percent were found to have articulation disorders. In their study of 400 randomly selected residents at a training school with a C.A. mean of 28;9 and a MA of 7;8, Schlanger and Gottsleben reported that 78 percent presented articulation delays ranging from slight to severe. Individuals with Down's Syndrome (DS) or whose etiologies were based upon central nervous system impairment demonstrated the most pronounced speech delay.

A review of specific phonologic errors (Bleile, 1982; Smith and Stoel-Gammon, 1983; Sommers, Reinhart, and Sistrunk, 1988) suggests that speech development and error patterns of persons with mental retardation are not qualitatively different from those of young normally developing children. Kumin, Council, and Goodman (1994) reported a great deal of variability in the age at which sounds emerge in the speech of children with DS. They also stated that these children do "not appear to follow the same order as the norms for acquisition for typically developing children" (300), and also that emergence of some sounds were as much as five years later than the age in which normally developing children acquire a sound.

Shriberg and Widder (1990) indicated that findings from nearly four decades of speech research in mental retardation can be summarized as follows:

1. Persons with mental retardation are likely to have articulation errors.
2. The most frequent type of articulation error is likely to be deletions of consonants.
3. Articulation errors are likely to be inconsistent.
4. The pattern of articulation errors is likely to be similar to that of very young children or children with "functional" articulation delay.

Several investigators have explored DS individuals, a genetically controlled subset of individuals with mental retardation. Sommers et al. (1988) reported that among the phonological errors evidenced by children with DS, ages 13 to 22 years, some were phonemes frequently seen in error in 5- and 6-year-olds of normal intelligence (i.e., /r/, /r/ clusters, /s/, /s/ clusters, /z/, /θ/, and /v/). The authors indicated that these errors would appear to support the assertion that the phonological development of children with DS follows the same general pattern as that of normal children. However, they also reported that DS children evidenced errors not typically seen in normal 5- and 6-year-olds (i.e., deletion of alveolar stops and nasals). They further reported that imitative and spontaneous single-word picture-naming responses of their subjects failed to identify many of the omission errors found in connected speech samples of their subjects.

Rosin, Swift, Bless, and Vetter (1988) studied the articulation of DS children as part of a study of overall communication profiles in this population. They compared a group of 10 DS male subjects (x C.A. = 14;7 years) with a control group of mentally retarded subjects, and two control groups of normals representing two age levels (x C.A. 6;1, 15;5).

They reported that as M.A. increased across subjects, intelligibility on a language sample increased. The DS group was also significantly different from the group of individuals with other forms of mental retardation and the younger age normal group (the older group was not compared) in terms of the percent of consonants correctly articulated on the *Goldman-Fristoe Test of Articulation.*

In addition to the speech measures mentioned above, Rosin and colleagues (1988) also included other language measures, an oral motor evaluation, and aerodynamic measures in their assessment. They reported that the DS group had difficulty with production measures as demands for sequencing increased (e.g., consonant-vowel repetitions, length of words). The DS group needed a significant amount of cueing in order to articulate the target /pataka/, and had more variable intraoral pressure when producing /papapaps/. The mean length of utterance of the DS group was also significantly shorter than the mentally retarded and normal groups. The authors indicated that these findings are in accord with observations of others and suggested that sequencing underlies both oral motor control and language problems evidenced in DS subjects.

Summary

Investigators concur that there is a low positive correlation between intelligence and articulatory function within the range of normal intelligence, and thus it can be inferred that intellectual functioning is of limited importance as a contributing factor to articulatory skill, and can be viewed as a poor predictor of articulation. On the other hand, a much higher correlation has been found between intelligence and articulation in the mentally retarded population. The articulatory skills in individuals with DS reflect error patterns similar to those seen in young normally developing children; however, they also evidence errors that are considered difficult or unusual when compared to normal developing children.

Language Development

Because phonology is one component of a child's developing linguistic system, there has been an interest in the relationship between phonologic development and development of other aspects of language (i.e., morphology/syntax, semantics, pragmatics). Of particular interest to clinical phonologists has been the extent to which delay or disorders in phonology may co-occur with delay or disorder in other aspects of language. Such co-occurrence of speech and language impairments has been reported in approximately 50 percent or more of a preschool population with phonological disorders (Tyler, Lewis, Haskill, and Tolbert, 2002).

Whitaker, Luper, and Pollio (1970) reported that children with articulation disorders were also impaired in language skills involving knowledge of phonological rules, form classes, and sentence structure. Subjects ranged in age from 6;1 to 7;7 and included both an articulation disorders group and a normal control group. All subjects in the disorders group failed to meet the cutoff score for 7-year-old children on the *Templin-Darley Articulation Screening Test.* The authors reported that the disordered group appeared to be developing language in the normal sequence but at a retarded rate.

Shriner, Holloway, and Daniloff (1969) compared the language skills of a normal control group with those of a group of 30 children between the ages of 5 and 8 who were considered to have severe articulation disorders (had at least seven articulatory errors and scored one standard deviation below the mean on the *Templin-Darley Tests of Articulation*). Subjects in the articulatory-defective group used significantly shorter and less complex utterances in their spontaneous conversation than members of the control group.

The relationship between articulation disorders and language comprehension was explored by Marquardt and Saxman (1972) using two groups of kindergarten children; one group performed one standard deviation or more below the norm for that age on the *Templin-Darley Tests of Articulation*, and the other (the control group) produced no more than one defective sound. The investigators administered the *Test of Auditory Comprehension of Language* and found that the impaired group made significantly more language comprehension errors than the control group. A correlation of scores obtained on both measures revealed that children who made the greatest number of articulation errors also made the greatest number of errors in language comprehension.

Gross, St. Louis, Ruscello, and Hull (1985) studied the language skills of three groups of school-age subjects: (1) a group with multiple articulation errors; defined as those with at least two errors in the final position; with /l/, /r/, and /s/ not included in this consideration; (2) a group with residual articulation errors; defined as two or more positional errors for at least one of the following phonemes: /l/, /r/, and /s/. Consonant cluster errors on these phonemes were allowed, but subjects could have no other phonemic errors; and (3) a normal control group. A total of 144 subjects from grades 1, 3, 5, and 7 were included in this retrospective study. The investigators reported that mean language structural scores for completeness and complexity were significantly lower for the multiple error group than the residual error and control groups. Scores for length of utterances were not significantly different among groups. The total number of language errors reduced progressively from multiple error to residual error to control groups.

Research investigations such as those cited above, which have attempted to explore the correlation between certain aspects of language and phonology, have generally reported a moderate correlation between phonologic and language disorders. After reviewing literature related to the language-phonology relationship, Tyler and Watterson (1991) indicated that one might expect to find disorders of language and phonology co-occurring in 60 to 80 percent of the young children who have been identified as having a disorder of one type or the other. Shriberg and Kwiatkowski (1994) reported that based on 178 children with developmental phonological disorders between 50 to 70 percent of the children will have productive language involvement and 10 to 40 percent will also have a delay in language comprehension.

Some investigators have attempted to further study and explain the interaction between phonology and other aspects of language, especially syntax. A common perception is that language is organized "from the top down"—in other words, a speaker goes from pragmatic intent, to semantic coding, to syntactic structure, to phonologic productions. Thus, higher-level linguistic formulations may ultimately be reflected in a child's phonologic productions. If this theory is accurate, it might be expected that the more complex the syntax, the more likely a child is to evidence linguistic breakdown, which may then be evidenced in phonologic productions. Schmauch, Panagos, and Klich (1978) conducted a study in which 5-year-old children with phonologic and language problems were required to produce certain nouns (drawn from phonologic inventories) in three syntactic contexts; that is, an isolated noun phrase (the simplest context), a declarative sentence, and a passive sentence (the most complex context). These investigators reported a 17 percent increase in articulatory errors between the noun phrase and each of the sentence contexts. They also reported that later developing consonants were those most influenced by syntactical complexity and that error productions reflected quantitative rather than qualitative changes.

A follow-up study of the top-down notion was conducted by Panagos, Quine, and Klich (1979). In this study, 5-year-old children were required to produce 15 target consonants in noun phrases, declarative sentences, and passive sentences; consonants appeared in the initial and final word-positions of one- and two-syllable words. Syntax was again found to significantly influence articulatory accuracy, as did number of syllables in target words. Word position did not influence phonologic accuracy. The authors further reported that two sources of complexity—phonologic (including difficulty with later developing consonants as well as specific contexts) and syntactic—combined additively to increase the number of phonologic errors. From the easiest context (final word position of one-syllable words in noun phrases) to the hardest (final word position of two-syllable word in passive sentences), there was a 36 percent increase in articulatory errors. The effects of grammatical complexity on articulatory accuracy were cumulative.

A second perspective on the language-phonology relationship suggests that linguistic influences operate "from the bottom up." In this view, language expression is regulated by feedback (internal and external) from phonologic performance. Feedback from phonologic performance is needed to maintain syntactic processing and accuracy, especially when errors occur and must be corrected.

Panagos and Prelock (1982) conducted a study to test the hypothesis that phonologic structure influences children's syntactic processing. Ten children with language disorders were required to produce sentences containing words with varying syllable complexity; that is, **simple**: "The (CV) kid (CVC) pushed (CVCC) the (CV) car (CVC) in (VC) the (CV) room (CVC)," and **complex**: "The (CV) chocolate (CVCVCVC) is (VC) in (VC) the (CV) napkin (CVCCVC)." In addition, sentence complexity was varied from unembedded ("The girl washed the doll in the tub") to right embedded ("The cook washed the pot the boy dropped") to center embedded ("The lady the uncle liked sewed the coat"). The results of the study supported the hypothesis. When subjects repeated sentences containing words of greater syllable complexity, they made 27 percent more syntactic errors. In addition to this bottom-up influence, Panagos and Prelock (1982) also reported that syntactic complexity further compounded production difficulties. From the unembedded to the center embedded, there was a 57 percent increase in phonologic errors.

These findings support the view that a simultaneous top-down bottom-up relationship exists between language and phonology. Another way of expressing this concept is to consider that children with disordered language-phonology have a limited encoding capacity; and the more this capacity is strained at one level or another, the greater the probability of delay in one component or more of language. It should be pointed out that the investigators who have examined the affect of complexity on the language-phonology relationship have typically employed elicited imitation tasks, and thus complexity of utterances was controlled by the investigators. It can be argued that with this type of performance task, structural simplifications are expected outcomes. Elicited imitation tasks do not reflect the conditions present when a child is engaged in conversation, and thus we cannot assume that constraints of the nature demonstrated by Panagos and Prelock (1982) can predict behavior in a conversational context (Paul and Shriberg, 1984).

In an investigation by Paul and Shriberg (1982) designed to study phonologic productions as they relate to particular morphophonemic structures, continuous speech samples were obtained from 30 speech-delayed children. They reported that certain of their subjects were able to produce complex morphosyntactic contexts spontaneously, which did not result in phonologic simplifications. In other words, some of their subjects were able to maintain a similar level of phonologic production in spite of producing more complex syntactic targets. They (Paul and Shriberg, 1984) suggested that children may "do things other than phonologic simplification in an attempt to control complexity in spontaneous speech" (319). They summarized by indicating that some speech-delayed children are sometimes able to allocate their limited linguistic resources to realize phonologic targets consistent with their linguistic knowledge in the context of free speech, even though at other times they may use avoidance strategies or other means of reducing the encoding load.

The simultaneous top-down bottom-up relationship between phonology and other aspects of language is reflected in the concept of a snyergistic view of language (Schwartz, Leonard, Folger, and Wilcox, 1980; Shriner et al., 1969). This perspective assumes a complex interaction and interdependency of various aspects of linguistic behaviors including language and phonology.

Several investigators have studied whether intervention focused on one aspect of the linguistic domain (e.g., morphosyntax), facilitates gains in an untreated domain (e.g., phonology). Matheny and Panagos (1978) looked at the effects of syntactic programming on phonologic improvement and the effects of phonologic programming on syntactic improvement in school-age children. Each group made the greatest gains in the treated domain as compared to a control group, but also made improvements in the untreated domain. Similar findings were reported by Wilcox and Morris (1995). They reported that children with phonological and language impairments who participated in a preschool language-focused program made gains not only in language, but in phonology as well, based on comparison to a control group. Hoffman, Norris, and Monjure (1990), in a study based on two siblings from a set of triplets, also found that a narrative intervention program facilitated gains in both language and phonology for one brother, while gains in phonology only were achieved by the brother who only received phonologic instruction.

One of the more comprehensive studies of cross-domain improvement between language (morphosyntax) and phonology was reported by Tyler and colleagues (2002). They compared treatment outcomes for three groups of children, all of whom evidenced both phonologic and morphosyntactic disorders: (1) Group 1 received morphosyntactic instruction for a 12-week block, followed by 12 weeks in phonology; (2) Group 2 reversed the order of the 12-week blocks; and (3) Group 3 served as a control group. These investigators reported that in comparison to the control group, both interventions were effective; however, only morphosyntactic instruction led to cross-domain improvement (i.e., language therapy improved phonology but not the reverse).

These findings have not been supported in all investigations of cross-domain improvements.

Tyler and Watterson (1991) reported that subjects with a severe overall language and phonological disorder made improvements in language when presented with language therapy; however, gains were not made in phonology (they actually reported a tendency for performance to become slightly worse). On the other hand, subjects with mild-moderate but unequal impairments in phonology and language improved in both areas when presented with phonologic therapy. The authors suggested that a language-based intervention program may not result in improvement in phonologic as well as other language skills for children whose disorders are severe and comparable in each domain. However, children with less severe problems in one or both domains may benefit from therapy with either a language or phonology focus.

Fey, Cleave, Ravida, Long, Dejmal, and Easton (1994) conducted an experimental treatment program with 26 subjects, ages 44–70 months, with impairments in both grammar and phonology. Eighteen children received language intervention (grammar facilitation) in accord with one or another of two designated teaching approaches and eight children served as controls. Results indicated that despite a strong effect for intervention on the children's grammatical output, there were no direct effects on the subjects' phonologic productions. The authors indicated that trying to improve intelligibility by focusing on grammar is not defensible for children in the age and severity range of their subjects. They further indicated that for most children who have impairments in both speech and language, intervention will need to be focused on both areas. While this study only examined one form of language intervention that anticipated phonologic effects, these data provide strong evidence that in children aged 4–6 treatment approaches should address phonologic problems directly if changes in phonologic performance are to be expected.

Tyler and colleagues (2002) have indicated that differences in findings between the their study and that of the Fey and colleagues (1994) study may be due to differences in goal selection, intervention techniques, or measures used to determine changes in phonology. Further clinical studies are needed to clarify the synergistic relationship between language and phonology, including cross-domain improvements. The influence of age, nature and severity of both language and phonologic disorders, treatment approaches employed, and measures used to ascertain progress all need further study.

Summary

Research has shown that younger children with severe phonologic disorders are more likely to evidence language problems than those with mild-moderate delay and that between 60 to 80 percent of moderate to severely involved phonologically delayed children are likely to also have language delay. Language and phonology may be related in what has been termed a synergistic relationship. Investigators face the challenge of further defining the intricacies of the relationship between phonology and other linguistic behaviors in terms of both development and clinical management of disorders. It appears that for children with language impairment and moderate to severe phonologic delay, direct phonologic intervention may be required in order to impact phonology. Further research in cross-domain generalization is needed to guide clinical practice in this area.

Academic Performance

The relationship between phonologic disorders and academic performance is of interest to clinicians working with school-age children since oral language skills are fundamental to the development of many literacy related academic skills such as reading and spelling. Because the use of sounds in symbolic lexical units is a task common to learning to speak, read, and write, researchers for many years have studied the co-occurrence of reading and articulation disorders, and have discussed possible common factors underlying the acquisition of literacy and other language-related skills.

Hall (1938) compared 21 children with functional articulation disorders with a normal control group on the *Gates Silent Reading Test* and the *Iowa Silent Reading Test* and reported no significant differences in silent reading achievement between the two groups. Everhart (1953) also used the *Gates Silent Reading Test* and reported no significant relationship between articulatory disorders and reading ability, although boys with normal articulation tended to obtain higher reading scores than the overall group of children with articulation disorders.

The relationship between reading readiness and articulation development in children with and without defective articulation was studied by Fitzsimons (1958) and Weaver, Furbee, and Everhart (1960). Fitzsimons used the *Metropolitan Reading Readiness Test* to determine the status of reading readiness and reported that below grade-level scores were more frequent among children with articulation disorders than among those with normally developing articulation. Weaver and colleagues (1960) reported a significant relationship between articulatory performance and reading readiness as well as between articulatory performance and reading scores.

Flynn and Byrne (1970) took a different approach to exploring the relationship between articulation disorders and reading. They compared articulatory performance of 52 advanced and 42 delayed third-grade readers on the *Templin-Darley Tests of Articulation*. Those who scored 4.2 or higher on the *Iowa Test of Basic Skills* were classified as advanced readers; those who scored 2.2 or lower were classified as delayed readers. The authors reported no significant difference between the two groups in articulation test scores.

Lewis and Freebairn-Far (1991) conducted a cross-sectional study designed to examine the performance of individuals with a history of a preschool phonologic disorder on measures of phonology, reading, and spelling. Groups of subjects included at least 17 individuals from each of the following categories: preschool, school age, adolescence, and adulthood. Normal comparison groups at each age level were also tested. Significant differences between the disordered and normal groups were reported on the reading and spelling measures for the school-age group, and on the reading measure for the adult group. Although the reading and spelling measures for the adolescent group and the spelling measure for the adult group did not reach significance, the trend was for the individuals with histories of disorders to perform more poorly than normals. Data also indicated that subjects who evidenced a phonologic disorder accompanied by additional language problems performed more poorly on measures of reading and spelling than subjects with phonologic disorders only. The authors indicated that children evidencing phonologic impairment are at-risk for reading and spelling problems in school and may have special educational needs.

Felsenfeld, McGue, and Broen (1995) conducted a comparison study of the children of 24 adults with a documented history of a phonologic-language disorder that persisted from childhood until at least grade 11 (proband group), and 28 adults who were known to have had normal articulation abilities as children (control group). Included among the comparison variables were several categorized under "educational performance." Results revealed that 28 percent of the children of the proband group repeated at least one grade, compared to 0 percent from the control group. Likewise, 22 percent of the proband children compared to 4 percent of the controls had received academic tutoring. Speech treatment had been received by 33 percent of the proband group and 0 percent of the control group. They also reported that half of the school-age children who were receiving speech treatment were also either participating in remedial academic services and/or had repeated a grade.

While interest has traditionally focused on the co-occurrence of reading-spelling and phonologic disorders in children, more recently there has also been interest in children's ability to process phonology as part of various reading tasks. More specifically, some reading-disabled students may lack awareness of individual sounds, have difficulty dividing words into sounds, and recalling sound-symbol relationships (phonologic awareness). Catts (1986) found that reading-disabled children may have problems with these linguistically oriented tasks and yet not reflect phonologic impairment.

Investigators have attempted to apply phonologic concepts to aid in the understanding of reading and spelling disorders. This activity is based on the assumption that acquisition of speaking, reading, and writing skills involves the analysis of sounds in lexical units, which may be related to underlying cognitive-linguistic processes. In particular, the concepts of phonologic processes and underlying internal knowledge of the sound system have been employed to aid in understanding the development of spelling and reading skills (Hoffman and Norris, 1989).

Liberman and Shankweiler (1985), in a discussion of the phonologic basis of literacy, indicated that reading success was related to the degree to which children were aware of "underlying phonologic structure" and that poor readers often were unable to segment words into their phonologic constituents. They suggested that a relationship exists between children's readiness for reading and spelling and their metalinguistic awareness of the internal structure of words. O'Conner and Jenkins (1999) reported that performance on phonological awareness tasks (e.g., initial sound identification, rhyme production, phoneme segmentation) in kindergarten predicted differences in reading achievement at the end of first grade, and was reliable in identifying children who would later be diagnosed as having a reading disability.

Catts (1991) suggested that speech-language pathologists working in school systems should seek to develop programs designed to facilitate "phonologic awareness" in children, particularly those at risk for reading disabilities. Catts suggested that "phonologic awareness" activities might include activities designed to increase awareness of syllables, phonemes, manner of phoneme production, and sound positions in words. Activities to accomplish these goals could include sound play, rhyming, alliteration, and segmentation tasks. This topic, including how it relates to phonologic disorders, is discussed in greater detail in Chapter 9.

Hoffman and Norris (1989) analyzed spelling errors of 45 elementary school children for evidence of phonologic process patterns. They reported that many of the spelling errors involved both syllable reduction and feature changes similar to the sound simplifications seen in the speech of young children with normal speech development. They further indicated that even though children had acquired normal speech, they exhibited spelling errors similar to those seen in the speech simplifications of younger children. Hoffman (1990) related specific types of developmental spelling patterns to stages of normal phonologic acquisition. For example, "precommunicative spellings" (seemingly random selection of letters of the alphabet to represent words), were described as parallel to the random sound productions of babbling. "Semiphonetic spellings" (letters used to represent sounds, but only some of the sounds are represented, e.g., *E* for *eagle*), were described as parallel to the stage where children delete syllables or segments and substitute sound classes for one another. He also indicated that because the speech-language pathologist is the school-based professional who has the most detailed knowledge of sound perception and production, phonologic organization, stages of acquisition, and methods of phonologic description, he or she is in a good position to serve as a resource to teachers regarding the application of phonologic concepts to the understanding of spelling errors. Chapter 9 focuses on phonological awareness and its relationship to literacy and the role of the speech-language pathologist in literacy.

Summary

Research investigations that have focused on the co-occurrence of phonologic and literacy impairments indicate a possible relationship between these disorders in some children. Data indicate that young children with severe phonologic and/or other language disorders are at risk for academic problems, and there may be a familial propensity for such difficulties. The role of "phonologic awareness" in the development of reading and spelling skills has been the focus of a lot study in the last decade. Parallels have been made between the use of phonologic processes and stages in the acquisition of oral language and acquisition of reading and spelling skills. It has been suggested that speech-language pathologists are in a unique position to offer assistance to the classroom teacher in their efforts to assist children at risk for reading and/or spelling problems.

Psychosocial Factors

Psychosocial factors represent a third cluster of variables that have long fascinated clinicians in terms of their potential relationship to phonology. Age, gender, family history, and socioeconomic status have been studied in an effort to better understand factors that may precipitate or otherwise be associated with phonologic impairment.

Age

Chapters 2 and 3 reviewed the literature on phonologic acquisition. Investigations of phonologic development have revealed that children's articulatory and phonologic skills continue to improve until approximately 8 years of age, by which time the normal child has acquired most aspects of the adult sound system. In fact, it appears that by age 4 normally developing children have articulation skills that closely resemble that of adults.

Speech-language pathologists use normative information concerning phonologic development as a guide in case selection and for determining treatment goals. Clinicians should keep in mind that the order in which sounds are incorporated into speech varies from child to child and does not necessarily follow a specific sequence. There is no indication that one sound is dependent on any other for its development.

Speech-language pathologists have shown a particular interest in the effect of maturation on children identified as having phonologic disorders. Roe and Milisen (1942) sampled 1,989 children in grades 1 through 6 and found that the children's mean number of articulation errors decreased between grades 1 and 2, grades 2 and 3, and grades 3 and 4. In contrast, the difference in the mean number of errors between grades 4 and 5 and grades 5 and 6 was not significant. The authors concluded that maturation was responsible for improvement in articulation performance between grades 1 and 4 but was not an appreciable factor in articulation improvement in grades 5 and 6.

Sayler (1949) assessed articulation in 1,998 students in grades 7 through 12 as they read sentences orally. His findings indicated a slight decrease in the mean number of articulation errors at each subsequent grade level, but because the improvement in speech sound productions was so small, he concluded that maturation does not appear to be an appreciable factor in improvement in the secondary grades. Children in upper elementary and secondary grades appear to be more consistent in their phonologic patterns than children in the lower elementary grades.

Factors that relate to normal phonologic variations during the school years include refinement of the timing of sequential articulatory gestures, the influence of reading and spelling, and peer influence (Vihman, Chapter 3 of this book). These factors, however, would only result in, at most, minor phonologic variations within this age group.

Summary

Acquisition by a child of the adult speech sound system has been shown to be related to maturation. There is a direct correlation between improvement in articulation skills and age through approximately age 8, when phonologic mastering is essentially complete in normally developing, children. Maturation generally is not a factor in speech sound acquisition after age 9 in normally developing children.

Gender

Child development specialists have long been interested in contrasts between males and females in phonologic acquisition, and, likewise, speech-language pathologists have investigated the relationship between gender and articulation status. Research in this area has focused on (1) a comparison of phoneme acquisition in males and females, and (2) a comparison of the incidence of phonologic disorders in males and females.

Dawson (1929) examined the articulatory skills of 200 children from grades 1 through 12 on six measures of articulation. He reported that until approximately age 12, girls were slightly superior to boys in their articulatory skills. Templin (1963) reported similar findings: "In articulation development, girls consistently are found to be slightly accelerated . . . in all instances the differences are relatively small and often are not statistically significant" (13).

Smit, Hand, Freilinger, Bernthal, and Bird (1990) conducted a large-scale normative study of phonologic development in children ages 3 through 9 from Iowa and Nebraska. They reported that the Iowa-Nebraska girls appeared to acquire sounds at somewhat earlier ages than boys through age 6. The differences reached statistical significance only at age 6 and younger and not in every preschool age group. Kenney and Prather (1986), who elicited multiple productions of frequent error sounds, reported significant differences favoring girls in the age range 3 through 5.

Speech surveys conducted by Hall (1938), Mills and Streit (1942), Morley (1952), Everhart (1960), and Hull, Mielke, Timmons, and Willeford (1971) indicated that the incidence of articulation disorder was higher in males than females, regardless of the age group studied. Smit and colleagues (1990) stated that "it is a well-known fact that boys are at much greater risk than girls for delayed speech, and this propensity continues to be reported" (790).

Summary

The sex of a child does not appear to be a significant factor in phonologic acquisition. It should be recognized, however, that at certain ages females tend to be slightly ahead of males in phonologic acquisition, and significantly more male than female children are identified as being phonologically delayed.

Family Background

Researchers have been interested in the influence of family background, both environmental and biological, and how it may affect a child's speech and language development. In the paragraphs below we will review literature related to family background and phonology organized around three topics: (1) socioeconomic status, (2) family transmission, and (3) sibling influences.

Socioeconomic Status

The socioeconomic status of a child's family, as measured by parents' educational background, parental occupation, income, and location of family residence, is a significant part of the child's environment. Since some behavioral deficiencies occur more frequently in lower socioeconomic environments, socioeconomic status has been of interest to speech-language clinicians as a possible factor in language development.

Everhart (1953, 1956) explored the variable of parental occupational status in an investigation of the relationship between articulation and other developmental factors in children. In speech surveys of children in grades 1 through 6, those classified as having articulation disorders were compared to children with normal articulation development with respect to parental occupation. No significant differences were found, and Everhart concluded that the occurrence of articulation disorders in children was not related to parental occupation.

Templin (1957) analyzed developmental language data from children aged 3 to 8 years in terms of parental occupation and reached a somewhat different conclusion. She used the *Minnesota Scale for Parental Occupations* to categorize parental occupation. At each age level, children whose parents were in the upper occupational group had fewer misarticulations than the children in the lower occupational group. In particular, 4-, 4½-, and 7-year-old children whose parents were in the lower occupational group had significantly more articulation errors than those whose parents were in the upper group. Templin concluded that parental occupation seemed to be a factor in children's articulation skill until about age 4 but that parental occupation no longer seemed to influence articulation development by the time children were 8 years old.

Weaver and colleagues (1960) also investigated the relationship between parental occupation and articulation proficiency in 592 first-grade children and found that a greater number of children with normal articulation skills came from homes in the upper occupational group, whereas more children with articulation errors came from homes in the lower occupational group. The poorest articulation proficiency, as judged by number of articulation errors, was found among children from the two lowest occupational classes.

Prins (1962a) found no significant correlation between articulation and socioeconomic level for 92 articulatory defective children between the ages of 2 and 6 years. Likewise, Smit and colleagues (1990) in the Iowa-Nebraska normative study reported that socioeconomic level did not have a significant relationship to articulatory performance. After an extensive review of the literature on the relationship between articulation and socioeconomic status, Winitz (1969) concluded that "more misarticulating children and more articulatory errors are found in the lower socioeconomic groups than in the upper socioeconomic groups. However, when a correlational index is used, the relationship is low or nonsignificant" (147).

Familial Tendencies

It is not uncommon for speech-language pathologists to observe a family history of developmental speech and language disorders. While information of this nature is often noted in diagnostic reports, until the 1980s few systematic attempts were made to study phonologic disorders as they related to family history. Neils and Aram (1986) obtained reports from the parents of 74 preschool language-disordered children and indicated that 46 percent reported that other family members had histories of speech and language disorders. Of this group, 55 percent were reported to have articulation disorders, the most prevalent type of familial disorder reported. Shriberg and Kwiatkowski (1994) reported data from sixty-two 3- to 6-year-old children with developmental phonologic disorders. They found that 39 percent of the children had one member of the family with the same speech problem, while an additional 17 percent (total = 56 percent) had more than one family member with the same speech problem.

Two twin studies have been reported that contribute to our understanding of familial influences, including genetic factors that may relate to phonologic disorders. Matheny and Bruggeman (1973) studied 101 same-sex twin sets, 22 opposite-sex twin sets, and 94 siblings between the ages of 3 and 8 years. An articulation screening test was administered to each child. Monozygotic twins' articulation screening correlated more closely with each other than did dizygotic twins' scores. The authors concluded that there is a strong hereditary influence on articulation status. In addition, sex differences were found to favor females. Locke and Mather (1987) examined speech sound productions in 13 monozygotic and 13 dizygotic twin sets. They reported more phonetic concordance in the monozygotic than the dizygotic twins.

Lewis, Ekelman, and Aram (1989) examined the familial basis of phonologic disorders by comparing sibling articulation status for a group of children identified as evidencing a severe phonologic disorder, and a group who reflected normal phonologic development. Phonologic measures included the *Natural Process Analysis*, repetition of 50 multisyllabic words, and the *Screening Test for Developmental Verbal Apraxia*. In addition, language, gross and fine motor skills, and reading were assessed. Family histories of communication disorders and/or learning disabilities were noted. Results revealed that the siblings of the disordered children performed more poorly than control siblings on phonology and reading measures. Disordered subjects' phonologic skills correlated positively with those of their siblings, whereas controls' scores did not. Families of disordered children reported significantly more members with speech and language disorders and dyslexia than did families of controls. Sex differences were reflected in the incidence but not in the severity or type of disorder present. The authors concluded that their findings suggested a familial basis for at least some forms of severe phonologic disorders.

One of the most interesting studies of the familial basis of phonologic impairments was conducted by Felsenfeld and colleagues (1995). These investigators utilized speech and academic development data involving 400 normally developing children that was gathered between 1960 and 1972 by Templin and Glaman (1976). From this sample, two follow-up groups were identified consisting of 24 adults with a history of a moderate phonologic-language disorder as children, and a control group of 28 adults with a documented history of normal articulation development. Results demonstrated that in comparison to the children of controls, the children of the "disordered" subjects performed significantly more poorly on all tests of articulation and expressive language functioning and were significantly more likely to have received articulation treatment. There was, however, no evidence that specific misarticulations or phonologic processes could be identified with the "disorders" families.

It may be inferred from the studies reviewed above that genetic or biological inheritance factors may precipitate phonologic impairment, yet it is often difficult to separate environmental from genetic/biological influences. A study that examined environmental influences was reported by Parlour and Broen (1991). Their research was predicated on the possibility that individuals who themselves experienced significant speech and language disorders as children are likely to become adults who will provide a less than optimal cultural or linguistic milieu for their own families.

Parlour and Broen (1991) collected follow-up family data of adults with and without a childhood history of delayed phonologic development. Both groups of subjects were originally part of the large normative study that was conducted by Mildred Templin (1968), 28 years earlier. The group who had displayed a moderate to moderately severe phonologic disorder in early elementary school was comprised of 24 individuals. The control group was comprised of 28 adults who had evidenced average or better articulation during the same time period. Two environmental measures, the *Preschool HOME Scale* and the *Mod-*

ified Templin Child-Rearing Questionnaire, were employed to ascertain qualitative aspects of a child's environment including physical, emotional, and cognitive support available to preschool children, and child-rearing practices. These two measures included direct observation of the examiner, parental reports, and parental responses to a written questionnaire.

The two groups performed in a generally comparable manner for all of the environmental domains sampled, with one exception, acceptance, which assessed disciplinary practices. Parlour and Broen (1991) reported that families with a history of phonologic disorders were more reliant on physical punishment than were control families. In terms of future research efforts, the authors suggested that although differences were generally not significant between the groups, the disordered group received lower mean scores than controls on each of the Home subscales, suggesting that some subtle differences may have been present, particularly for domains involving the use of punishment, learning, and language stimulation.

Sibling Influence

Another factor of interest to investigators of phonologic acquisition has been sibling number and birth order. Since the amount of time that parents can spend with each child decreases with each child added to a family, some clinicians have questioned whether sibling status is related to articulatory development. Koch (1956) studied the relationships between certain speech and voice characteristics in young children and siblings in two-child families. In this study, 384 children between 5 and 6 years old were divided into 24 subgroups matched individual by individual on the basis of age, socioeconomic class, and residence. Data on speech and voice characteristics consisted of teachers' ratings. Koch reported that firstborn children had better articulation than secondborn, and the wider the age difference between a child and his or her sibling, the better the child's articulation. Likewise, Davis (1937) reported that children without siblings demonstrated superior articulatory performance to children with siblings and to twins. On the other hand, Wellman, Case, Mengert, and Bradbury (1931) did not find a significant relationship between the number of siblings and level of articulation skill for 3-year-olds.

Twins have been reported to present unique patterns of speech sound acquisition (Perkins, 1977; Powers, 1971; Winitz, 1969). From birth, twins receive speech stimulation not only from others within their environment but also from each other. Powers (1971) indicated that the "emotional ties of twins, too, are likely to be closer than those of singled siblings, which further augments their interdependence in speech" (868). It is not uncommon for twins to reflect common phonologic patterns and use similar phonologic processes. Schwartz and colleagues (1980) reported, however, that in the very early stages of phonologic acquisition (the first 50 words), similarities in phonemes used, including phonologic patterns and lexical items, were not present. Unique patterns of speech occasionally found in twins 2 years and older that have little resemblance to adult models and have meaning only to the twins are termed *idioglossia*.

Summary

Little relationship exists between socioeconomic and articulation status based on available reports. Although greater numbers of misarticulating children tend to be found in lower socioeconomic groups (especially children under 4 years), socioeconomic status does not appear to contribute significantly to the presence of a phonologic disorder.

Studies of phonologic development in twins, as well as in families with a history of phonologic impairment, suggest some sort of familial propensity toward the presence of such a disorder. Investigations examining phonologic status and sibling relationships are limited, but findings have been fairly consistent. Firstborn and only children exhibit better articulation performance than children with older siblings or twins. The age span between siblings also appears to affect phonologic proficiency, with better articulation associated with wider age differences. One can speculate that the firstborn or only child receives better speech models and greater stimulation than the child who has older siblings. The possibility also exists that older siblings produce "normal" developmental phonologic errors and, thus at points in time present imperfect speech models to younger siblings. Unique patterns of sound productions have been reported in twins; reasons for these patterns are speculative and tend to focus on the stimulation each twin receives from the other. Unique speech patterns have, however, been reported, even in very young twins.

Personality

The relationship between personality characteristics and phonologic behavior has been investigated to determine if particular personality patterns are likely to be associated with phonologic disorders. Researchers have examined not only the child's personality traits but also those of the child's parents, using various assessment tools.

Bloch and Goodstein (1971) concluded, in a review of the literature, that personality traits and emotional adjustment of individuals with articulatory disorders have shown contradictory findings and attributed this to two major problems with the investigations: (1) the criteria for defining articulatory impairment has varied from one study to the next, and (2) the tools or instruments used to assess personality and adjustment have varied in their validity and reliability.

In a causal-correlates profile based on 178 children with developmental phonologic disorders, Shriberg and Kwiatkowski (1994) presented data on psychosocial inputs (parental behaviors) and psychosocial behaviors (child characteristics) that were descriptive of this population. Twenty-seven (27) percent of the parents were judged to be either somewhat or considerably ineffective in terms of behavioral management, and 17 percent were either somewhat or considerably overconcerned about their child's problem. An even smaller percentage of parents indicated that it was their perception that their child had difficulty with initial acceptance by peers. Over half the children (51 percent) were described as somewhat too sensitive (easily hurt feelings), and an additional 14 percent were described as overly sensitive (very easily hurt feelings). They reported that their descriptive data indicated that "a significant number of children with developmental phonologic disorders experience psychosocial difficulties" (1115). They indicated, however, that one cannot be completely certain that sampling biases did not inflate the magnitudes of the findings, or whether the subjects would differ significantly from data in a nonspeech-delayed group.

Parlour and Broen (1991) studied environmental factors in the homes of 24 adults who as children evidenced moderate to moderately severe phonologic disorders, and a control group of adults who as children evidenced average or better articulation. Two environmental measures, the *Preschool HOME Scale* and the *Modified Templin Child-Rearing Questionnaire*, were used to study and rate aspects of the home presumed to reflect the quality of physical, emotional, and cognitive support available to a preschool child. While the findings for the two groups were generally similar, mean scores for the group with a history of phonologic disorders were lower than for the normal group. A significant difference between the two groups was found in disciplinary practices, suggesting that some children with phonologic disorders came from families that were more reliant on physical punishment than were control families.

Summary

While certain personality characteristics have been linked to some children with developmental phonologic impairments, no clear picture of personality variance from normals has emerged in this population. Likewise, certain parental/home variables have been associated with this population, but the strength of that association is unclear. Further studies involving normal–disordered child comparisons are necessary before a definitive statement regarding this causal-correlate can be made.

Conclusion

The speech-language pathologist must have a basic knowledge of factors related to phonologic disorders in order to assess phonologic status, plan remediation programs, and counsel clients and their parents. This is particularly true when there is impairment in the structure and function of the speech and hearing mechanism. Despite the large body of literature reflecting investigations of a wide variety of variables potentially related to articulation impairments, many questions remain unanswered. One truth that emerges from the literature, however, is the absence of any one-to-one correspondence between the presence of a particular etiological factor and the precise nature of most individuals' phonologic status. Prediction of cause-effect relationships represents a scientific ideal, but determination of such relationships in the realm of human behavior, including communication disorders, is often difficult.

QUESTIONS FOR CHAPTER 4

1. Cite specific examples wherein knowledge of etiology is highly important, if not essential, to developing an effective and efficient intervention program.

2. What is the relationship of speech sound perception and speech sound errors?

3. What is the relationship between phonological disorders and morphosyntactic language impairments?

4. What is the relationship of phonological delay, phonological awareness, and a child's acquisition of literacy?

5. Explain "correlation does not imply causation."

6. How is each of the following factors related to clinical phonology and speech production?

A. Otitis media

B. Tongue thrusting

C. Missing teeth

D. Apraxia

E. Mental retardation

F. Severe language impairment in young children

G. Poor literacy skills

H. Lower socioeconomic status

I. Dental braces

J. Significant hearing loss

K. Family history of phonological difficulties

L. Removal of part of the tongue

REFERENCES

American Speech-Language-Hearing Association, "Report of ad hoc committee on labial-lingual posturing function." *Asha*, 31 (1989): 92–94.

American Speech-Language-Hearing Association, "The role of the speech-language pathologist in management of oral myofunctional disorders." *Asha*, 33 (Suppl. 5) (1991): 7.

Arndt, W., M. Elbert, and R. Shelton, "Standardization of a test of oral stereognosis." In J. Bosman (Ed.), *Second Symposium on Oral Sensation and Perception*. Springfield, Ill: Chas. C. Thomas, 1970.

Arnst, D., and D. Fucci, "Vibrotactile sensitivity of the tongue in hearing impaired subjects." *Journal of Auditory Research*, 15 (1975): 115–118.

Aungst, L., and J. Frick, "Auditory discrimination ability and consistency of articulation of /r/." *Journal of Speech and Hearing Disorders*, 29 (1964): 76–85.

Backus, O., "Speech rehabilitation following excision of tip of the tongue." *American Journal of the Disabled Child*, 60 (1940): 368–370.

Bankson, N., and M. Byrne, "The relationship between missing teeth and selected consonant sounds." *Journal of Speech and Hearing Disorders*, 24 (1962): 341–348.

Barton, D., "The role of perception in the acquisition of phonology." Ph.D. Dissertation, University of London, 1976.

Bernstein, M., "The relation of speech defects and malocclusion." *American Journal of Orthodontia*, 40 (1954): 149–150.

Bishop, M., R. Ringel, and H. House, "Orosensory perception, speech production and deafness." *Journal of Speech and Hearing Research*, 16 (1973): 257–266.

Bleile, K., "Consonant ordering in Down's Syndrome," *Journal of Communicative Disorders*, 15 (1982): 275–285.

Bloch, R., and L. Goodstein, "Functional speech disorders and personality: A decade of research," *Journal of Speech and Hearing Disorders*, 36 (1971): 295–314.

Bloomer, H., and A. Hawk, "Speech considerations: Speech disorders associated with ablative surgery of the face, mouth and pharynx—ablative approaches to learning." In *ASHA Report #8: Orofacial Anomalies*. Washington, DC: ASHA, 1973.

Bordon, G., "Consideration of motor-sensory targets and a problem of perception." In H. Winitz (Ed.), *Treating Articulation Disorders: For Clinicians by Clinicians*. Austin, Tex.: Pro-Ed, 1984.

Butterfield, E., and G. Cairns, "Discussion-summary of infant reception research." In R. Schiefulbusch and L. Lloyd (Eds.), *Language Perspectives: Acquisition, Retardation and Intervention*. Baltimore, Md.: University Park Press, 1974.

Calvert, D., "Articulation and hearing impairments." In L. Lass, J. Northern, D. Yoder, and L. McReynolds (Eds.), *Speech, Language and Hearing*. Vol. 2. Philadelphia: Saunders, 1982.

Canning, B., and M. Rose, "Clinical measurements of the speech, tongue and lip movements in British children with normal speech." *British Journal of Disorders of Communication, 9* (1974): 45–50.

Carrell, J., and K. Pendergast, "An experimental study of the possible relation between errors of speech and spelling." *Journal of Speech and Hearing Disorders, 19* (1954): 327–334.

Catts, H. W., "Speech, production/phonological deficits in reading-disordered children." *Learning Disabilities, 19* (1986): 504–508.

Catts, H. W., "Facilitating phonological awareness: Role of speech-language pathologists." *Language, Speech, and Hearing Services in Schools, 22* (1991): 196–203.

Chaney, C., and P. Menyuk, "Production and identification of /w, l, r/ in normal and articulation-impaired children." Paper presented at the convention of the American Speech and Hearing Association, Washington, D.C., 1975.

Churchill, J., B. Hodson, B. Jones, and R. Novak, "A preliminary investigation comparing phonological systems of speech disordered clients with and without histories of recurrent otitis media." Paper presented at the annual convention of the American Speech-Language-Hearing Association, Washington, D.C., 1985.

Crary, M., and R. Towne, "The asynergistic nature of developmental verbal dyspraxia." *Australian Journal of Human Communication Disorders, 12* (1984): 27–28.

Darley, F., A. Aronson, and J. Brown, "Differential diagnostic patterns of dysarthria." *Journal of Speech and Hearing Research, 12* (1969): 246–269.

Darley, F., A. Aronson, and J. Brown, *Motor Speech Disorders*. Philadelphia: Saunders, 1975.

Davis, E., "The development of linguistic skills in twins, singletons with siblings, and only children from age five to ten years." *Institute of Child Welfare Monograph Series, 14*, Minneapolis: University of Minnesota Press, 1937.

Dawson, L., "A study of the development of the rate of articulation." *Elementary School Journal, 29* (1929): 610–615.

De Renzi, E., A. Pieczuro, and L. Vignolo, "Oral apraxia and aphasia." *Cortex, 2* (1966): 50–73.

Dubois, E., and J. Bernthal, "A comparison of three methods for obtaining articulatory responses." *Journal of Speech and Hearing Disorders, 43* (1978): 295–305.

Dunn, C., and L. Newton, "A comprehensive model for speech development in hearing-impaired children." *Topics in Language Disorders: Hearing Impairment: Implications from Normal Child Language, 6* (1986): 25–46.

Dworkin, J., "Protrusive lingual force and lingual diadochokinetic rates: A comparative analysis between normal and lisping speakers." *Language, Speech, and Hearing Services in Schools, 9* (1978): 8–16.

Dworkin, J., and R. Culatta, "Tongue strength: Its relationship to tongue thrusting, open-bite, and articulatory

proficiency." *Journal of Speech and Hearing Disorders, 45* (1980): 227–282.

Eilers, R. E., and D. K. Oller, "The role of speech discrimination in developmental sound substitutions." *Journal of Child Language, 3* (1976): 319–329.

Eimas, P., E. Siqueland, P. Jusczyk, and J. Vigorito, "Speech perception in infants." *Science, 171* (1971): 303–306.

Everhart, R., "The relationship between articulation and other developmental factors in children." *Journal of Speech and Hearing Disorders, 18* (1953): 332–338.

Everhart, R., "Paternal occupational classification and the maturation of articulation." *Speech Monographs, 23* (1956): 75–77.

Everhart, R., "Literature survey of growth and developmental factors in articulation maturation." *Journal of Speech and Hearing Disorders, 25* (1960): 59–69.

Fairbanks, G., and E. Green, "A study of minor organic deviations in 'functional' disorders of articulation; 2. Dimension and relationships of the lips." *Journal of Speech and Hearing Disorders, 15* (1950): 165–168.

Fairbanks, G., and M. Lintner, "A study of minor organic deviations in functional disorders of articulation." *Journal of Speech and Hearing Disorders, 16* (1951): 273–279.

Felsenfeld, S., M. McGue, and P. A. Broen, "Familial aggregation of phonological disorders: Results from a 28-year follow-up." *Journal of Speech and Hearing Research, 38* (1995): 1091–1107.

Fey, M. E., P. L. Cleave, A. I. Ravida, S. H. Long, A. E. Dejmal, and D. L. Easton, "Effects of grammar facilitation on the phonological performance of children with speech and language impairments." *Journal of Speech and Hearing Research, 37* (1994): 594–607.

Fitzsimons, R., "Developmental, psychosocial and educational factors in children with nonorganic articulation problems." *Child Development, 29* (1958): 481–489.

Fletcher, S., "Time-by-count measurement of diadochokinetic syllable rate." *Journal of Speech and Hearing Research, 15* (1972): 763–780.

Fletcher, S., R. Casteel, and D. Bradley, "Tongue thrust swallow, speech articulation and age." *Journal of Speech and Hearing Disorders, 26* (1961): 201–208.

Fletcher, S., and J. Meldrum, "Lingual function and relative length of the lingual frenulum." *Journal of Speech and Hearing Research, 11* (1968): 382–399.

Flynn, P., and M. Byrne, "Relationship between reading and selected auditory abilities of third-grade children." *Journal of Speech and Hearing Research, 13* (1970): 731–740.

Fucci, D., "Oral vibrotactile sensation: An evaluation of normal and defective speakers." *Journal of Speech and Hearing Research, 15* (1972): 179–184.

Gammon, S., P. Smith, R. Daniloff, and C. Kim, "Articulation and stress juncture production under oral anesthetization and masking." *Journal of Speech and Hearing Research, 14* (1971): 271–282.

Garrett, R., "A study of children's discrimination of phonetic variations of the /s/ phoneme." Ph.D. Dissertation, Ohio University, 1969.

Gray, S. I., and R. L. Shelton, "Self-monitoring effects on articulation carryover in school-age children." *Language, Speech, and Hearing Services in Schools, 23* (1992): 334–342.

Gross, G., K. St. Louis, D. Ruscello, and F. Hull, "Language abilities of articulatory-disordered school children with multiple or residual errors." *Language, Speech, and Hearing Services in Schools, 16* (1985): 174–186.

Hall, M., "Auditory factors in functional articulatory speech defects." *Journal of Experimental Education, 7* (1938): 110–132.

Hansen, B., "The application of sound discrimination tests to functional articulatory defectives with normal hearing." *Journal of Speech Disorders, 9* (1944): 347–355.

Hanson, M. L., "Orofacial myofunctional disorders: Guidelines for assessment and treatment." *International Journal of Orofacial Myology, 14* (1988a): 27–32.

Hanson, M. L., "Orofacial myofunctional therapy: Historical and philosophical considerations." *International Journal of Orofacial Myology, 14* (1988b): 3–10.

Hanson, M. L., "Oral myofunctional disorders and articulatory patterns." In J. Bernthal and N. Bankson (Eds.), *Child Phonology: Characteristics, Assessment, and Intervention with Special Populations* (pp. 29–53). New York: Thieme Medical Publishers, 1994.

Haynes, S., D. Johns, and E. May, "Assessment and therapeutic management of an adult patient with developmental apraxia of speech and orosensory perceptual deficits." *Tejas, 3* (1978): 6–9.

Hilton, L., "Treatment of deviant phonologic systems: Tongue thrust." In W. Perkins (Ed.), *Phonological-articulatory Disorders*. New York: Thieme-Stratton, 1984.

Hodson, B., "Phonological remediation: A cycles approach." In N. Creaghead, P. Newman, and W. Secord (Eds.), *Assessment and Remediation of Articulatory and Phonological Disorders*. Columbus, Ohio: Charles E. Merrill, 1989.

Hoffman, P., "Spelling, phonology, and the speech pathologist: A whole language perspective." *Language, Speech, and Hearing Services in Schools, 21* (1990): 238–243.

Hoffman, P., and J. Norris, "On the nature of phonological development: Evidence from normal children's spelling errors." *Journal of Speech and Hearing Research, 32* (1989): 787–794.

Hoffman, P., J. Norris, and J. Monjure, "Comparison of process targeting and whole language treatments of phonologically delayed children. *Language, Speech, and Hearing Services in Schools, 21* (1990): 102–109.

Hoffman, P., S. Stager, and R. Daniloff, "Perception and production of misarticulated /r/." *Journal of Speech and Hearing Disorders, 48* (1983): 210–214.

Holland, A., "Training speech sound discrimination in children who misarticulate. A demonstration of teaching machine technique in speech correction." Project No. 5007. Washington, DC: U.S. Department of Health, Education and Welfare, 1967.

Hull, F., P. Mielke, R. Timmons, and J. Willeford, "The national speech and hearing survey: Preliminary results." *Asha, 13* (1971): 501–509.

Itoh, M., and S. Sasanuma, "Articulatory movements in apraxia of speech." In J. Rosenbek, M. McNeil, and A. Aronson (Eds.), *Apraxia of Speech: Physiology, Acoustics, Linguistics, Management*. San Diego: College-Hill Press, 1984.

Jaffe, M., "Neurological impairment of speech production: Assessment and treatment." In J. Costello and A. Holland (Eds.) *Handbook of Speech and Language Disorders* (pp. 157–186). San Diego: College Hill Press, 1986.

Jann, G., M. Ward, and H. Jann, "A longitudinal study of articulation, deglutition and malocclusion." *Journal of Speech and Hearing Disorders, 29* (1964): 424–435.

Johns, D., and F. Darley, "Phonemic variability in apraxia of speech." *Journal of Speech and Hearing Research, 13* (1970): 556–583.

Johns, D., and K. Salyer, "Surgical and prosthetic management of neurogenic speech disorders." In D. Johns (Ed.), *Clinical Management of Neurogenic Communicative Disorders*. Boston: Little, Brown, 1978.

Jordan, L., J. Hardy, and H. Morris, "Performance of children with good and poor articulation on tasks of tongue placement." *Journal of Speech and Hearing Research, 21* (1978): 429–439.

Jusczyk, P. W., and P. A. Luce, "Speech perception and spoken word recognition: Past and present." *Ear & Hearing, 23* (2002): 2–40.

Kenny, K., and E. Prather, "Articulation in preschool children: Consistency of productions." *Journal of Speech and Hearing Research, 29* (1986): 29–36.

Koch, H., "Sibling influence on children's speech." *Journal of Speech and Hearing Disorders, 21* (1956): 322–329.

Koegel, L. K., R. L. Koegel, and J. C. Ingham, "Programming rapid generalization of correct articulation through self-monitoring procedures." *Journal of Speech and Hearing Disorders, 51* (1986): 24–32.

Koegel, R., L. Koegel, K. Van Voy, and J. Ingham, "Within-clinic versus outside-of-clinic self-monitoring of articulation to promote generalization." *Journal of Speech and Hearing Disorders, 53* (1988): 392–399.

Kronvall, E., and C. Diehl, "The relationship of auditory discrimination to articulatory defects of children with no known organic impairment." *Journal of Speech and Hearing Disorders, 19* (1954): 335–338.

Kumin, L., C. Council, and M. Goodman, "A longitudinal study of emergence of phonemes in children with Down syndrome." *Journal of Communication Disorders, 27* (1994): 293–303.

Lapko, L., and N. Bankson, "Relationship between auditory discrimination, articulation stimulability and consistency of misarticulation." *Perceptual and Motor Skills, 40* (1975): 171–177.

Lapointe, L., and R. Wertz, "Oral-movement abilities and articulatory characteristics of brain-injured adults." *Perceptual Motor Skills, 39* (1974): 39–46.

Leonard, R. J., "Characteristics of speech in speakers with oral/oralpharyngeal ablation." In J. Bernthal and N. Bankson (Eds.), *Child Phonology: Characteristics, Assessment, and Intervention with Special Populations* (pp 54–78). New York: Thieme Medical Publishers, 1994.

Levitt, H., and H. Stromberg, "Segmental characteristics of speech of hearing-impaired children: Factors affecting intelligibility." In I. Hochberg, H. Levitt, and M. Osberger (Eds.), *Speech of the Hearing Impaired* (pp 53–73). Baltimore, Md.: University Park Press, 1983.

Lewis, B., B. Ekelman, and D. Aram, "A familial study of severe phonological disorders." *Journal of Speech and Hearing Research, 32* (1989): 713–724.

Lewis, B., and L. Freebairn-Farr, "Preschool phonology disorders at school age, adolescence, and adulthood." Paper presented at the annual convention of the American Speech-Language-Hearing Association, Atlanta, 1991.

Liberman, I., and D. Shankweiler, "Phonology and problems of learning to read and write." *Remedial and Special Education, 6* (1985): 8–17.

Ling, D., *Foundations of Spoken Language for Hearing-Impaired Children*. Washington, DC: Alexander Graham Bell Association for the Deaf, 1989.

Locke, J., "Oral perception and articulation learning." *Perceptual and Motor Skills, 26* (1968): 1259–1264.

Locke, J. L., "The inference of speech perception in the phonologically disordered child, part I: A rationale, some criteria, the conventional tests." *Journal of Speech and Hearing Disorders, 4* (1980): 431–444.

Locke, J., and K. Kutz, "Memory for speech and speech for memory." *Journal of Speech and Hearing Research, 18* (1975): 179–191.

Locke, J., and P. Mather, "Genetic factors in phonology. Evidence from monozygotic and dizygotic twins." Paper presented at the annual convention of the American Speech-Language-Hearing Association, New Orleans, 1987.

Lof, G. and S. Synan, "Is there a speech discrimination/perception link to disordered articulation and phonology? A review of 80 years of literature." *Contemporary Issues in Communication Science and Disorders, 24* (1997): 63–77.

Love, R., *Childhood Motor Speech Disability*. New York: Macmillan Publishing Co., 1992.

Lundeen, C., "Prevalence of hearing impairment among school children." *Language, Speech, and Hearing Services in Schools, 22* (1991): 269–271.

Marquardt, T., and J. Saxman, "Language comprehension and auditory discrimination in articulation deficient kindergarten children." *Journal of Speech and Hearing Research, 15* (1972): 382–389.

Marshall, P. "Oral-motor techniques in articulation therapy." Videotapes. Seattle, Wash.: Innovative Concepts, 1992.

Mase, D., "Etiology of articulatory speech defects." *Teacher's College Contribution to Education*, No. 921. New York: Columbia University, 1946.

Mason, R. M., "Orthodontic perspectives on orofacial myofunctional therapy." *International Journal of Orofacial Myology, 14* (1988): 49–55.

Mason, R., and W. Proffit, "The tongue-thrust controversy: Background and recommendations." *Journal of Speech and Hearing Disorders, 39* (1974): 115–132.

Massengill, R., S. Maxwell, and K. Picknell, "An analysis of articulation following partial and total glossectomy." *Journal of Speech and Hearing Disorders, 35* (1970): 170–173.

Matheny, A., and C. Bruggeman, "Children's speech: Heredity components and sex differences." *Folia Phoniatrica, 25* (1973): 442–449.

Matheny, N., and J. Panagos, "Comparing the effects of articulation and syntax programs on syntax and articulation improvement." *Language, Speech, and Hearing Services in Schools, 9* (1978): 57–61.

McDonald, E. T., *Articulation Testing and Treatment: A Sensory Motor Approach*. Pittsburgh, Penn.: Stanwix House, 1964.

McDonald, E. T., and L. Aungst, "Apparent impedence of oral sensory functions and articulatory proficiency." In J. Bosma (Ed.), *Second Symposium on Oral Sensation and Perception*. Springfield, Ill.: Chas. C. Thomas, 1970.

McEnery, E., and F. Gaines, "Tongue-tie in infants and children." *Journal of Pediatrics, 18* (1941): 252–255.

McNutt, J., "Oral sensory and motor behaviors of children with /s/ or /r/ misarticulations." *Journal of Speech and Hearing Research, 20* (1977): 694–703.

Mills, A., and H. Streit, "Report of a speech survey, Holyoke, Massachusetts." *Journal of Speech Disorders, 7* (1942): 161–167.

Monson, R., "The oral speech intelligibility of hearing-impaired talkers." *Journal of Speech and Hearing Disorders, 48* (1983): 286–296.

Morley, D., "A ten-year survey of speech disorders among university students." *Journal of Speech and Hearing Disorders, 17* (1952): 25–31.

Morley, M. E., *The Development and Disorders of Speech in Childhood*, (1st Ed.). London: Livingston, 1957.

Mowrer, D., R. Baker, and R. Schutz, "Operant procedures in the control of speech articulation." In H. Sloane and B. MacAulay (Eds.), *Operant Procedures in Remedial Speech and Language Training*. Boston: Houghton Mifflin, 1968.

Neils, J., and D. Aram, "Family history of children with developmental language disorders," *Perceptual and Motor Skills, 63* (1986): 655–658.

Neiva, F. S., and H. F. Wertzner, "A protocol for oral myofunctional assessment: For application with children. *International Journal of Orofacial Myology, 2* (1996): 8–19.

Netsell, R. A., *A Neurobiologic View of Speech Production and the Dysarthrias*. Boston, Mass.: College-Hill Press, 1986.

O'Conner, R. E., and J. R. Jenkins, "Prediction of reading disabilities in kindergarten and first grade." *Scientific Studies of Reading, 3* (1999): 159–197.

Paden, E. P., M. L. Matthies, and M. A. Novak, "Recovery from OME-related phonologic delay following tube placement." *Journal of Speech and Hearing Disorders, 54* (1989): 94–100.

Paden, E. P., M. A. Novak, and A. L. Beiter, "Predictors of phonological inadequacy in young children prone to otitis media." *Journal of Speech and Hearing Disorders, 52* (1987): 232–242.

Palmer, J., "Tongue-thrusting: A clinical hypothesis." *Journal of Speech and Hearing Disorders, 27* (1962): 323–333.

Panagos, J., and P. Prelock, "Phonological constraints on the sentence productions of language disordered children." *Journal of Speech and Hearing Research, 25* (1982): 171–176.

Panagos, J., M. Quine, and R. Klich, "Syntactic and phonological influences on children's articulation." *Journal of Speech and Hearing Research, 22* (1979): 841–848.

Parlour, S., and P. Broen, "Environmental factors in familial phonological disorders: Preliminary home scale results." Paper presented at the annual convention of the American Speech-Language-Hearing Association, Atlanta, 1991.

Paterson, M., "Articulation and phonological disorders in hearing-impaired school-aged children with severe and profound sensorineural losses." In J. Bernthal and N. Bankson (Eds.), *Child Phonology: Characteristics, Assessment, and Intervention with Special Populations* (pp 199–224). New York: Thieme Medical Publishers, 1994.

Paul, R., and L. D. Shriberg, "Associations between phonology and syntax in speech delayed children." *Journal of Speech and Hearing Research, 25* (1982): 536–546.

Paul, R., and L. D. Shriberg, "Reply to Panagos and Prelock (Letter)." *Journal of Speech and Hearing Research, 27* (1984): 319–320.

Perkins, W., *Speech Pathology: An Applied Behavioral Science*. St. Louis: Mosby, 1977.

Powers, M., "Functional disorders of articulation-symptomatology and etiology." In L. Travis (Ed.), *Handbook of Speech Pathology and Audiology*. Engelwood Cliffs, NJ: Prentice-Hall, 1957, 1971.

Prins, D., "Analysis of correlations among various articulatory deviations." *Journal of Speech and Hearing Research, 5* (1962a): 151–160.

Prins, D., "Motor and auditory abilities in different groups of children with articulatory deviations." *Journal of Speech and Hearing Research, 5* (1962b): 161–168.

Proffit, W. R., *Contemporary Orthodontics*. St. Louis, MO: C.V. Mosby, 1986.

Prosek, R., and A. House, "Intraoral air pressure as a feedback cue in consonant production." *Journal of Speech and Hearing Research, 18* (1975): 133–147.

Reid, G., "The efficiency of speech re-education of functional articulatory defectives in elementary school." *Journal of Speech and Hearing Disorders, 12* (1947a): 301–313.

Reid, G., "The etiology and nature of functional articulatory defects in elementary school children." *Journal of Speech and Hearing Disorders, 12* (1947b): 143–150.

Ringel, R., K. Burk, and C. Scott, "Tactile perception: Form discrimination in the mouth." In J. Bosma (Ed.), *Second Symposium on Oral Sensation and Perception*. Springfield, Ill.: Chas. C. Thomas, 1970.

Ringel, R., and S. Ewanowski, "Oral perception: I. Two-point discrimination." *Journal of Speech and Hearing Research, 8* (1965): 389–400.

Ringel, R., A. House, K. Burk, J. Dolinsky, and C. Scott, "Some relations between orosensory discrimination and articulatory aspects of speech production." *Journal of Speech and Hearing Disorders, 35* (1970): 3–11.

Roberts, J. E., M. R. Burchinal, M. A. Koch, M. M. Footo, and F. W. Henderson, "Otitis media in early childhood and its relationship to later phonological development." *Journal of Speech and Hearing Disorders, 53* (1988): 424–432.

Roberts, J. E., and S. Clarke-Klein, "Otitis media." In J. Bernthal and N. Bankson (Eds.), *Child Phonology: Characteristics, Assessment, and Intervention with Special Populations* (pp 182–198). New York: Thieme Medical Publishers, 1994.

Roe, V., and R. Milisen, "The effect of maturation upon defective articulation in elementary grades." *Journal of Speech Disorders, 7* (1942): 37–50.

Rosenbek, J., and R. Wertz, "A review of fifty cases of developmental apraxia of speech." *Language, Speech and Hearing Services in Schools, 1* (1972): 23–33.

Rosin, M., E. Swift, D. Bless, and D. K. Vetter, "Communication profiles of adolescents with Down's Syndrome." *Journal of Childhood Communication Disorders, 12* (1988): 49–62.

Ruscello, D. M., "Articulation improvement and oral tactile changes in children." Thesis, University of West Virginia, 1972.

Rvachew, S., "Speech perception training can facilitate sound production learning." *Journal of Speech and Hearing Research, 37* (1994): 347–357.

Rvachew, S., S. Rafaat, and M. Martin, "Stimulability, speech perception skills, and the treatment of phonological disorders." *American Journal of Speech-Language Pathology, 8* (1999): 33–43.

SAILS: Speech Assessment and Interactive Learning System (Computer Software). (1995). London, Ontario, Canada: AVAAZ Innovations.

Sayler, H., "The effect of maturation upon defective articulation in grades seven through twelve." *Journal of Speech and Hearing Disorders, 14* (1949): 202–207.

Schlanger, B., "Speech examination of a group of institutionalized mentally handicapped children." *Journal of Speech and Hearing Disorders, 18* (1953): 339–349.

Schlanger, B., and R. Gottsleben, "Analysis of speech defects among the institutionalized mentally retarded." *Journal of Speech and Hearing Disorders, 22* (1957): 98–103.

Schmauch, V., J. Panagos, and R. Klich, "Syntax influences the accuracy of consonant production in language-disordered children." *Journal of Communication Disorders, 11* (1978): 315–323.

Schwartz, A., and R. Goldman, "Variables influencing performance on speech sound discrimination tests." *Journal of Speech and Hearing Research, 17* (1974): 25–32.

Schwartz, R., L. Leonard, M. K. Folger, and M. J. Wilcox, "Evidence for a synergistic view of linguistic disorders: Early phonological behavior in normal and language disordered children." *Journal of Speech and Hearing Disorders, 45* (1980): 357–377.

Scott, C., and R. Ringel, "Articulation without oral sensory control." *Journal of Speech and Hearing Research, 14* (1971): 804–818.

Shelton, R., "Science, clinical art, and speech pathology." Paper presented at Kansas University, Spring 1989.

Shelton, R., A. Johnson, and W. Arndt, "Delayed judgment speech sound discrimination and /r/ or /s/ articulation status and improvement." *Journal of Speech and Hearing Research, 20* (1977): 704–717.

Shelton, R. L., V. Willis, A. F. Johnson, and W. B. Arndt, "Oral form recognition training and articulation change." *Perceptual Motor Skills, 36* (1973): 523–531.

Sherman, D., and A. Geith, "Speech sound discrimination and articulation skill." *Journal of Speech and Hearing Disorders, 10* (1967): 277–280.

Shriberg, L. D., and J. Kwiatkowski, "Phonological disorders I: A diagnostic classification system." *Journal of Speech and Hearing Disorders, 47* (1982): 226–241.

Shriberg, L., and J. Kwiatkowski, "Developmental phonological disorders I: A clinical profile." *Journal of Speech and Hearing Research, 37* (1994): 1100–1126.

Shriberg, L., and C. Widder, "Speech and prosody characteristics of adults with mental retardation." *Journal of Speech and Hearing Research, 33* (1990): 627–653.

Shriberg, L. D., D. M. Aram, and J. Kwiatkowski. "Developmental apraxia of speech: II. Toward a diagnostic marker." *Journal of Speech, Language, and Hearing Research, 40* (1997): 286–312.

Shriberg, L. D., and A. J. Smith, "Phonological correlates of middle-ear involvement in speech-delayed children: A methodological note." *Journal of Speech and Hearing Research, 26* (1983): 293–297.

Shriner, T., M. Holloway, and R. Daniloff, "The relationship between articulatory deficits and syntax in speech defective children." *Journal of Speech and Hearing Research, 12* (1969): 319–325.

Skelly, M., D. Spector, R. Donaldson, A. Brodeur, and F. Paletta, "Compensatory physiologic phonetics for the glossectomee." *Journal of Speech and Hearing Disorders, 36* (1971): 101–114.

Smit, A., L. Hand, J. Freilinger, J. Bernthal, and A. Bird, "The Iowa articulation norms project and its Nebraska replication." *Journal of Speech and Hearing Disorders, 55* (1990): 779–798.

Smith, B., and C. Stoel-Gammon, "A longitudinal study of the development of stop consonant production in normal and Down's Syndrome children." *Journal of Speech and Hearing Disorders, 48* (1983): 114–118.

Snow, K., "Articulation proficiency in relation to certain dental abnormalities." *Journal of Speech and Hearing Disorders, 26* (1961): 209–212.

Sommers, R., R. Reinhart, and D. Sistrunk, "Traditional articulation measures of Down's Syndrome speakers, ages 13–22." *Journal of Childhood Communication Disorders, 12* (1988): 93–108.

Sonderman, J., "An experimental study of clinical relationships between auditory discrimination and articulation skills." Paper presented at the annual convention of the American Speech and Hearing Association, San Francisco, 1971.

Starr, C., "Dental and occlusal hazards to normal speech production." In K. Bzoch (Ed.), *Communicative Disorders Related to Cleft Lip and Palate.* Boston: Little, Brown, 1972.

Stelcik, J., "An investigation of internal versus external discrimination and general versus phoneme-specific discrimination." Unpublished Thesis, University of Maryland, 1972.

Stoel-Gammon, C., and M. Kehoe, "Hearing impairment in infants and toddlers: Identification, vocal development, and intervention in child phonology" (pp 163–181). In J. Bernthal and N. Bankson (Eds.), *Child Phonology: Characteristics, Assessment, and Intervention with Special Populations.* New York: Thieme Medical Publishers, 1994.

Strange, W., and P. Broen, "Perception and production of approximant consonants by 3 year olds: A first study." In G. Yeni-Komshian, J. Kavanaugh, and C. A. Ferguson (Eds.), *Child Phonology*, Vol. 2, *Perception.* New York: Academic Press, 1980.

Subtelny, J. D., "Malocclusions, orthodontic corrections and orofacial muscle adaptation." *Angle Orthod, 40* (1970): 170.

Subtelny, J., J. Mestre, and J. Subtelny, "Comparative study of normal and defective articulation of /s/ as related to malocclusion and deglutition." *Journal of Speech and Hearing Disorders, 29* (1964): 269–285.

Sullivan, M., C. Gaebler, D. Beukelman, G. Mahanna, J. Marshall, D. Lydiatt, and W. Lydiatt, "Impact of palatal prosthodontic intervention on communication performance of patients' maxillectomy defects: A multi-level outcome study." *Head and Neck, 24* (6) (2002): 530–538.

Templin, M., *Certain Language Skills in Children.* Institute of Child Welfare Monograph Series 26. Minneapolis: University of Minnesota, 1957.

Templin, M., "Development of speech." *Journal of Pediatrics, 62* (1963): 11–14.

Templin, M., *Longitudinal Study Through the 4th Grade of Language Skills of Children with Varying Speech Sound Articulation in Kindergarten.* (Final Report, Project 2220). Washington, DC: U.S. Department of Health, Education, and Welfare, Office of Education, 1968.

Templin, M., and G. Glaman, "A longitudinal study of correlations of predictive measures obtained in prekindergarten and first grade with achievement measures through eleventh grade" (Unpublished report #101). Washington, D.C.: U.S. Department of Health, Education, and Welfare, Office of Education, 1976.

Tiffany, W., "Effects of syllable structure on diadochokinetic and reading rates." *Journal of Speech and Hearing Research, 23* (1980): 894–908.

Travis, L., and B. Rasmus, "The speech sound discrimination ability of cases with functional disorders of articulation." *Quarterly Journal of Speech, 17* (1931): 217–226.

Tye-Murray, N., "The establishment of open articulatory postures by deaf and hearing talkers." *Journal of Speech and Hearing Research, 34* (1991): 453–458.

Tyler, A. A., K. E. Lewis, A. Haskill, and L. C. Tolbert, "Efficacy of cross-domain effects of a morphosyntax and a phonologic intervention." *Language, Speech, and Hearing Services in Schools, 33* (2002): 52–66.

Tyler, A., and K. Watterson, "Effects of phonological versus language intervention in preschoolers with both phonological and language impairment." *Child Language Teaching and Therapy, 7* (1991): 141–160.

Umberger, F. G., and R. G. Johnston, "The efficacy of oral myofunctional and coarticulation therapy." *International Journal of Orofacial Myology, 23* (1997): 3–9.

Veatch, J., "An experimental investigation of a motor theory of auditory discrimination." Ph.D. Dissertation, University of Idaho, 1970.

Velleman, S. L., "Children's production and perception of English voiceless fricatives." Unpublished Ph.D. Dissertation, University of Texas at Austin, 1983.

Velleman, S., and K. Strand, "Developmental verbal dyspraxia." In J. Bernthal and N. Bankson (Eds.), *Child Phonology: Characteristics, Assessment, and Intervention with Special Populations* (pp. 110–139). New York: Thieme Medical Publishers, 1994.

Wadsworth, S. D., C. A. Maul, and E. J. Stevens, "The prevalence of orofacial myofunctional disorders among children identified with speech and language disorders in grades kindergarten through six." *International Journal of Orofacial Myology, 24* (1998): 1–19.

Weaver, C., C. Furbee, and R. Everhart, "Paternal occupational class and articulatory defects in children." *Journal of Speech and Hearing Disorders, 25* (1960) 171–175.

Weiner, P., "Auditory discrimination and articulation." *Journal of Speech and Hearing Disorders, 32* (1967): 19–28.

Wellman, B., I. Case, I. Mengert, and D. Bradbury, "Speech sounds of young children." *University of Iowa Studies in Child Welfare, 5* (1931).

Whitaker, J., H. Luper, and H. Pollio, "General language deficits in children with articulation problems." *Language and Speech, 3* (1970): 231–239.

Wilcox, K. A., and S. E. Morris, "Speech outcomes of the language-focused curriculum." In M. Rice and K. Wilcox (Eds.), *Building a Language-Focused Curriculum for the Preschool Classroom: A Foundation for Lifelong Communication* (pp. 73–79). Baltimore, Md.: Brookes, 1995.

Wilhelm, C. L., "The effects of oral form recognition training on articulation in children." Dissertation, University of Kansas, 1971.

Williams, G., and L. McReynolds, "The relationship between discrimination and articulation training in children with misarticulations." *Journal of Speech and Hearing Research, 18* (1975): 401–412.

Wilson, F., "Efficacy of speech therapy with educable mentally retarded children." *Journal of Speech and Hearing Research, 9* (1966): 423–433.

Winitz, H., "Language skills of male and female kindergarten children." *Journal of Speech and Hearing Research*, 2 (1959a): 377–386.

Winitz, H., "Relationship between language and nonlanguage measures of kindergarten children." *Journal of Speech and Hearing Research*, 2 (1959b): 387–391.

Winitz, H., *Articulatory Acquisition and Behavior*. Englewood Cliffs, NJ: Prentice-Hall, 1969.

Winitz, H., "Auditory considerations in articulation training." In H. Winitz (Ed.), *Treating Articulation Disorders: For Clinicians By Clinicians*. Baltimore: University Park Press, 1984.

Wolfe, V., and R. Irwin, "Sound discrimination ability of children with misarticulation of the /r/ sound." *Perceptual and Motor Skills*, 37 (1973): 415–420.

Wolk, S., and A. N. Schildroth, "Deaf children and speech intelligibility: A national study." In A. N. Schildroth and M. A. Karchmer (Eds.), *Deaf Children in America* (pp 139–159). San Diego: College-Hill, 1986.

Woolf, G., and M. Pilberg, "A comparison of three tests of auditory discrimination and their relationship to performance on a deep test of articulation." *Journal of Communication Disorders*, 3 (1971): 239–249.

Yorkston, K. M., D. R. Beukelman, E. A. Strand, and K. R. Bell, *Management of Motor Speech Disorders in Children and Adults* (2nd ed.). Austin, Tex.: PRO-ED, 1999.

Yoss, K., and F. Darley, "Developmental apraxia of speech in children with defective articulation." *Journal of Speech and Hearing Research*, 17 (1974): 399–416.

5

Phonological Assessment Procedures

NICHOLAS W. BANKSON
James Madison University

JOHN E. BERNTHAL
University of Nebraska—Lincoln

Phonological Sampling

Introduction

One of the unique contributions of the field of speech-language pathology to the assessment of verbal behavior is the development of **phonological assessment** instruments. For several decades, phonological/articulation assessment procedures have remained almost the exclusive domain of speech-language clinicians, although linguists, child development specialists, psychologists, pediatricians, and special educators also use such tools.

Evaluation of an individual's phonological status typically involves description of his or her speech sound production system and comparing this system to the adult standard of the speaker's linguistic community (**relational analysis**). For speakers with limited phonological repertoires, the speech sound system is often described independent of the adult standard (**independent analysis**). Phonological assessment is often done in the context of a communication evaluation that also includes assessment of voice quality, resonance, fluency, syntax, semantics, pragmatics, discourse, and prosodic aspects of language. Additional related measures such as hearing testing and an oral mechanism examination are usually included in a comprehensive communication evaluation/assessment. Although some clinicians have differentiated between phonological delay (children whose speech sound errors are similar to those found in younger normally developing children) and phonological disorders (children whose speech sound errors differ from normal developing children), in this text we will not differentiate between the two. In reality, most children with multiple misarticulations will have errors that fall into both categories.

Phonological assessment is used to describe the phonological status of an individual and:

1. Determine whether his or her speech sound system is sufficiently different from normal development to warrant intervention.
2. Determine treatment direction, including target behaviors and strategies to be used in the management of the client.
3. Make prognostic statements relative to phonological change with or without intervention/therapy.
4. Monitor change in phonological performance across time.
5. Identify factors that may be related to the presence or maintenance of a phonological disability.

In addition, the speech-language pathologist may be called on to identify and describe dialectal variations of Standard American English. The need to describe such differences usually follows a request or inquiry for accent reduction by individuals who speak a regional or cultural dialect or for whom English is a second language. In the case of a client referred for a phonologic evaluation whose speech reflects dialectal differences, the speech-language pathologist must be able to differentiate which phonological characteristics reflect dialect differences and which reflect a speech disorder.

The primary purposes of a phonological assessment are to determine whether an individual needs phonological instruction, and if so, the direction of such treatment. To make these determinations, the clinician engages in a multistep process that involves sampling the client's speech through a variety of procedures, analyzing the data gathered, interpreting the data that have been analyzed, and then making clinical recommendations. In this chapter, we will discuss various sampling and testing procedures and discuss factors and issues that should be taken into consideration when analyzing and interpreting phonological samples. This chapter will focus on impairments rather than accent/dialect reduction since the latter will be discussed in detail in Chapter 8. At the end of this chapter, you will find a case history of a child to whom procedures discussed in this chapter are applied.

Screening for Phonological Disorders

A complete phonological assessment, including analysis and interpretation of results is not something that can be done quickly. Because of this time expenditure, clinicians will often do a *screening* to determine if a more comprehensive phonological assessment is warranted. Screening procedures are not designed to determine the need or direction of therapy, but rather to identify individuals who merit further evaluation from those for whom further assessment is not indicated. Screening might include (1) screening children at a preschool or "kindergarten roundup" to determine whether they have age-appropriate phonological skills, (2) screening children in grade 3 (by which time maturation should have resolved most developmental errors), (3) screening individuals preparing for occupations, such as broadcast journalism, which require specific speech performance standards, and (4) screening the phonological status of clients referred for a suspected communication impairment.

In screening, individuals are not identified as candidates for therapy, but rather are simply identified as needing further assessment. Additional testing is often required before statements about the presence or absence of a phonological disorder can be made, and it is certainly required for determining the direction for treatment. Instruments used for screening consist of a limited sampling of speech sound productions, which can usually be administered in five minutes or less. Screening measures can be categorized as informal or formal. *Informal measures* are often used when people wish to develop their own screening tools in order to meet their particular needs. *Formal measures* are often employed when users desire established norms or testing methodologies that are more uniform.

Informal Screening Measures

Informal screening measures are usually devised by the examiner and are tailored to the population being screened. While informal procedures can be easily and economically devised, they do not include standardized administration procedures or normative data, which are characteristics of formal screening measures. For example, with a group of kindergarten children, the examiner might ask each child to

1. state his or her name and address.
2. count to ten; name the days of the week.
3. tell about a television show.

If the subjects are adults, the examiner might ask them to do one or both of the following:

1. Read sentences designed to elicit several productions of frequently misarticulated sounds, such as /s/, /r/, /l/, and /θ/. For example, "I saw Sally at her seaside house; Rob ran around the orange car."
2. Read a passage with a representative sample of English speech sounds, such as the "Grandfather Passage."

   Grandfather Passage.   You wish to know all about my grandfather. Well, he is nearly 93 years old, yet he still thinks as swiftly as ever. He dresses himself in an old black frock coat, usually several buttons missing. A long beard clings to his chin, giving those who observe him a pronounced feeling of the utmost respect. When he speaks, his voice is just a bit cracked and quivers a bit. Twice each day he plays skillfully and with zest upon a small organ. Except in winter when the snow or ice prevents, he slowly takes a short walk in the open air each day. We have often urged him to walk more and smoke less, but he always answers, "Banana oil." Grandfather likes to be modern in his language.

Criteria for failure of informal screening are determined by the examiner. An often-used rule of thumb is "if in doubt, refer." In other words, an examiner who suspects that the client's speech sound system is not appropriate for his or her age and/or linguistic community should be referred for a more complete assessment. The examiner may also choose to determine or establish performance standards on the screening instrument that will help to identify those referred for further testing. Those individuals with the greatest need for additional testing and probable intervention will usually be obvious to the examiner from even a small sample of their speech and language.

Formal Screening Measures

Formal screening measures include published elicitation procedures for which normative data and/or cut-off scores are often available. These formal measures are of three types: (1) tests that are part of a single-word (citation) articulation test, (2) tests designed solely for screening phonology, and (3) tests which screen phonology as well as other aspects of language. Tests designed explicitly for screening phonology are most frequently used when screening phonology is the primary goal. Those instruments that combine phonological screening with other aspects of language screening are most commonly used for more general communication disorders screening.

The following are formal phonology screening tests:

Quick Screen of Phonology (QSP) (Bankson and Bernthal, 1990a)

This test consists of 28 picture-naming items, with each word assessing sounds in more than one context (usually initial and final). Twenty-three phonemes plus three consonant clusters are screened. These items were selected because of their correlation with the overall performance on the *Bankson-Bernthal Test of Phonology*. Percentile ranks and standard scores are provided for children ages 3;0 through 7;11 years on the QSP.

Denver Articulation Screening Test (Drumwright, 1971)

This instrument was designed specifically for screening phonological status in Anglo, black, and Mexican-American children. Responses are elicited imitatively. The examiner is asked to judge intelligibility on a 4-point scale, with 1 being "easy to understand" and 4 being "can't evaluate." Children are ranked "normal to abnormal," depending on composite articulation and intelligibility scores.

The following tests include screening of phonology as part of a speech and language screening:

Fluharty Preschool Speech and Language Screening Test—Second Edition (Fluharty, 2000)

This test was designed for children, ages 3 through 6 years. The articulation portion of the test uses 15 pictured objects to elicit 30 target sounds. Some stimulus items are designed to assess two sounds. Standard scores and percentiles for the subtests are included.

Speech-Ease Screening Inventory (K–1) (Pigott, Barry, Hughes, Eastin, Titus, Stensil, Metcalf, and Porter, 1985)

This test was designed for kindergarteners and first graders. The overall test takes 7–10 minutes to administer, with the articulation section being comprised of 12 items. Fourteen phonemes and three blends are assessed through sentence completion items. Cut-off scores for phoneme error counts indicative of the need for further testing are provided.

Preschool Language Scale (Zimmerman, Steiner, and Pond, 1992)

This test was designed for children, ages 1 through 7. The "articulation screener" portion of the test consists of 37 items that test 18 speech sounds plus one consonant cluster. Performance levels expected for children are provided.

Summary

Screening procedures are not designed to determine the need or direction of treatment. Rather, their purpose is to identify individuals for further testing. The criteria for failure on informal screening tests are often left up to the examiner. When available, standard scores and percentile ranks aid the examiner in establishing such criteria. It is not uncommon for a score one standard deviation below the mean to be used as a cut-off score. For some instruments, cut-off scores or age expectation scores are provided.

Comprehensive Phonological Assessment: Assessment Battery

Sampling procedures involved in phonological assessment are more in-depth and detailed than those described for screening. When doing a phonological analysis, the clinician usually employs a battery of assessment instruments and sampling procedures since no one sampling procedure or test provides all a clinician needs to know when making case selection decisions and determining the direction that an intervention program should take. A phonological evaluation typically involves phonological productions in samples of varying lengths, phonetic contexts, and in response to various elicitation procedures. This collection of samples is often referred to as an **assessment battery**.

As stated above, the two major purposes of a phonological assessment are to determine the need for and direction of treatment. It is to these purposes that most of the writings, research, and testing materials on phonological disorders have been addressed. In the following pages, components of a phonological evaluation battery, with an emphasis on procedures for obtaining phonological samples, are presented. Following this, analysis and interpretation of data collected through sampling procedures are discussed. Throughout this chapter, an attempt is made to synthesize the available literature and make suggestions based upon the authors' clinical experience.

Phonological Samples Included in the Test Battery

Connected/Conversational Speech Sampling

Rationale. All phonological evaluations should include a sample of connected speech. Since the ultimate objective of phonological treatment is correct production of sounds in spontaneous conversation, it is important that the examiner observe sound productions in as "natural" a speaking context as possible. Such samples allow one to transcribe phoneme productions in a variety of phonetic contexts, to observe error patterns, and to judge the severity of the problem and the intelligibility of the speaker in continuous discourse.

Sounds produced in connected speech may also be studied in relation to other factors such as speech rate, intonation, stress, and syllable structure. In addition, connected speech samples allow for multiple productions of sounds across lexical items.

Because spontaneous connected speech samples are the most valid or representative sample of phonological performance, some clinicians suggest that phonological analyses should be exclusively based on this type of sample (Shriberg and Kwiatkowski, 1980; Stoel-Gammon and Dunn, 1985; Morrison and Shriberg, 1992). Connected speech samples have the advantage of allowing the examiner to transcribe sound productions within the context of the child's own vocabulary and in running speech which includes his natural prosodic patterns. In addition, these samples can be used for other types of language analysis. Sometimes, however, there are practical problems associated with relying solely on such samples. Many individuals with severe phonological problems may be almost unintelligible, and it may be impossible or very difficult to reliably determine and/or transcribe what they are attempting to say in conversational speech. Some children may be reluctant to engage in conversational dialogue with an adult they do not know. It may also be an almost impossible task to obtain a spontaneous speech corpus that contains a representative sample of English phonemes.

Ingram (1989) suggested that difficulty in obtaining a "cross-section of the sounds in English" (representative sample) may not be a critical issue. He argued that if a spontaneous sample is of "sufficient size," the child's preference for sounds is revealed. Sounds missing from the sample may reflect a "selective avoidance" by the child; that is, the child chooses not to produce them. However, the absence of specific sounds in a child's spontaneous speech may reflect an infrequent occurrence of those sounds in English rather than selective avoidance; and even if the inference of selective avoidance is valid, clinicians may want the benefit of information about other productions. In summary, while connected speech samples are an essential part of an assessment battery, most clinicians do not rely on this type sample exclusively.

Elicitation Procedures.   The customary and preferred method for obtaining a sample of connected speech is to engage a client in spontaneous conversation. The clinician may talk with the client about such things as their family, television shows, or places the client has visited. The samples should be recorded so that the clinician can play them back as often as required to accurately transcribe the client's utterances. Clinicians should make notes about topics covered and errors noted to facilitate later transcription.

Some clinicians have the client read a passage orally as an alternative method for obtaining a connected sample of speech. Although this procedure provides a sample of connected speech, it has been demonstrated that usually fewer errors occur in a reading sample obtained in this manner than in a corpus of conversational speech (Wright, Shelton, and Arndt, 1969). Moreover, clinicians frequently test children who have not yet learned to read, in which case this procedure is obviously not a viable option.

Some speech sound tests specify procedures for obtaining a sample of connected speech. For example, in the "Sounds-in-Sentences" subtest of the *Goldman-Fristoe Test of Articulation* (Goldman and Fristoe, 2000), the client listens to a story while viewing the accompanying pictures and is then asked to repeat the story. Such a *delayed imitation task* is designed to elicit particular sounds in certain phonetic contexts.

A more spontaneous method than either the immediate or delayed imitation technique is for the client to tell a story about a series of pictures selected to elicit target words and sounds. Dubois and Bernthal (1978) compared productions in the same word stimuli elicited through a picture-naming task, a delayed imitation task, and a storytelling task. They reported that the greatest number of errors was found on the storytelling task and the smallest number on the picture-naming task. These findings were not surprising since the task of naming single words requires different skills than the sequencing of words in phrases and sentences. Although the differences between the methods were statistically significant, the authors interpreted the differences as clinically nonsignificant. They did, however, report that some individuals varied from group trends in their production of certain sounds, depending on the task; for example, some children made significantly more errors on the delayed imitation task than on the picture-naming task.

Summary. A connected speech sample is a crucial part of any phonological assessment battery because it allows (1) assessment of overall intelligibility and severity, (2) determination of speech sound usage in its natural form, and (3) a database from which to judge the accuracy of individual sounds, patterns of errors, and consistency of misarticulations. The preferred method for obtaining connected speech samples is to engage the client in spontaneous conversation. If, for some reason, this cannot be accomplished, alternate procedures that can be used include: (1) conversational responses elicited via picture stimuli or toys, (2) utilization of a reading passage, and (3) telling a story following the clinician's model (delayed imitation).

Single-Word/Citation Form Sampling

Rationale. From the standpoint of widespread usage, analyzing phoneme productions in a corpus of single-word productions (usually elicited by having an examinee name pictures) has been a common method for assessing speech sounds. Single words provide a discrete, identifiable unit of production that examiners can usually readily transcribe. Since transcribers often are interested in observing the production of only one or perhaps two segments per word, they are thus able to transcribe and analyze single-word samples more quickly than multiple or connected word samples. Even though a test may prescribe the scoring of only one or two sounds, the tester should transcribe the entire word, including vowels. The efficiency of analyzing sound productions from single-word productions has resulted in widespread usage of such stimuli. As suggested earlier, this type of sampling provides data that is supplemental to information obtained from the connected speech sample.

When sampling single words, it is typical for only one or two consonants to be scored in a word. Sound-positions include sounds in the *initial* position (sound at the beginning of a word, e.g., /b/ in /bot/), *final* position (sound at the end of a word, e.g., /t/ in /ræbɪt/), and *medial* position (all sounds between the initial and final sounds, e.g., /ɔ/, /k/, and /ɪ/ in /wɔkɪŋ/).

In some instances, the prefixes *pre-*, *inter-*, and *post-* are each combined with the term *vocalic* to describe the location of a consonant sound within syllables. Prevocalic position refers to consonants that precede a vowel (CV) and, therefore, initiate the syllable (e.g., *s*oap, *c*at). Postvocalic position refers to consonants that follow the vowel (VC) and, therefore, terminate the syllable (e.g., so*ap*, ca*t*). Intervocalic position involves a consonant that is embedded (VCV) between two vowels (e.g., ca*m*el, ea*g*er). A singleton consonant in the initial position of a word is prevocalic. Likewise a singleton sound in word-final position is postvocalic. A consonant in the intervocalic position serves the dual function of ending the preceding syllable and initiating the following syllable. Ingram (1981) suggested that when one consonant occurs between two vowel nuclei, such "ambisyllabic" consonants may be viewed as being shared by both syllables. The intervocalic consonant would be in the word-medial position since medial refers to somewhere between the first and the last sounds of the word. A medial consonant may stand next to another consonant and serve to initiate (release) or terminate (arrest) a syllable and, therefore, is not necessarily intervocalic. Thus, references to initial, medial, and final positions refer to location of consonants in a word, whereas the terms *prevocalic, intervocalic, postvocalic, releasor,* and *arrestor* refer to consonant position relative to syllables.

Speech sound productions are influenced by the complexity of the syllables and words in which they are produced. We know that the number and juxtaposition of phonemes make some syllables more difficult to produce than others. For example, a syllable such as /go/ is easier to produce than /grop/. The first syllable shapes to develop are generally CV, VC, and CVCV, which constitute the simplest syllable shapes.

One of the key issues in assessment concerns the correlation between phonological productions that occur in citation form (single words) and those that occur in connected speech. Research findings support a positive correlation between responses obtained from naming pictures and speech sound productions in spontaneous speaking situations. It should be noted, however, that in some clients, differences are frequently observed between these two types of measures. Clinicians need to be aware that sound productions in single words may not accurately reflect the same sounds produced in a spontaneous speech context.

Morrison and Shriberg (1992) reviewed 40 years of studies which were designed to compare citation-form testing with continuous-speech sampling. They reported that, in general, more errors occur in spontaneous connected speech as compared to production of single words although there were instances in which speech sound errors were more frequent in word naming. However, in their own research they reported that children produced sounds more accurately in connected speech than they did in citation-form testing.

Single-word testing does not provide the tester an opportunity to thoroughly evaluate the effect of context on speech sound productions (coarticulation). As discussed in Chapter 1, coarticulatory effects transcend phonetic, syllabic, and lexical (word) boundaries. Gallagher and Shriner (1975) reported that children's /s/ productions were affected by position in CCV consonant clusters. Curtis and Hardy (1959) reported that /r/ was more likely to be produced correctly in consonant clusters than in single phoneme productions. Hoffman, Schuckers, and Ratusnik (1977) reported that /r/ was influenced by factors such as lexical constraints (within vs. across word boundaries) and phonetic contexts. For example, when *r* was embedded in nonlexically constrained contexts (e.g., "the sick *r*at dies"), production was facilitated in the environment of /s/ as compared to /m/, /p/, and /t/. Variations in consonant production when sounds are elicited in consonant plus vowel contexts rather than in consonant clusters are widely recognized.

Despite reservations concerning some of the inferences that can be made about conversational speech on the basis of single-word samples, most clinicians value and include single-word productions in the assessment battery. Single-word tests, which can provide the clinician with information concerning phonetic skills, typically include all consonant phonemes in a language, and can provide phonological data in a relatively short time. In addition, for unintelligible clients, the tester has the advantage of knowing the productions the client has attempted to say. Because of the variations and because of the different kinds of data each sample provides in productions of single words versus connected speech, both should be included in the assessment battery.

Elicitation Procedures.   The customary way to elicit single-word productions is through the administration of a single-word articulation test (sometimes called a speech sound inventory), where a client names single words in response to picture stimuli. Single words may also be obtained by having a child name toys or objects. For young children, the clinician may simply wish to transcribe single-word productions the child produced spontaneously. Since picture-naming tests are the typical method for sampling single words, the following discussion will focus on this type of sampling procedure.

Speech sound inventories typically sample consonants, consonant clusters, and occasionally vowels and diphthongs. Consonants are often assessed in the initial, medial, and final positions of words. For example, /s/ in *s*aw, pen*c*il, hou*s*e; /ʃ/ in *s*hoe, sta*t*ion, fi*sh*, or in word-initial and final positions. Some instruments elicit sounds only in the initial and final positions (see Figure 5.1). The specific sounds included in inventories vary from test to test but almost always include those sounds that have a high frequency of error in children's speech. Studies have shown the following as the most frequently misarticulated sounds: /s, z, θ, ð, ʃ, ʒ, tʃ, dʒ, v, r, hw/. With the exception of the /hw/ (a phoneme that is often collapsed with /w/ in English), these sounds are among those items usually included in single-word tests.

As stated previously, speech sound inventories have traditionally placed little emphasis on the assessment of vowels. Undoubtedly this is a reflection of the fact that most preschool and school-age children with phonological disorders have problems primarily with consonants and that vowels are typically mastered at a relatively early age. As speech pathologists are increasingly involved in early intervention programs for children at risk for communication impairments, vowel productions have, however, been increasingly scrutinized. While some speech sound tests do target vowels, the examiner is encouraged to transcribe vowel productions even though a test is designed to examine only consonants.

Pollock (1991) delineated the following suggestions regarding vowel sampling:

1. Clients should be provided with multiple opportunities to produce each vowel.
2. Vowels should be assessed in a variety of different contexts, including (a) monosyllabic and multisyllabic words, (b) stressed and unstressed syllables, and (c) a variety of adjacent preceding and especially following consonants.
3. Limits for the range of responses considered correct or acceptable should be established since cultural influences may affect what is considered "correct."
4. Recommended vowels and diphthongs to be assessed include the following:

Target Word/ Phonetic Transcription	Word Correct	Transcription of Child's Production	Modeled
1. cat / kæt /	☐	_____	☐
2. gate / get /	☐	_____	☐
3. cup / kʌp /	☐	_____	☐
4. candy / kændi /	☐	_____	☐
5. dog / dɔg /	☐	_____	☐
6. bed / bɛd /	☐	_____	☐
7. boat / bot /	☐	_____	☐
8. goat / got /	☐	_____	☐
9. gun / gʌn /	☐	_____	☐
10. cow / kaʊ /	☐	_____	☐
11. crab / kræb /	☐	_____	☐
12. coat / kot /	☐	_____	☐
13. wagon / wægən /	☐	_____	☐
14. cake / kek /	☐	_____	☐
15. knife / naɪf /	☐	_____	☐
16. hat / hæt /	☐	_____	☐
17. rabbit / ræbɪt /	☐	_____	☐
18. balloon / bəlun /	☐	_____	☐
19. lamp / læmp /	☐	_____	☐
20. radio / redio [redɪo] /	☐	_____	☐
21. rain / ren /	☐	_____	☐
22. carrot / kɛrət /	☐	_____	☐
23. lion / laɪən /	☐	_____	☐
24. leaf / lif /	☐	_____	☐
25. bus / bʌs /	☐	_____	☐
26. seal / sil /	☐	_____	☐
27. fish / fiʃ /	☐	_____	☐
28. sun / sʌn /	☐	_____	☐

Consonant Inventory

Circle the I or F to indicate an error on an initial or final consonant or consonant cluster

#	p	b	m	w	f	v	θ	ð	t	d	s	z	n	l	ʃ	tʃ	dʒ	j	r	k	g	h	ɚ	clusters
1									F											I				
2									F											I				
3	F																			I				
4																				I				
5										I											F			
6		I								F														
7		I							F															
8									F												I			
9													F								I			
10																				I				
11	F																							cl
12									F											I				
13				I									F											
14																				I/F				
15					F																			(I at n)
16									F													I		
17									F										I					
18		I												F										
19														I										F (cl)
20																			I					
21													F						I					
22									F										I					
23													F	I										
24					F									I										
25		I									F													
26											I			F										
27					I										F									
28											I		F											

	p	b	m	w	f	v	θ	ð	t	d	s	z	n	l	ʃ	tʃ	dʒ	j	r	k	g	h	ɚ	cl.
Page 3 Subtotals Initial Errors																								
Page 3 Subtotals Final Errors																								

Page 3 Subtotal Words Correct ☐

FIGURE 5.1 Two-position Speech Sound Test which samples words in initial and final position.

Source: Sample items from phonetic inventory portion of the *Bankson-Bernthal Test of Phonology (BBTOP)*,1990b. Used with permission of PRO-ED.

Non-rhotic

/i/	/ou/
/ɪ/	/ɔ/
/ei/	/ɑ/
/ɛ/	/ʌ/ə/
/ae/	/aɪ/
/u/	/aʊ/
/ʊ/	/ɔi/

Rhotic

/ɝ, ɚ/	/ɔɚ/
/ɪɚ/	/ɑɚ/
/ɛɚ/	

To compensate for the lack of formal vowel assessment procedures, it is suggested that clinicians transcribe whole-word responses to the stimuli from commonly used phonological tests. In order to conduct a comprehensive review of vowels and diphthongs, it may be necessary, however, to supplement existing stimuli with additional vowels, diphthongs, and contexts not included in standard tests. For a comprehensive review of vowel disorders, the reader is referred to Ball and Gibbon (2001).

A number of phonological/articulation tests are commercially available. Despite the similarities between such tests, certain stimulus and response features differentiate one test from another. For example, one test may present items in a developmental sequence, another may organize the analysis according to place and manner of articulation. A third test may emphasize colored line drawings that are especially attractive to young children or include actual photographs.

Although phonological tests usually use pictures or photographs to elicit spontaneous responses, in some instances, toys or imitation tasks are used to elicit responses. Studies comparing responses elicited via imitation with those elicited through spontaneous picture naming have produced inconsistent results. Investigators studying children between the ages of 5 and 8 years have reported that responses elicited via imitation tasks yield a greater number of correct responses than those elicited via spontaneous picture naming (Siegel, Winitz, and Conkey, 1963; Smith and Ainsworth, 1967; Carter and Buck, 1958; Snow and Milisen, 1954). Other investigators who studied children ranging in age from 2 to 6 years reported no significant differences in results from elicitation via picture naming and imitation (Templin, 1947; Paynter and Bumpas, 1977).

Harrington, Lux, and Higgins (1984) studied responses to different types of picture-naming tasks and reported that children produced fewer errors when items were elicited via photographs as compared to line drawings. These data again suggest that different response elicitation procedures frequently produce different findings; however, the clinical significance of such differences tends to be minimal. The clinician should be mindful that for a given client, the nature of the test stimuli may have a bearing on responses obtained.

In spite of their widespread use, single-word tests have a number of limitations. Such measures do not allow children to use their "own" words but rather a set of predetermined and sometimes complex syllable and word shapes. The use of multisyllabic test words may make more demands on a child's productions and elicit more errors than would monosyllabic words or the words used in a child's own spontaneous speech. Ingram (1976) reported that when initial occurring fricative and affricate word pairs were similar in stress pattern and syllable structure, phoneme productions tended to be similar, but when syllable structure and/or stress of the pairs differed, monosyllabic words were more likely to be produced correctly than were multisyllabic words. Clinicians should recognize that syllable shape and stress patterns of stimulus words may affect speech sound productions. The clinician should keep in mind that citation tests primarily consist of nouns since they can be pictured; thus citation tests do not reflect the parts of speech used in connected conversational speech.

Another difficulty with tests designed to elicit a sample via picture-naming is that they often elicit only a single production of a given sound in each of either two or three word positions. During phonological development, inconsistency in production is common, even in the same stimulus word. Since the production of a sound may fluctuate, the client's customary articulatory patterns may be difficult to determine with only one to three samples of a sound. The clinician can increase the number of sound samples obtained through a single-word test by transcribing all the sounds in each stimulus (lexical) item, instead of focusing only on one or two sounds in each stimulus item.

As a supplement to standard phonological analyses that are segmentally oriented, Ingram and Ingram (2001) outlined two measures based on whole-word productions. They pointed out that during the acquisition process children attempt to learn and say words, not phonemes/segments, and thus word-oriented measures can assist the clinician to better understand a child's phonological system and the child's learning. They suggest that selection of target words for instruction should include an assessment of the complexity of the words to ensure that new sounds are introduced in word forms within the child's word system, that is, words within his or her vocabulary or those he or she can approximate. The goal of therapy is to expand not only the sound system and syllable shapes, but also increase the child's overall word complexity. They proposed a metric called "phonological mean length of utterance" (PMLU) that attempts to do what mean length of utterance does in language assessment. This metric examines the number of correct consonants produced at the word level, a number that increases with the length of the child's productions. A second metric—proportion of whole-word proximity (PWP)—was assumed to be highly correlated with word intelligibility. The PWP is calculated by dividing the PMLU of a word into the PMLU of the child's production of the same word. Ingram and Ingram (2001) give the example of zucchini [zukini], with a PMLU of 9, i.e., one point for each segment and one extra point for each of the three consonants. The child produces [zim] with a PMLU score of 6, i.e., four segments plus two points for each consonant. The PWP is then .67, i.e., 9 divided by 6. These two alternative measures are used to determine whole word correctness, complexity, intelligibility, and variations. It is of note that although Schmitt, Howard, and Schmitt (1983) reported a significant correlation between score on whole-word accuracy and articulation scores; Bankson and Bernthal (1990b) reported that many children's "whole-word correct" score varied from what would have been predicted from segmental and process scores, although no statistical analysis of the correlation was reported.

Summary.   Single-word samples, including speech sound tests, provide an efficient and relatively easy method for obtaining a sample of speech sound productions. Although they can be a valuable part of the phonological assessment battery, they should not constitute the only sampling procedure. Among their limitations are the small number of phonetic contexts sampled, the failure to fully reflect the effects of conversational context, the questionable representativeness of single-word naming responses, and the lack of consistency in factors such as syllable shape, prosody, word familiarity, and parts of speech (e.g., nouns, verbs). To increase the number of phonetic contexts sampled through such tests, the clinician is encouraged to transcribe entire stimulus words rather than just the target sound in the word.

Stimulability Testing

Rationale. Another sample of speech sound productions frequently included in a test battery is obtained through *stimulability testing*—that is, sampling the client's ability to repeat the correct form (adult standard) of error sounds when provided with "stimulation." In essence, this testing examines how well an individual imitates models of speech sounds that he or she produced incorrectly in single-word productions or in a connected speech sample. Although descriptions of what constitutes stimulability testing have varied, a commonly used procedure is one in which the examiner asks the respondent to imitate an auditory and/or visual model of a sound. Examiners typically seek to elicit imitative productions at one or more of three levels: sound in isolation, sound in initial, medial, and final positions of syllables and words. The examiner may tell the client to "watch and listen to what I am going to say, and then you say it." It should be recognized, however, that there are few standardized procedures for conducting this type of testing. Some tests, such as the *Goldman-Fristoe Test of Articulation* include a stimulability subtest. See Figure 5.2 for an example of a stimulability test for sounds in isolation and syllable productions.

Stimulability testing has been used (1) to determine whether or not a sound is likely to be acquired without intervention, (2) to determine the level and/or type of production at which instruction might begin, and (3) to predict the occurrence and nature of generalization. In other words, these data are often used when making decisions regarding case selection and determining which speech sounds to target in treatment.

Investigators have reported that the ability of a child to imitate syllables or words is related to normal phonological acquisition as well as to the probability of a child's spontaneously correcting his or her misarticulations (Miccio, Elbert, and Forrest, 1999). Pre-test and post-test comparisons with kindergarten and first-grade children have indicated that untreated children with high stimulability skills tended to perform better than children with low stimulability scores. For subjects who were not stimulable, direct instruction on speech sounds was found to be necessary as children would not self correct their errors. It has also been reported that good stimulability suggests more rapid progress in treatment (Irwin, West, and Trombetta, 1966; Carter and Buck, 1958; Farquhar, 1961; Sommers, Leiss, Delp, Gerber, Fundrella, Smith, Revucky, Ellis, and Haley, 1967). Carter and Buck (1958) reported, in a study of first-grade children, that stimulability testing can be used for such prognostic purposes. They inferred that first-grade children who correctly imitated error sounds in nonsense syllables were more likely to correct those sounds without instruction than children who were not able to imitate their error sounds. Kisatsky (1967) compared the pre- to post-test gains in articulation accuracy over a six-month period of two groups of kindergarten children, one identified as a high stimulability group and the other as a low

Stimulability Probe										
Name:										
Transcriber:										
Date:										
Sound	Iso	#__i	i__i	i__#	#__ɑ	ɑ__ɑ	ɑ__#	#__u	u__u	u__#	% Correct
b											
w				▓			▓			▓	
tʃ											
k											
s											
h				▓			▓			▓	
r											
d											
f											
θ											
l											
ʃ											
v											
z											
ð											
m											
p											
n											
g											
j				▓			▓			▓	
dʒ											
t											
Probe: "Look at me, listen, and say what I say."											

FIGURE 5.2   Example probe for stimulability of sounds absent from a child's phonetic inventory. Used with permission of Adele Miccio.

stimulability group. Although neither group received articulation instruction, results indicated that significantly more speech sounds were self corrected by the high stimulability group in the six-month post-test when compared to the low stimulability group.

It can be inferred from these studies that individuals with poor stimulability skills should be seen for treatment as it is unlikely that such children will self correct their speech sound errors. While children with good stimulability skills tend to show more self-correction on their speech sound errors, this finding is not true for all children. As a result, stimulability is but one factor used in determining treatment decisions and targets for treatment. In summary, the prognosis for individuals who are stimulable is more favorable than that for individuals who are not stimulable or who initiate their error sounds. Likewise, a child can be expected to make faster progress on sounds in which he or she is stimulable than on sounds that are not stimulable.

Stimulability has also been found to be an important factor in generalization. Elbert and McReynolds (1978) noted that generalization of correct /s/ production to a variety of contexts occurred as soon as the children learned to imitate the sound. In addition, Powell, Elbert, and Dinnsen (1991) reported that stimulability was the most decisive variable that they examined in explaining generalization patterns and could be used to explain and predict generalization patterns. They concluded that clinicians should target nonstimulable sounds first, as nonstimulable sounds are unlikely to change while many stimulable sounds may self-correct during treatment, even without direct instruction on those stimulable sounds.

Elicitation Procedures.   As stated above, the examiner typically asks the client to look at the examiner's mouth or watch it in a mirror, listen to what is said, and then imitate the production. The examiner does not point out where teeth, tongue, or lips may be during production; the examinee is simply encouraged to listen and observe a production. If the client is unsuccessful at imitating the sound, some examiners engage in cueing or trial instruction, providing directions for how to make sounds. The latter information is also used in selecting targets and determining the direction of treatment.

Stimulability testing usually includes imitative testing of those sounds produced in error in word and/or conversational samples. Some articulation tests include a place on the scoring form to record stimulability results, particularly for sounds in isolation. Clinicians will usually want to assess imitation in isolation, nonsense syllables (usually prevocalic, intervocalic, and postvocalic positions), and monosyllabic words (again in across word-positions). The number of productions required at each level will vary from one client and/or examiner to the next. Cooperation of the child, number of sounds produced in error, and success with the imitative task are factors the clinician should consider when deciding how extensive the stimulability assessment will be.

For example, in the case of a client with a /θ/ for /s/ error or ([θʌn] for [sʌn]), the client could be asked to initiate /s/ as follows:

1. Isolation: /s/ 6 tries
2. Nonsense syllables:

*s*i	i*s*i	i*s*
*s*a	a*s*a	a*s*
*s*u	u*s*u	u*s*

3. Words:

sail	bicycle	ice
sun	baseball	horse
seal	missile	bus

For a client with multiple errors, individual sounds may be assessed only in isolation (two productions), with two syllables, and with one or two words because of time constraints.

Summary.   Stimulability testing is useful in identifying those individuals most likely to need phonological intervention (those with poor stimulability scores), and for determining stimulus items for initiation of instruction. Stimulability scores have been found to have prognostic value for identifying those speech sound errors a child will likely self-correct, and/or which will generalize most quickly in therapy.

Contextual Testing

Rationale.   As indicated earlier, speech sound errors, especially in children, are often variable and inconsistent. Sounds are often easier to produce in some contexts as opposed to others, thus accounting for some of the inconsistency in production during the phonological acquisition period. Knowledge of the consistency of phonological errors is often a factor taken into consideration when deciding on the need for therapy and for making treatment decisions such as choosing sounds or sound patterns to work on in therapy or deciding on a particular phonetic context that may facilitate accurate sound production.

Assessing contextual influences is based on the concept that sound productions influence each other in the ongoing stream of speech. McDonald (1964) and others have suggested that valuable clinical information can be gained by systematically examining a sound as it is produced in varying contexts. McDonald coined the term *deep test* to refer to the practice of testing a sound in a variety of phonetic contexts. Coarticulatory effects consist of mechanical constraints associated with adjacent sounds and simultaneous preprogramming adjustments for segments later in the speech stream. This overlapping of movements (preprogramming) may extend as far as six phonetic segments away from a given sound (Kent and Minifie, 1977). Though the primary influence would appear to be sounds immediately preceding or following a target sound (Zehel, Shelton, Arndt, Wright, and Elbert (1972), the result is that segments may be perceived by a listener as being produced correctly in one context but not in another. Such information is of value to the clinician who seeks to establish a particular segment in a client's repertoire.

Elicitation Procedures.   The first published instrument for sampling contextual influences on sounds was the *Deep Test of Articulation* (McDonald, 1964), a series of phoneme-specific tasks designed to assess individual speech sounds in approximately 50 phonetic contexts. Deep testing is predicated on the hypothesis that when the consonants preceding or following the sound of interest are systematically varied, the client will usually produce the target sound correctly in at least one phonetic context.

More recent materials that have been developed to assess consistency-contextual influences include the *Secord Contextual Articulation Tests (S-CAT)* (Secord and Shine,

1997), and the *Contextual Test of Articulation* (Aase, Hovre, Krause, Shelfhout, Smith, and Carpenter, 2000). The S-CAT consists of three components: (1) Contextual Probes of Artic-ulation Competence (CPAC), (2) Storytelling Probes of Articulation Competence (SPAC), and (3) Target Words for Contextual Training (TWAC). The CPAC and SPAC are designed to assess 23 consonants and vocalic ɝ in various phonetic contexts through word and connected speech, samples, and can be used with clients from preschool through adult. The *Contextual Test of Articulation* tests 5 consonant sounds and 15 consonant clusters through sentence completion items in 7 vowel contexts.

In addition to published contextual tests, an informal contextual analysis may be done by reviewing a connected speech sample for contexts in which a target sound is pro-duced correctly. Occasionally facilitating contexts can be found in conversation that are not observed in single words or word-pairs. Phonemes may also be examined in various mor-phophonemic alterations to determine the effect of morpheme structure on phonological productions. Such alterations may be examined by having the client produce a sound in dif-fering morphophonemic structures. For example, if word-final obstruent /g/ has been deleted in /dɔg/ (i.e., [dɔ]), the examiner might assess whether or not /g/ is produced in the diminutive /dɔgi/. Likewise, if the child misarticulates /z/ in the word /roz/, the examiner might observe /z/ production in the morphophonemic context of /rozəz/. In addition, such testing may allow the clinician to determine whether the error is a sound production prob-lem or a problem marking plurality.

Consonants may also be examined for correct phoneme productions in the context of consonant clusters. While it is true that in most instances a consonant is more likely to be produced correctly as a singleton rather than in consonant clusters, it is not unusual for sounds to be produced correctly in the context of a cluster even when misarticulated in a singleton context. For example, one may find a correct /r/ or /s/ production in a cluster, even though it may consistently be in error in a singleton context.

Summary. Contextual testing is conducted to determine phonetic contexts in which a sound error may be produced correctly. These contexts may then be used to identify a start-ing point for remediation. Contextual testing is also used as a measure of consistency of misarticulation.

Error Pattern Identification

For children with multiple errors, the assessment battery often includes a formal measure designed to identify phonological patterns and error sounds.

Rationale. Many clinicians employ a phonological process analysis to facilitate error pat-tern delineation in clients who evidence multiple phonological errors. A phonological *process* or *pattern* is typically defined as a systematic sound change or simplification that affects a class of sounds, a particular sequence of sounds, or the syllable structure of words. Response elicitation procedures are often identical to that employed in citation testing (i.e., the client names pictures to produce single word responses), but may also involve engaging a client in conversational speech. The type of scoring and analysis of either type of sample is designed to identify the presence of phonological process/phonological patterns among errors. This type of analysis is based on the assumption that children's speech sound errors are not random, but represent systematic variations from the adult standard. Phonologic patterns that describe several individual speech sound errors are identified through such procedures. When doing a pattern analysis, clinicians compare the child's productions with the adult standard and then categorize individual errors into phonologic patterns.

One of the reasons pattern analysis procedures have appeal is that they provide a description of the child's overall phonological system. Khan (1985) furnished the following illustration of this point. A child who substitutes /wawa/ for *water* might be described in a traditional substitution analysis as substituting [w] for /t/ and substituting [a] for final /ɚ/. On the basis of what we know about phonological acquisition, the [wawa] for *water* substitution is more accurately described as syllable reduplication. The child in this instance is probably repeating the first syllable of the word *water* rather than using sound substitutions for target sounds in the second syllable. In this example, the child is also demonstrating knowledge of syllable structure.

A second reason for doing a pattern analysis is the potential for facilitating treatment efficacy. When a pattern reflecting several sound errors is targeted for treatment, there is the potential for enhancing rapid generalization across sounds related to that pattern.

Systems of pattern analysis, whether based on a place-manner-voicing analysis, distinctive feature analysis, or the more commonly employed phonological process analysis procedures, are most appropriate for the client who has multiple errors. The intent of the analysis is to determine if there are patterns or relationships among speech sound error productions which differ from the adult standard. If only a few speech sounds are in error, one need not do a pattern analysis of a child's speech. For example, if a client is misarticulating only two consonants, /s/ and /ʃ/, the clinician would not do a pattern analysis. In this instance, the clinician would develop a remediation plan where both consonants are targeted for direct instruction.

Phonological patterns identified during analysis are used for target selection in treatment. For example, if a child has eight speech sound substitutions reflecting three error patterns (e.g., stopping of fricatives, gliding of liquids, and fronting), remediation would likely focus on the reduction of one or more of these phonological patterns. The modification of one or more speech sounds (exemplars) reflecting a particular error pattern frequently results in generalization to other speech sounds reflecting the same error pattern. For example, establishment of final /p/ and /f/ may generalize to other stops and fricatives deleted in word-final position. Another example of a pattern-oriented remediation strategy would be to target for instruction all speech sounds that appear to be simplified in a similar manner, such as fricatives being replaced with stops (i.e., stopping). In this instance, the clinician might focus on the contrast between stops and fricatives. By focusing on sounds that reflect a similar error pattern, treatment should be more efficient than if it focuses on individual sounds without regard to phonological patterns.

Elicitation Procedures.   Since the late 1970s, several analysis procedures have been published that are based on identifying phonologic processes/patterns. Phonologic analysis procedures have been published by Hodson (2003), Dawson and Tattersall (2001), Khan and Lewis (1986; 2002), Bankson and Bernthal (1990b), and Smit and Hand (1997). Through each of these single word measures, phonologic patterns can be identified. In addition to these published analysis procedures, phonologic productions recorded during connected speech sampling and/or single word testing can be analyzed for the presence of error patterns.

Summary

Instruments, designed to identify phonological pattern processes, facilitate identification of commonalities among error production. The unique nature of these tests is in the type of / analysis they facilitate, as opposed to the type of samples obtained. Further discussion of such analyses will be presented later in this chapter under analysis procedures.

Criteria for Selecting Phonological Assessment Instruments

Formal test instruments selected by the clinician should be appropriate to the individual being tested and provide the information desired by the clinician. When selecting commercially available test instruments for phonological assessment, the clinician will want to consider the sample the instrument is designed to obtain, the nature of the stimulus materials (e.g., how easily recognized are the target pictures and objects), the scoring system, and the type of analysis facilitated by the instrument. A practical consideration in test selection is the amount of time required to administer the instrument and analyze the sample obtained. The following variables need to be taken into consideration when selecting a test instrument to include in the battery.

Sample Obtained

A factor to consider in selecting a test instrument is the adequacy or representativeness of the speech sample obtained. Variables to consider include the specific consonants, consonant clusters, vowels, and diphthongs tested; as well as the units in which sounds are to be produced (i.e., syllables, words, sentences). In addition, stimulus presentation and type of sample elicited (e.g., picture naming, sentence completion, imitation, delayed imitation, conversation) should also be considered in selecting instruments.

Material Presentation

Another practical factor in selecting commercially available tests is the attractiveness, compactness, and manipulability of materials. Size, familiarity, and color of stimulus pictures and appropriateness to the age of the client may influence the ease with which the clinician obtains responses to test stimuli. In addition, the organization and format of the scoring sheet are important for information retrieval. Tests with familiar and attractive stimulus items and score sheets that facilitate analysis are desirable.

Scoring and Analysis

Because the scoring and analysis procedures that accompany a test instrument determine the type of information obtained from the instrument, they are important considerations in test selection. Different assessment instruments currently available are designed to facilitate one or more of the following types of analysis: (1) phonetic and/or phoneme analysis of consonant and vowel sounds of the language; (2) sound productions in a variety of word positions and phonetic contexts; (3) place, manner, voice analysis; (4) phonological pattern/process analysis; and (5) age appropriateness of phonological productions.

Transcription and Scoring Procedures

Methods for Recording Responses

The recording systems used by clinicians vary according to the purposes of testing, the transcription skills of the examiner, and personal preferences. The type of response recording the examiner employs will, however, determine the type of analysis the clinician is able to do with the sample obtained. In turn, management decisions, which frequently include a recommended treatment approach, may be significantly influenced by the type of analysis conducted.

In the least sophisticated scoring procedure, phonological productions are simply scored as correct or incorrect, based on the examiner's perception of whether the sound produced is within the acceptable adult phoneme boundary. This type of scoring is sometime used to assess day-to-day process but is not recommended when doing a phonological assessment designed to determine the direction of treatment because in this instance more detailed description is required.

The most common transcription system to identify speech productions is the *International Phonetic Alphabet* (IPA), which includes a different symbol for each phoneme. As indicated in Chapter 1, more than 40 such symbols are utilized to identify the phonemes of the English language. This broad transcription system supplemented with a set of **diacritics** (narrow markers) usually provides sufficient detail for speech-language clinicians to adequately describe speech sound productions. For example, in a broad transcription of the word *key*, one would transcribe the initial segment with the symbol /k/. A more precise transcription of the initial /k/ would include the diacritic for aspiration [ʰ] following word-initial [kʰ] because aspiration occurs in production of /k/ in word-initial contexts. The aspiration modifier [ʰ] in this transcription represents one example of a diacritic. Use of diacritics, sometimes called a *close transcription system*, allows for recording specific topographical dimensions of individual segments. Such a transcription system is recommended when broad transcription does not adequately describe the errors. An example of diacritics that reflects an error seen in disordered phonology is the following: If /t/ in the word /tɪp/ is dentalized, the diacritic for dentalization [̪] is placed under the /t/, thus [t̪ɪp]; if /s/ in the word /sʌn/ is lateralized, the diacritic for lateralization is placed under the /s/, thus [s̞ʌn]. A list of common symbols and diacritics for clinical use is presented in Table 5.1.

Diacritic markers are used to describe the speech of individuals whose speech sound productions cannot be adequately described by broad phonetic symbols. For example, in assessing the phonological status of an individual with a cleft condition who is unable to achieve velopharyngeal closure for certain speech sounds, diacritics indicating nasal emission (s̃nail), or nasalization (bæ̃n), may be useful in the description of the client's production of such segments. Similarly, when assessing the articulation of an individual with impaired hearing, symbols to indicate appropriate vowel duration (e.g., [si:] for lengthened, devoicing (e.g., [b̥]), and denasalization (e.g., ræn) are recommended if these characteristics are present in productions. Likewise, with developmental articulation errors characterized by lateralization (e.g., [s̞]), dentalization (e.g., [s̪]), and devoicing (e.g., [n̥]), diacritics should be utilized.

TABLE 5.1 Symbols and Diacritics.

[x]	voiceless velar fricative, as in *Bach*
[Φ]	voiceless bilabial fricative
[β]	voiced bilabial fricative
[ʔ]	glottal stop, as in [mʌʔi]
ɾ̞[w]	r with [w] like quality

Stop Release Diacritics

[ʰ]	aspirated, as in [tʰap]
[⁼]	unaspirated, as in [p⁼un]

Diacritics for Nasality

[˜]	nasalized, as in [fæ̃n]
[˝]	denasalized
[˟]	produced with nasal emission

Diacritics for Length

[:]	lengthened

Diacritics for Voicing

[̥]	partially devoiced, as in [spuṋ]

Diacritics for Tongue Position or Shape

[̪]	dentalized, as in [tɛṋθ]
[̺]	lateralized, as in [ṣop]

Accuracy of Transcriptions

One of the major concerns regarding transcription of responses relates to accuracy. Clinicians must be concerned with whether or not their transcriptions are a valid representation of a client's productions. In making transcriptions, clinicians rely primarily upon auditory perceptual judgments. These judgments are sometimes supplemented with physiological measures (such as air pressure and flow information) and acoustical measures (such as that obtained from spectrographic analysis). These three types of data may not always be consistent with each other. For example, a glottal substitution for a stop in word-final position may be identified via a spectrographic analysis, and yet the glottal production may not be heard by a listener and thus will be transcribed as a deletion (omission). It must be recognized, however, that even the more objective measures of speech segments (i.e., acoustical and physiological recordings) are not devoid of human interpretation and no one-to-one correspondence exists between a phoneme production, perception, and/or acoustical and physiological measurements. For most aspects of clinical phonology, auditory perceptual judgments by the examiner remain the primary basis for intervention decisions although air pressure and spectrographic analysis can be useful on occasion. Because of the dependence on perceptual judgments, it is important for clinicians to establish the reliability of their perceptual judgments.

Interjudge Reliability.   Traditionally, clinicians have used agreement between two independent transcribers as a means of establishing reliability of judgments. *Interjudge agreement* or *reliability* is determined by the comparison of one examiner's transcriptions with those of another and is essential for reporting the results of phonological research. In addition, for students beginning to make judgments about accuracy of phonological productions, establishing interjudge reliability with a more experienced person can assist in the development of accurate judgments. A commonly used method to determine interjudge reliability, called *point-to-point agreement*, compares the clinicians' judgments on each test item. The number of items judged the same is divided by the total number of items to determine a percentage of agreement between judges. As an example, if two judges were to agree on 17 of 20 items and disagree on 3, they would divide 17 by 20 and get 0.85, which would then be multiplied by 100 to obtain an interjudge reliability index of 85 percent agreement. Such point-to-point or item-by-item reliability is a typically employed method for establishing agreement between judges in phonological research.

Sometimes transcriptions are made by two or more examiners independently but simultaneously, with the final transcript arrived at by consensus (Shriberg, Kwiatkowski, and Hoffman, 1984). Discussion between examiners regarding what is heard occurs prior to a "final" judgment. This procedure, which typically involves a panel of examiners listening to tape-recorded responses, is used in situations that are difficult to judge. Obviously, some independence of judgment is lost in such a procedure.

Shriberg and Lof (1991), in a study of point-to-point reliability of judgments of broad and narrow phonetic transcription, reported that for interjudge and intrajudge reliability, average agreement for broad transcriptions exceeded 90 percent, and for narrow transcriptions, between 65 percent and 75 percent.

Intrajudge Reliability.   Along with knowing that his or her judgments are in agreement with those of another examiner, the clinician will also want to know that his or her standards for judgments are consistent over time. Comparison of judgment made when scoring the same data on two separate occasions is referred to as *intrajudge reliability*. High reliability on such a measure is an indication that the examiner is consistent in his or her judgments. Recordings of responses are used to determine this type of reliability, because two judgments are made of the same responses.

Phonologic Assessment in Young Children

Phonologic evaluation of young children (infants and toddlers) must be done within the broader context of evaluating overall communicative behavior. Since phonologic development is integrally related to development of cognition, language, and motor skills, obviously phonological development reflects other aspects of a child's development. However, for purposes of this text, it is useful to isolate phonologic considerations from the overall communication process. The following paragraphs will present information related to this component of communication development that is not discussed elsewhere in our discussion of phonologic assessment.

There is much variability among young children in terms of the speech sounds and/or specific phonemes produced at a given age. Such variability makes it difficult to formulate strict developmental expectations and guidelines for phonology in infants and toddlers. One of the first assessments of phonologic development, especially with children at risk for developmental delay, involves determining whether or not the infant is progressing normally through the stages of infant vocalization. Speech sound productions emerge within the context of infant vocalizations at the prelinguistic level. Information presented in Chapter 2 regarding the characteristics of these stages is helpful in knowing about sound productions that typically occur during this developmental period, including the gradual shift from prelinguistic to linguistic behavior that usually occurs during the first year.

The point in time and/or development when clinicians frequently become involved in assessing phonology in young children occurs after they have acquired approximately 50 words (completion of the transition stage), or are putting two words together. This usually occurs between 18 and 24 months. For these children, clinicians are usually interested in determining how a child is doing in comparison to age, peers, and/or the adult standard. For younger children, or those with limited vocal repertoires, the interest is directed to describing whatever sounds they may employ for communication regardless of correct usage. In normal developing children, first words typically occur about 12 months of age, the transition stage occurs between 12 and 18 months, and words are put together around 24 months. In children with *phonological delay*, obviously these stages may occur at a later chronological age. Phonologic analysis in young children is inextricably bound to development of the child's lexicon. Procedures for eliciting vocalizations from young children depend on the level of the child's development, and can include a range of activities such as stimulating vocalizations during caregiving and feeding activities; informal play with a caregiver, sibling, or clinician; structured play; interactive storytelling; sentence repetition; delayed imitation of a story told by the clinician; narrative generation (about a favorite book); and spontaneous conversation.

Stoel-Gammon (1994) indicated that at 24 months children may be categorized into three groups: (1) those who are normal in terms of linguistic development (85 percent of children); (2) those who are slow developing (late talkers), but evidence no major deviations from patterns of normal acquisition; and (3) those whose developmental patterns deviate substantially from the broadest interpretation of norms in terms of order of acquisition or achievement of certain milestones. She indicated that the second and third groups together constitute 15 percent of the population. Children in the second group should be monitored to be certain that they "catch up" with the normal group. Stoel-Gammon indicated that children falling into this category would likely be those who, at 24 months, have a vocabulary smaller than 50 words, have a phonetic inventory with only 4–5 consonants and a limited variety of vowels, and who, otherwise, are following the normal order of phoneme acquisition and do not have unusual error types. Children in the third group are those who need an early intervention program.

The type of phonological analysis often employed during the early stages of speech sound acquisition is termed an **independent analysis** of **phonological behavior**. An independent analysis identifies the speech sounds produced by a child without reference to appropriateness of usage relative to the adult standard. This type of analysis is appropriate for the assessment of both normal and delayed phoneme acquisition. For those children who have progressed to the point where they have enough language that intelligibility is a concern (beyond 50 words in their vocabulary), a **relational analysis** may also be employed. In such analyses, the child's phonological productions are compared with the adult standard.

An independent analysis of phonology is typically based on a continuous speech sample and is designed to describe a child's productions without reference to adult usage. Analysis of a child's productions as a self-contained system include the following (Stoel-Gammon and Dunn, 1985):

1. An inventory of sounds (consonants and vowels) classified by word position and articulatory features (e.g., place, manner, voicing).
2. An inventory of syllables and word shapes produced (e.g., CVC, CV, VC, CCV).
3. Sequential constraints on particular sound sequences.

As stated earlier, a relational analysis of phonological productions is typically used with children in the two year age range evidencing normal language development, as well as with older children with phonological delay. Most of the assessment information presented elsewhere in this chapter pertains to relational analyses.

Summary.   Phonological evaluations in infants and toddlers are done within the context of an overall communication assessment since phonological development is integrally related to other aspects of development such as cognition, motor development, other aspects of linguistic development. Informal assessment involving independent analyses is typically done with very young children and for those with limited verbal repertoires. Usually these include an inventory of sounds, syllables and word shapes produced, phonological contrasts employed, and sequential contrasts. Once a child has a vocabulary of at least 50 words, relational analysis may also be employed.

Related Assessment Procedures

The assessment of a child with a phonologic problem includes testing and data gathering procedures supplemental to those focusing directly on phonologic behavior, often preceding phonologic assessment. Information is gathered in order to provide a more comprehensive picture of an individual client and thereby contribute to a better understanding of his or her phonological status. It may also influence management recommendations that are made regarding a given client.

These additional assessment procedures often include a case history; an oral cavity examination; and hearing, language, fluency, and voice screenings. These procedures can aid the clinician in the identification of factors that may contribute to or be related to the delay or impairment of phonology, and may influence treatment recommendations. Data gathered from these additional measures may lead to referral to other specialists and/or influence remediation decisions. If, for example, a child has a problem with closure of the velopharyngeal port, referral to a cleft palate team may result in pharyngeal flap surgery prior to speech intervention.

Presence of suspected sensory, structural, or neurological deficiencies must be corroborated by appropriate related personnel (e.g., audiological, medical) and recommendations from those sources must be taken into consideration as part of the assessment. Any of these factors may be important in decisions regarding the need for therapy, the point at which therapy should begin, and the treatment to be prescribed. Although they are routinely screened in phonologic evaluations, language, fluency, and voice screening will not be covered in this text.

Case History

To facilitate an efficient and effective assessment, a case history is obtained from the client or a parent prior to the phonological assessment. This allows the clinician to identify (1) possible etiological factors; (2) the family's or client's perception of the problem; (3) the academic, work, home, and social environment of the client; and (4) medical, developmental, and social information about the client. Case history information is usually obtained through a written form completed by the client or parents. It is frequently supplemented, by an oral interview. Specific questions on the phonological status of a young child might include the following: (1) Did your child babble? Can you describe it? (2) When did your child say his or her first words? What were they? When did he or she start putting words together? (3) Describe your child's communication problem, and your concerns about it. (4) How easy is your child to understand? By the family? By strangers? (5) What sounds does your child say? (6) What do you think caused your child's speech difficulty? While case histories obtained from the client or the client's family are products of memory and perception and thus may not reflect total accuracy, parents and clients in general are reliable informants. In spite of shortcomings, the case history provides the clinician with important background information that frequently influences assessment decisions and subsequent management recommendations.

Oral Cavity Examination

Oral cavity (oral peripheral) examinations are administered to describe the structure and function of the oral mechanism for normal speech purposes. In particular, dentition is observed for bite and missing teeth; hard and soft palates are examined for clefts, submucous clefts, fistulas, and fissures. Size, symmetry, and movement of the lips; size and movement of the tongue; and symmetry, movement, and functional length of the soft palate are assessed.

To examine the intraoral structures, it is recommended that the client be seated immediately in front of the clinician with his or her head in a natural upright position and at a level that allows easy viewing. The examiner should wear surgical gloves. If the client is a child, the examiner may have the child sit on a table or the examiner can kneel on the floor. Although it might seem that the oral cavity would be viewed best when the client extends his or her head backward, such a position can distort normal relationships of the head and neck. The client's mouth usually should be at the examiner's eye level. A flashlight or other light source, together with a tongue blade will aid in the examination. Observations should start at the front of the oral cavity and progress to the back. Since the oral cavity examination is important in identifying possible etiological factors, a description of how an examination is conducted is presented below. For a more complete presentation of procedures for conducting an oral-mechanism examination, see St. Louis and Ruscello (2000).

Dentition

For the examiner to evaluate the occlusal relationship (i.e., alignment of upper and lower jaws), the client should have the first molars in contact with each other since the occlusal relationship of the upper and lower dental arch are made with reference to these molar contacts. The upper dental arch is normally longer and wider than the lower dental arch; therefore, the upper teeth normally extend horizontally around the lower dental arch; and the maxillary (upper) incisors protrude about one-quarter inch in front of the lower teeth and cover about one-third of the crown of the mandibular incisors. Such dental overjet or overbite is the normal relationship of the dental arches in occlusion.

The teeth are said to be in open bite when the upper teeth do not cover part of the lower teeth at any given point along the dental arch. Mason and Wickwire (1978) recommended that, when evaluating occlusal relationships, the clinician should instruct the client to bite on the back teeth and to separate the lips. They further stated that

> while in occlusion, the client should be asked to produce several speech sounds in isolation, especially /s/, /z/, /f/, and /v/. Although these sounds may not normally be produced by the client with teeth in occlusion, the standardization of airspace dimensions and increases in pressure in the oral cavity can unmask a variety of functional relationships. For example, the child who usually exhibits an interdental lisp may be able to articulate /s/ surprisingly well with teeth together. This occluded position can also unmask and/or counteract habit patterns related to the protrusion of tongue and mandible on selected sounds. (15)

Mason and Wickwire also suggested that when an individual with excessive overjet has difficulty with /s/, he or she should be instructed to rotate the mandible forward as a means of adaptation to the excessive overjet. As pointed out in Chapter 4, however, dental abnormality and speech problems are frequently unrelated, and thus a cause-and-effect relationship between occlusion deviation and articulation problems should not be assumed.

Hard Palate

The hard palate (i.e., the bony portion of the oral cavity roof) is best viewed when the client extends his or her head backward. Normal midline coloration is pink and white. When a blue tint on the midline is observed, further investigation of the integrity of the bony framework is indicated. Such discoloration may be caused by a blood supply close to the surface of the palate and is sometimes associated with a submucous cleft (an opening in the bony palatal shelf). But when a blue tint is seen lateral to the midline of the hard palate, it usually suggests only an extra bony growth, which occurs in approximately 20 percent of the population.

Where a submucous cleft of the hard palate is suspected, palpation (rubbing) of the mucous membrane at the midline of the most posterior portion of the hard palate (nasal spine) is recommended. Although many speech-language pathologists note the height of the hard palatal vault, it probably has little relationship to articulation deviations. The contour or height of the palatal vault may influence certain articulatory contacts, but most individuals with high palatal vaults use compensatory movements that allow for adequate speech sound production.

Soft Palate or Velum

The soft palate should be evaluated with the head in a natural upright position. When the head is not in that position, changes in the structural relationship in the oral cavity area may prevent the viewing of velar function as it occurs during speech.

Mason and Wickwire cautioned that the assessment of velar function, especially velar elevation, should not be done with the tongue protruded or with the mandible positioned for maximum mouth opening. They recommended a mouth opening of about three quarters of the maximum opening since velar elevation may be less than maximum when the mouth is open maximally.

The coloration of the soft palate, like that of the hard palate, should be pink and white. A midline bluish tint should alert the clinician to the possibility of a submucous cleft of the velum, in which case the surface of the velum is covered with mucous membrane, but the underling layer of periosteum is absent.

The critical factor in velar function is the effective or functional length of the velum, not the velar length per se. Effective velar length is the portion of tissue that fills the space between the posterior border of the hard palate and the pharyngeal closure. Effective velar length is only one factor in adequate velopharyngeal sphincter function and provides little or no information concerning the function of the sphincter's pharyngeal component (described below), another critical factor for adequate velopharyngeal valving.

The final velar observation typically made is velar symmetry and evaluation. The elevation and posterior movement of the velum is also partially obstructed from view in an intraoral exam. But when the velum does not elevate to the plane of the hard palate during sustained vowel phonation, an inadequately functioning velopharyngeal sphincter should be suspected. It should also be remembered that if the observation is made with the tongue protruded, velar elevation can be restricted.

The posterior-most appendage or extension of the velum is the uvula, which has little or no role in speech production. However, a *bifid* uvula should alert the clinician to other possible anatomical deviations. A bifid uvula appears as two appendages rather than one and is occasionally seen in the presence of submucous clefts and other abnormal anatomical findings.

Fauces

The next area to observe in the oral cavity is the faucial pillars and the tonsillar masses. Only in rare instances are these structures a factor in speech production. The presence or absence of tonsillar masses is noted and, if present, their size and coloration are observed. Redness or inflammation may be evidence of tonsillitis, and large tonsillar masses may displace the faucial pillars and reduce the isthmus.

Pharynx

The oropharyngeal area is difficult to view in an intraoral examination. The pharyngeal contribution to velopharyngeal closure cannot be assessed through intraoral viewing because pharyngeal valving occurs at the level of the nasopharynx, a level superior to that which can be observed through the oral cavity. In some individuals, movement of tissue to form a prominence or ridge (Passavant's Pad) can be seen on the posterior wall of the pharynx; Passavant's Pad is not visible at rest but can usually be seen during sustained phonation. Passavant's Pad is present in approximately one-third of the individuals with cleft palates but is otherwise rare. Since its presence reflects a compensatory mechanism, the examiner should be alert to possible velopharyngeal valving problems. The presence of Passavant's Pad may suggest that adenoidal tissue is needed for velopharyngeal closure, and this factor should be considered in surgical decisions regarding adenoidectomies.

The pharyngeal gag response has been identified as a useful procedure to obtain an idea of the functional potential of the velum. Gagging usually results in maximum velar excursion and maximum movement of the pharyngeal walls. Gagging can be induced by pressing firmly on the base of the tongue or by touching the velum with a tongue blade. We recommend that the gag response be used only in very rare instances since many clients have a strong aversion to the procedure, and velar function during gagging generally has little relationship to velopharyngeal valving during speech. Elicitation of a gag may provide some useful information in cases where lack of innervation and a paresis of the pharyngeal or palatal function is suspected.

Considerable research has been conducted in the development of instrumental measures that can help in the assessment of velopharyngeal adequacy and function. Such measures are used to supplement clinical perceptions related to the adequacy of velopharyngeal function. Inadequate velopharyngeal function frequently is associated with hypernasal resonance, weak production of pressured consonants, i.e., stops, fricatives and affricates, and nasal emission of air. A number of direct and indirect instrumental procedures can help to assess velopharyngeal function, for example, nasometer, videofluoroscopy, nasopharyngoscopy, and airflow (aerodynamic) measures. For more information about such techniques see chapters in Bzoch (1997).

Tongue

As pointed out in Chapter 4, the tongue is a primary articulator, and individuals are able to modify tongue movements to compensate for many structural variations in the oral cavity. In terms of tongue size, two problematic conditions are occasionally found. The first, termed *macroglossia*, is an abnormally large tongue. Although this characteristic occurs frequently in certain populations (for example, those with Down's Syndrome), the overall incidence is relatively low and research data do not point to the tongue as the cause of speech problems in Down's children. The condition where the tongue is abnormally small in relation to the oral cavity is termed *microglossia*, but this condition rarely, if ever, causes a speech problem.

It has been pointed out that tongue movements for speech activities show little relationship to tongue movements for nonspeech activities. Unless motor problems are suspected, little is gained by having the client perform a series of tongue movements used for nonspeech activities. Protrusion of the tongue or moving the tongue laterally from one corner of the mouth to the other may provide information about possible motor limitations or problems in control of the tongue.

The rapid speech movements observed in diadochokinetic tasks (syllabic repetition— e.g., pʌ pʌ pʌ, pʌ tʌ kʌ) provide some information with respect to speech function. The absolute number of syllables that an individual can produce in a given unit of time usually bears little relationship to articulatory proficiency except when gross motor problems are present. For a discussion of the relationship between diadochokinetic testing and articulation, see Chapter 4. Mason and Wickwire (1978) suggested that the clinician focus on the pattern of tongue movement and the consistency of contacts during diadochokinetic tasks.

A short lingual frenum can restrict movement of the tongue tip. Most individuals, however, acquire normal speech in spite of a short lingual frenum. If the client can touch the alveolar ridge with the tongue tip, the length of the frenum is probably adequate for speech purposes. In the rare instance where this is not possible, surgical intervention may be necessary.

Summary

In an oral cavity examination, in which the clinician notes an inadequacy of structure or function that might contribute to the articulation disorders, he or she has several options: (1) refer the client to other professionals (e.g., otolaryngologist, orthodontist, cleft palate team) for assessment and possible intervention, (2) engage in further observation and testing to verify the earlier observation and note its impact upon speaking skills, and (3) provide instruction related to compensatory or remedial behaviors.

Audiological Screening

The primary purpose of audiological screening is to determine whether a client exhibits a loss of auditory function, which could be an etiological factor associated with a phonological disorder. Audiological screening is usually conducted with pure tones and/or impedance audiometry prior to phonological assessment.

Pure tone screening typically involves presentation of pure tone stimuli at 500, 1000, 2000, and 4000 Hz at a predetermined intensity level. Usually, a 20 dB HL is used for screening, but this level may be altered to compensate for ambient noise in the room. The pure tone frequencies used in screening are those considered most important for receiving speech stimuli. The loudness of the pure tone stimuli reflects threshold levels needed to function adequately in the classroom.

Impedance screening measures eardrum compliance (movement of the eardrum) and middle-ear pressure as air pressure is altered in the external auditory canal. This screening test yields basic information about the functioning of the tympanic membrane by eliciting the acoustic reflex. The acoustic reflex can be measured by presenting a relatively loud signal to the ear and observing the presence or absence of a change in the compliance of the eardrum. Screening of the acoustic reflex usually involves the presentation of a 1000 Hz signal at 70 dB above a person's threshold. The acoustic reflex is a contraction of the stapedial muscle when the ear is stimulated by a loud sound and serves as a protective device for the inner ear. The client who fails a pure tone or impedance screening test should be referred to an audiologist for a complete audiological assessment.

Summary

As indicated in Chapter 4 in the discussion of hearing as it relates to speech sound productions, it is critical to know the status of a client's hearing. There is some indication that recurrent middle ear problems can contribute to phonological delay. In the case of more severe auditory impairments, there is frequently a correlation between extent of hearing loss and level of speech and language development. Given this relationship, audiological screening must be a routine part of phonological assessment procedures.

Speech Sound Perception/Discrimination Testing

A review of the literature concerning the relationship between speech sound discrimination and articulation is presented in Chapter 4. The information presented there provides background for the assessment of speech sound perception, which is discussed below.

In earlier years, clinicians assumed that children with articulation errors were unable to perceive the difference between the standard adult production and their own error production, and then inferred that many phonological problems were the result of faulty perception. As a result of this assumption, speech sound discrimination testing that covered a wide variety of sound contrasts became a standard procedure in the assessment battery. These general discrimination tests did not examine contrasts relevant to a particular child's error productions (e.g., target sound vs. error sound—*wabbit* vs. *rabbit*), but as indicated, sampled a wide variety of contrasts. An example of a general test of discrimination is the *Goldman-Fristoe-Woodcock Test of Auditory Discrimination* (Goldman, Fristoe, and Woodcock, 1970). Research findings have cast doubt on the relationship between general speech sound discrimination and phonological disorders. The result has been that general speech sound discrimination tests are rarely used in clinical assessment. This testing is, however, recommended for those few clients suspected of having a generalized perceptual problem (e.g., inability to differentiate a wide variety of minimal pair sound contrasts). The type of testing recommended for clinical use is a phoneme task based on error production.

Locke's Speech Perception/Discrimination Testing

The *Speech Production Perception Task* (Locke, 1980) is a perceptual measure designed to assess a child's perception of his or her articulatory errors and involves no preselected stimuli, but rather stimuli based on the child's error productions. The format for this task, along with an example of the scoring sheet, appear in Table 5.2.

Preliminary to the presentation of the *Speech Production Perception Task*, the child's speech sound errors must be identified. The child's error productions and the corresponding adult standard (correct) forms are then used to construct the perception task. In this procedure, the adult norm is identified as the *stimulus phoneme* (SP), the child's substitution or deletion as the *response phoneme* (RP), and a perceptually similar "control phoneme" is identified as (CP). For example, if the client substitutes [wek] for /rek/, the stimulus production (SP) would be *rake* /r/, the response production (RP) would be *wake* /w/, and an appropriate control production (CP) would be *lake* /l/, since /l/ is a liquid as is /r/.

To administer the task, the examiner presents a picture or an object to the child and names it, either the correct or stimulus phoneme (SP), the client's incorrect response phoneme (RP), or a control phoneme. The number of correct responses to the three types of stimulus items (SP, RP, CP) are tabulated. A similar 18-item test is constructed for each sound substitution in which perception is to be examined in-depth.

TABLE 5.2   Speech Production Perception Task.

Child's Name _____ Sex: M F Birthdate: _____ Age: ____ Yrs. ____ Mos. ____

Date _____			Date _____			Date _____		
Production Task			Production Task			Production Task		
Stimulus		Response*	Stimulus		Response	Stimulus		Response
/θ ʌ m/	→	/f ʌ m/	/r e i k/	→	/w e i k/	/ʃ u/	→	/s u/
SP /θ/ RP /f/ CP /s/			SP /r/ RP /w/ CP /l/			SP /ʃ/ RP /s/ CP /t/		
Stimulus-Class		Response	Stimulus-Class		Response	Stimulus-Class		Response
1 /s/ - CP		yes NO	1 /r/ - SP		YES no	1 /s/ - RP		yes NO
2 /f/ - RP		yes NO	2 /l/ - CP		yes NO	2 /t/ - CP		yes NO
3 /θ/ - SP		YES no	3 /r/ - SP		YES no	3 /t/ - CP		yes NO
4 /θ/ - SP		YES no	4 /l/ - CP		yes NO	4 /ʃ/ - SP		YES no
5 /f/ - RP		yes NO	5 /w/ - RP		yes NO	5 /ʃ/ - SP		YES no
6 /s/ - CP		yes NO	6 /w/ - RP		yes NO	6 /s/ - RP		yes NO
7 /s/ - CP		yes NO	7 /r/ - SP		YES no	7 /s/ - RP		yes NO
8 /θ/ - SP		YES no	8 /w/ - RP		yes NO	8 /ʃ/ - SP		YES no
9 /f/ - RP		yes NO	9 /r/ - SP		YES no	9 /t/ - CP		yes NO
10 /θ/ - SP		YES no	10 /l/ - CP		yes NO	10 /ʃ/ - SP		YES no
11 /f/ - RP		yes NO	11 /l/ - CP		yes NO	11 /t/ - CP		yes NO
12 /s/ - CP		yes NO	12 /w/ - RP		yes NO	12 /s/ - RP		yes NO
13 /f/ - RP		yes NO	13 /t/ - SP		YES no	13 /ʃ/ - SP		YES no
14 /θ/ - SP		YES no	14 /l/ - CP		yes NO	14 /s/ - RP		yes NO
15 /s/ - CP		yes NO	15 /w/ - SP		YES no	15 /ʃ/ - SP		YES no
16 /f/ - RP		yes NO	16 /r/ - SP		YES no	16 /t/ - CP		yes NO
17 /θ/ - SP		YES no	17 /w/ - RP		yes NO	17 /t/ - CP		yes NO
18 /s/ - CP		yes NO	18 /l/ - CP		yes NO	18 /s/ - RP		yes NO
RP ____ CP ____ SP ____			RP ____ CP ____ SP ____			RP ____ CP ____ SP ____		

Source: Adapted by permission from J. Locke, "The Inference of Speech Perception in the Phonologically Disordered Child Part II: Some Clinically Novel Procedures, Their Use, Some Findings." *Journal of Speech and Hearing Disorders*, 45 (1980): 447.

*The correct response is in upper case letters.

Phonological Contrast Testing

The type of perceptual testing recommended is the assessment of a client's perception of phonological contrasts related to his/her error productions. Perceptual testing usually involves the client's differentiating the adult standard production from his or her error production and/or assessment of the child's perception of minimal pair phonological contrasts related to his or her error sound. In-depth perceptual testing of an error sound requires numerous phonemic pairings, all focusing on contrasts with the target sound.

Contrast testing is also useful with individuals learning English as a second language. Frequently it is difficult for such people to hear sound differences that involve sounds not used in their native language. For example, native Japanese have trouble differentiating /r/ and /l/, and Spanish speakers sometimes have trouble differentiating /ɪ/ and /i/.

Assessment of a child's awareness of phonological contrasts provides the clinician with data relative to the child's phonemic system at a perceptual level. Most clinicians improvise assessment tasks requiring the child to indicate awareness that certain contrasts are in his or her perceptual repertoire. For example, a child may be shown pictures of the following pairs of words which contrast s/t, s/ʃ, and s/θ, and be asked to pick up one picture from each pair as it is named.

sea	sea	some
tea	she	thumb

Summary

If it is suspected that a child's phonological errors may be related to faulty perception, perceptual testing is appropriate. The primary concern relates to the child's ability to differentiate between the adult standard and his or her error productions. Tests based on the child's specific errors and tests of phonemic contrasts are recommended for this purpose. While our understanding of the relationship between phonological productions and perception is incomplete, it appears that improving perceptual skills may be useful in helping some children to improve their phonological productions. For individuals who are second language learners, perception testing is also a useful component to the assessment battery.

Determining the Need for Intervention

After the clinician has collected various types of phonological samples, the data gathered during the assessment are analyzed and interpreted to determine (1) whether or not there is a phonological problem; (2) the nature of the problem, if there is one; (3) whether or not the client should be seen for treatment; and (4) if treatment is indicated, a recommended plan of action. The primary goals of *analyses* are to score, sort, or otherwise organize data collected in order to describe phonological performance. The purpose of *interpretation* is to examine the results of the phonological analyses and determine what course of action should be taken. Based on the interpretation of the phonological analyses, the clinician must determine whether or not the client needs instruction, and, if so, select target behaviors for treatment and appropriate intervention strategies. In summary, the clinician reviews responses to the phonological assessment tasks and interprets the analysis of these data in order to make appropriate and efficacious decisions.

In the case of children who will likely be receiving phonological therapy in the school under the provision of the Individual with Disabilities Education Act (IDEA), services are mandated only for those children whose speech and language interferes with their academic performance. As a result, in some school districts, services for a child with speech-language disorders may be directly tied to whether or not the speech-language impairment interferes with academic performance and, in some school districts, social acceptability. Qualifying children for phonological intervention requires the school-based speech-language pathologist to collaborate with a school-based diagnostic team to establish the need for services consistent with state and local eligibility criteria.

Intelligibility

An important consideration for determining the phonological status of an individual is the intelligibility or understandability of the client's spontaneous speech. The intelligibility of spontaneous speech is a reflection of the client's verbal communication competence and is a most important factor when determining the need for intervention and for evaluating the effectiveness of intervention strategies. Intelligibility of the speaker is the factor most frequently cited by both speech-language pathologists and naive listeners when judging the severity of a phonological problem (Shriberg and Kwiatkowski, 1982). It should be pointed out that severity, which will be discussed later, and intelligibility, are different though related concepts.

Degree of speech intelligibility is a perceptual judgment made by a listener and is based, to a large extent, on the percentage of words in a speech sample which are understood. Intelligibility of speech reflects a continuum of judgments ranging from unintelligible (where the message is not understood) to totally intelligible (where the message is completely understood by the listener). Intermediate points along such a continuum might include the following: speech is usually unintelligible, speech is partially intelligible, speech is intelligible although noticeably in error, or speech sound errors are occasionally noticed in continuous speech. Furthermore, intelligibility varies according to level of communication and the listener; single words with an unfamiliar listener; conversation with a familiar listener; conversation with an unfamiliar listener.

There is no standard procedure for quantifying the intelligibility of young children. Gordon-Brannan (1994) identified three general approaches for measuring intelligibility: (1) *open-set word identification* procedure, which calculates the percentage of words understood in a sample where the examiner transcribes a speech sample and determines the percentage of words identifiable; (2) *closed-set word identification*, wherein a listener identifies words read from prescribed word lists; and (3) *rating scale* procedures, which may take the form of either an *interval scaling* procedure, where a listener assigns a rating (number along a continuum of 5–9 points) or a *direct magnitude scale*, where a judgment of a speech sample is made relative to a standard stimulus.

Factors influencing speech sound intelligibility include the number and types of speech sound errors, consistency of sound errors, frequency of occurrence of error sounds, and phonological patterns used. In general, the larger the number of a speaker's productions which differ from the adult standard, the more intelligibility is reduced. However, a simple tally of the number of sounds in error is not an adequate index of intelligibility. As Shriberg and Kwiatkowski (1982) reported, there is a low correlation (r=.42) between the percentage of consonants correct and the intelligibility of a speech sample.

As stated, other factors in addition to the numbers of errors impact intelligibility. The nature of the clients' errors relative to the target is one such factor. For example, deleting a sound will affect intelligibility more than a distortion of the same sound will. Intelligibility is also affected by the consistency of misarticulated sounds and by the frequency with which an error sound occurs in the language. The more consistently a target sound is produced in error, and, likewise, the more frequently target sounds occur in the language, the more likely the listener will perceive the speaker's speech as defective.

Extraneous factors may influence intelligibility judgments. These factors include the listeners' familiarity with the speaker's speech pattern; prosodic factors such as speaker's rate, inflection, stress patterns, pauses, voice quality, loudness, and fluency; the linguistic experience of the listener; the social environment of the communication act; the message content; the communication cues available to the listener; and the characteristics of the transmission media. The complexity of these factors probably accounts for the finding that intelligibility ratings are not highly correlated with the percentage of consonants correct.

In case selection, a general principle of operation is that the poorer the ratings of intelligibility the more likely the need for intervention. According to parent reports, normal developing 2-year-old children can be understood by a stranger 50 percent of the time (Coplan and Gleason, 1988). Vihman reported in Chapter 2 a study of normal development wherein her 3-year-old subjects from well-educated families averaged over 70 percent intelligibility in conversation (range of 50–80 percent). Gordon-Brannan (1994) reported a mean intelligibility of 93 percent (range of 73–100 percent) with normal developing 4-year-old children. Commonly accepted standards for intelligibility expectations are as follows: 3 years, 75 percent intelligible, 4 years, 85 percent intelligible, 5 years, 95 percent intelligible. Bowen (2002) suggested the following intelligibility (percentage of words understood in conversation with an unfamiliar adult) expectations: 1 year, 25 percent intelligible; 2 years, 50 percent intelligible; 3 years, 75 percent intelligible; 4 years, 100 percent intelligible. She arrived at this percentage by dividing a child's age in years by 4. It should be pointed out that these percentages are in keeping with commonly accepted standards of intelligibility, particularly for 3- and 4-year-old children. These percentages do not reflect correct consonants, but simply the ability of a listener to understand what a speaker intended to say. It is generally recognized that a client 3 years of age or older who is unintelligible is a candidate for treatment.

Gordon-Brannan (1994), following a review of the literature concerning the assessment of intelligibility of children, suggested that calculating the actual percentage of words understood in a speech sample may be the most valid way to determine intelligibility. She suggested that the procedure could be enhanced by including orthographic transcription by a caregiver as a reliability check, and she also pointed out that while rating scales for judging speech intelligibility are less time consuming than determining percentage of words understood, such rating scales have not been validated or standardized for children with phonological deficits. For a review of procedures for evaluating the intelligibility of children's speech, see Kent, Miolo, and Bloedel (1994).

Severity

Severity of a phonological disorder refers to the degree of impairment or "handicap" in a particular client (Shriberg and Kwiatkowski, 1982). The severity of a phonological disorder is a second variable considered by speech-language clinicians in case selection decisions. Often school systems take severity ratings into consideration when determining caseload size for individual clinicians, since clients with more severe problems require more clinician time. Shriberg and Kwiatkowski developed a metric for quantifying the severity of involvement of children with a developmental phonological disorder which has become widely used. They recommended the calculation of **percentage of consonants correct** (PCC) as an index to quantify severity of involvement. Their research indicated that among several variables studied in relation to listeners' perceptions of severity, the PCC correlated most closely. The percentage of consonants correct requires the examiner to make correct-incorrect judgments of individual sounds produced in a continuous speech sample. Such judgments were found to be a fairly reliable measure for the classification of most children's phonological disorders as mild, mild-moderate, moderate-severe, or severe.

Procedures outlined by Shriberg and Kwiatkowski (1982; 267) for determining PCC are as follows:

> Tape record a continuous speech sample of a child following sampling procedures. Any means that yield continuous speech from the child are acceptable, provided that the clinician can tell the child that his exact words will be repeated onto the "tape machine" so that the clinician is sure to "get things right."

I. Sampling Rules
   A. Consider only intended (target) consonants in words. Intended vowels are not considered.
      1. Addition of a consonant before a vowel, for example, *on* [hon], is not scored because the target sound /ɔ/ is a vowel.
      2. Postvocalic /r/ in fair [feir] is a consonant, but stressed and unstressed vocalics [ɝ] and [ɚ], as in *furrier* [fɝiɚ], are considered vowels.
   B. Do not score target consonants in the second or successive repetitions of a syllable, for example, *ba-balloon*—score only the first /b/.
   C. Do not score target consonants in words that are completely or partially unintelligible or whose gloss is highly questionable.
   D. Do not score target consonants in the third or successive repetitions of adjacent words unless articulation changes. For example, the consonants in only the first two words of the series [kæt], [kæt], [kæt] are counted. However, the consonants in all three words are counted as if the series were [kæt], [kæk], [kæt].

II. Scoring Rules
   A. The following six types of consonant sound changes are scored as incorrect:
      1. Deletions of a target consonant
      2. Substitutions of another sound for a target consonant, including replacement by a glottal stop or a cognate
      3. Partial voicing of initial target consonants
      4. Distortions of a target sound, no matter how subtle
      5. Addition of a sound to a correct or incorrect target consonant, for example, *cars* said as [karks]
      6. Initial /h/ deletion (*he* [i]) and final n/ŋ substitutions (*ring* [rin]) are counted as errors only when they occur in stressed syllables; in unstressed syllables they are counted as correct, for example *feed her* [fidɚ]; *running* [rʌnin].
   B. Observe the following:
      1. The response definition for children who obviously have speech errors is "score as incorrect unless heard as correct." This response definition assigns questionable speech behaviors to an "incorrect" category.
      2. Dialectal variants should be glossed as intended in the child's dialect, for example, *picture* "piture," *ask* "aks," and so on.

3. Fast or casual speech sound changes should be glossed as the child intended, for example, *don't know* "dono," and "*n*," and the like.

4. Allophones should be scored as correct, for example, *water* [waɾɚ], *tail* [teɪl̩].

III. Calculation of Percentage of Consonants Correct (PCC)

$$PCC = \frac{\text{Number of Correct Consonants}}{\text{Number of Correct Plus Incorrect Consonants}} \times 100$$

Based on research that related PCC values to listeners' perception of degree of handicap, Shriberg and Kwiatkowski recommended the following scale of severity:

85–100%	- mild
65–85%	- mild/moderate
50–65%	- moderate/severe
<50%	- severe

Shriberg, Austin, Lewis, McSweeney, and Wilson (1997) have described modifications of this widely employed PCC metric. These extensions were developed to address concerns related to what some clinical phonologists perceived as limitations in the original procedure. Thus the authors have presented alternative PCC formulas that address such issues as frequency of occurrence of sounds; types of errors, including omissions and substitutions, and the nature of distortions; vowel and diphthong errors; and age and gender.

Quantitative estimates of severity, such as the PCC, provide the clinician with an objective means for determining the relative priority of those who may need intervention and a way to monitor progress/change.

Stimulability

As stated earlier in the discussion of the assessment battery, stimulability data are often used in making decisions regarding case selection. Investigators have reported that the ability of a child to imitate syllables and/or words containing a target sound is related to the probability that a child will spontaneously correct his/her misarticulations of that sound. The fact that a young child acquiring phonology can imitate error sounds correctly suggests that the child may be in the process of acquiring those sounds.

The use of stimulability testing for predicting spontaneous improvement or the rate of improvement in remediation has not been documented to the extent that definitive prognostic statements can be made, particularly with reference to an individual client.

Stimulability testing is only a general guide for the identification of clients who may correct their phonological errors without intervention. False positives (i.e., clients identified as needing instruction but who ultimately will outgrow their problems) and false negatives (i.e., clients identified as not needing instruction but who ultimately will require intervention) have been identified in all investigations focusing on stimulability as a prognostic indicator. These findings must be considered when results from stimulability testing are used to make predictive statements in clinical practice.

Error Patterns

After the examiner has reviewed a speaker's phonological productions in terms of intelligibility, severity, and stimulability, for those clients with multiple errors the next step is to further review the phonological samples for possible patterns of the error productions. Individual sound productions and error patterns are reviewed to determine if a child is using sounds and/or patterns at a level appropriate to their age. In such procedures, the clinician reviews and categorizes errors according to commonalities and/or phonological patterns/processes. As already suggested, determination of a child's phonological patterns may be based on a process assessment instrument, a connected speech sample, and/or productions obtained from a single-word articulation test.

Types of Pattern Analysis

Place-Manner-Voicing.   Perhaps the most simple type of pattern analysis involves classifying substitution errors according to place, manner, and voicing characteristics. A **place-manner-voicing analysis** facilitates the identification of patterns such as voiced for voiceless sound substitutions (e.g., voicing errors—/v/→[f] /d/→[t]), replacement of fricatives by stops (e.g., manner errors—/ð/→[d] /s/→/t/), or substitution of linguavelar sounds for linguaveolar sounds (e.g., place errors—/t/→[k] /d/→[g]).

Consider a child with several speech sound errors whose speech patterns reflect correct manner and voicing but produce errors in place of articulation, such as backing of consonants, for example, /t/→[k] /d/→[g] /b/→[g] /p/→[k]. In this instance, the clinician's strategy might be to teach the client to focus on the place of production. Some clinicians might choose to teach a single sound, for example, /t/, as an exemplar of the correct place of production and then probe for generalization to other sounds. Others might choose an alternative strategy and teach simultaneously all of the misarticulated stop sounds (same sound class) that reflect the place of articulation error pattern. When selected exemplars are taught, the assumption is that generalization will occur to other untrained sounds. The clinician should not assume that generalization will always occur, especially if the errors occur across sound classes. Generalization from trained to untrained sounds is difficult to predict. In addition, there is a great deal of individual variability in such generalization.

Distinctive feature and phonological process analysis procedures are extensions of analyses based on place, manner, and voicing. These procedures are discussed below.

Distinctive Feature Analysis.   In this type of pattern analysis, speech sound substitutions are reviewed for presence or absence of particular distinctive features. As presented in Chapter 1, the idea underlying **distinctive features** is that a combination of elements or features characterize a given sound segment and that such features can distinguish one sound from other sounds. Distinctive features are based on acoustic, perceptual, and/or articulatory characteristics. From a clinical perspective, distinctive features most easily adapted to assessment and treatment of phonological problems are those based primarily on articulatory characteristics. Distinctive feature systems typically include between 13 and 16 binary (plus or minus feature value) characteristics that are used to distinguish speech sound segments.

Some of the applications that speech-language pathologists have made of distinctive feature analysis have been the subject of criticism. It has been suggested that distinctive features, although helpful in classifying sounds of languages, may not be suited to the analysis of speech sound errors. Since distinctive feature systems were developed to classify the speech sounds of languages, they do not accurately describe many nonstandard (error) productions (e.g., certain sound distortions). The binary nature of the distinctive features may not reflect the varied productions seen in the speech of children with phonological disorders. A further problem is that the features of a deleted target sound are scored as errors although the sound and, as a result, the features were never attempted. Furthermore, those features that rely on acoustical characteristics are often impractical clinically. For a critical discussion of the issues regarding the application of distinctive features to clinical analysis and intervention, the reader is referred to the papers by Walsh (1974), Parker (1976), and Foster, Riley, and Parker (1985).

Phonological Pattern/Process Analysis.   A third type of pattern analysis, often called phonological process analysis, was described earlier in terms of case selection. Phonological pattern/process analysis is a method for identifying commonalities among errors, including the influence of sound position within word and syllable shapes. In other words, since speech sound productions are affected by such factors as phonetic context, position in words, and syllable structure of words, these factors are reviewed for any patterns that occur across the error sound productions. Before discussing interpretation of such analyses, we would like to review again some of the more common processes or patterns observed in the speech of young children. Although the process listings of different authors may vary (you will note some variance between those listed here and those identified by Vihman in Chapter 2), most resemble this listing.

Whole Word (and Syllable) Processes.   Whole word and syllable structure processes are changes that affect the syllabic structures of the target word.

1. *Final consonant deletion*. Deletion of the final consonant in a word.

   e.g. *book*   [bu]
      cap   [ka]
      fish   [fɪ]

2. *Unstressed syllable deletion* (weak syllable deletion). An unstressed syllable is deleted, often at the beginning of a word, sometimes in the middle.

   e.g. *potato*   [teto]
      telephone   [tɛfon]
      pajamas   [dʒæmiz]

3. *Reduplication.* A syllable or a portion of a syllable is repeated or duplicated usually becoming CVCV.

   e.g. *dad*   [dada]
      water   [wawa]
      cat   [kaka]

4. *Consonant cluster simplification.* A consonant cluster is simplified in some manner. The cluster can be reduced to one member of the consonant cluster (i.e., cluster reduction), or a substitution may occur for one or more members of the cluster.

e.g. *stop* [tap]   *brown* [bwon]   *milk* [mɪ]

    park [pak]   *snow* [n̥ou]

5. *Epenthesis.* A segment, usually the unstressed vowel [ə], is inserted.

e.g. *black* [bəlak]

    sweet [səwit]

    sun [sθʌn]

    long [lɔŋg]

6. *Metathesis.* There is a transposition or reversal of two segments (sounds) in a word.

e.g. *basket* [bæksɪt]

    spaghetti [pʌsgɛti]

    elephant [ɛfəlʌnt]

7. *Coalescence.* Characteristics of features from two adjacent sounds are combined so that one sound replaces two other sounds.

e.g. *swim* [fɪm]   *tree* [fɪ]

8. *Assimilatory (harmony) processes.* One sound is influenced by another sound such that a sound assumes features of a second sound. Thus, the two segments become more alike or similar (hence the term harmony) or, frequently identical. These sound changes are sometimes termed **progressive assimilation** if the sound that causes the sound change precedes the affected sound (*gate* [geɪk]) and **regressive assimilation** if the sound that causes the sound change follows the affected sound (*soup* [pup]).

   a. *Velar assimilation.* A nonvelar sound is assimilated (changed) to a velar sound because of the influence, or dominance, of the velar.

e.g. *duck* [gʌk] (regressive assimilation)

    take [kek] (regressive assimilation)

    coat [kok] (progressive assimilation)

   b. *Nasal assimilation.* A nonnasal sound is assimilated because of the influence, or dominance, of a nasal consonant.

e.g. *candy* [næni] (regressive assimilation)

    lamb [næm] (regressive assimilation)

    fun [nʌn] (regressive assimilation)

   c. *Labial assimilation.* A nonlabial sound is assimilated to a labial consonant because of the influence of a labial consonant.

e.g. *bed* [bɛb] (progressive assimilation)

    table [bebu] (regressive assimilation)

    pit [pip] (progressive assimilation)

Segment Change (Substitution) Processes. One sound is substituted for another, with the replacement sound reflecting changes in place of articulation, manner of articulation, or some other change in the way a sound is produced in a standard production.

1. *Velar fronting.* Substitutions are produced anterior, or forward of, the standard production.

   e.g. *key*   [ti]   (velar replaced by alveolar)
   monkey   [mʌnti]   (velar replaced by alveolar)
   go   [do]   (velar replaced by alveolar)

2. *Backing.* Sounds are substituted or replaced by segments produced posterior to, or further back in, the oral cavity than the standard production.

   e.g. *tan*   [kæn]
   do   [gu]
   sip   [ʃɪp]

3. *Stopping.* Fricatives or affricates are replaced by stops.

   e.g. *sun*   [tʌn]
   peach   [pit]
   that   [dæt]

4. *Gliding of liquids.* Prevocalic liquids are replaced by glides.

   e.g. *run*   [wʌn]
   yellow [jɛwo]
   leaf   [wif]

5. *Affrication.* Fricatives are replaced by affricates.

   e.g. *saw*   [tʃau]
   shoe [tʃu]
   sun   [tʃʌn]

6. *Vocalization.* Liquids or nasals are replaced by vowels.

   e.g. *bird*   [bʌd]
   table   [tebo]
   mother [mʌðo]

7. *Denasalization.* Nasals are replaced by homorganic stops (place of articulation is similar to target sound).

   e.g. *moon*   [bud]
   nice   [deis]
   man   [bæn]

8. *Deaffrication.* Affricates are replaced by fricatives.

   e.g. *chop*   [sap]
   chip   [ʃɪp]
   page   [pez]

9. *Glottal replacement.* Glottal stops replace sounds usually in either intervocalic or final position.

   e.g. *cat*   [kæʔ]
   tooth   [tuʔ]
   bottle [baʔl]

10. *Prevocalic voicing.* Voiceless consonants (obstruents) in the prevocalic position are voiced.

   e.g. *paper* [bepɚ]
   Tom [dam]
   table [debi]

11. *Devoicing of final consonants.* Voiced obstruents are devoiced in final position.

   e.g. *dog* [dɔk]
   nose [nos]
   bed [bɛt]

Multiple Pattern Occurrence.   The examples of phonological patterns given above typically included lexical items in which only a single pattern was used. In reality, the child may produce forms that reflect more than one process, including some that are not reflected in the definitions and descriptions above. A single lexical item may have two or even more processes interacting. When such productions occur, they are more complex and difficult to unravel than words which reflect a single process. For example, in the production of [du] for *shoe*, Edwards (1983) pointed out that the [d] for /ʃ/ replacement reflects the phonological pattern of (1) depalatalization, which changes the place of articulation; (2) stopping, which changes the manner of articulation; and (3) prevocalic voicing, which changes a voiceless consonant target to a voiced consonant. In the substitution of [dar] for *car*, the [d] for /k/ substitution is accounted for by the processes of velar fronting and prevocalic voicing. The identification of the sequence of steps describing how interacting processes account for substitutions is called a **derivation** or **process ordering**.

Unusual Pattern Occurrence.   As indicated throughout this book, a great deal of individual variation exists in the phonological acquisition of children. Although there are common developmental phonological patterns used by many children, the patterns observed across individuals vary. Unusual phonological patterns (e.g., use of a nasal sound for /s/ and /z/), called idiosyncratic processes or patterns, differ from the more common phonological patterns and are seen in both children with normal and delayed phonological development. The greatest variation in phonology occurs during the early stages of development and is probably influenced, in part, by the lexical items the child uses when acquiring his or her first words. When idiosyncratic patterns persist after age 3;0 to 3;5 years, they likely reflect a phonological disorder.

   The list of phonological processes presented above is not exhaustive but represents most of the common patterns seen in normally developing children. These phonological patterns have also been used in analyzing the sound errors of phonologically delayed children. Several procedures designed to assist the clinician in the identification of phonological patterns/processes in children's speech have been published in monograph or kit form. Included in these procedures are various groupings, as well as additions and deletions to the patterns/processes listed above. Table 5.3 reflects a modified version of Edwards' (1983) listing of the characteristics of published phonological assessment procedures.

TABLE 5.3 Characteristics of the Published Phonological Assessment Procedures.

Basis of Comparison by Authors	Hodson (2003)	Khan-Lewis (2002)	Bankson and Bernthal (1990b)	Smit and Hand (1997)	Lowe (1986)
Stimuli	3-dimensional objects	Pictures from the *Goldman-Fristoe Test of Articulation*	Pictures from the *Bankson-Bernthal Test of Phonology*	Photographs from the *Smit-Hand Articulation and Phonology Evaluation*	Embedded target words-picture stimuli
Elicitation procedures	Object-naming; no set order	Picture-naming in citation form	Picture-naming in citation form	Photograph-naming in citation form	Delayed sentence imitation-picture stimuli supplemental
Sample size	50 single words	44 single words	80 single words	80 single words	50 words
Transcription	Broad transcriptions modified; audiotaped for reference	Narrow "on-line" and from recordings	Live and from recordings	Live and from recordings check sheet with options delineated	Live
Number of processes	30 deviations	12 developmental processes 3 nondevelopmental processes	10 most frequently occurring processes in standardization samples	11 most frequently occurring processes in standardization samples	15
Target population	Children with multiple articulation errors; unintelligible speech	Normally developing and phonologically disordered children	Normally developing and phonologically disordered children ages 3–6	Normally developing and phonologically disordered children ages 3–9	Normally developing and phonologically disordered children ages 3–9
Time (total)	±50 minutes	±35 minutes	±30 minutes	Not specified	10-15 minutes
Number of processes per word	Allows for multiple processes	Allows for multiple processes	Allows for multiple processes	Allows for multiple processes	Allows for multiple processes
Process descriptions	Number of occurrences tabulated across sounds and positions	Organized by sounds and word-position	Organized by sounds and word-position	Number of occurrences in test words	Number of occurrences in test words
Frequency of occurrence	Calculation for 10 basic deviations	Frequency of each of the 15 processes calculated	Frequency of each of the 10 processes calculated	Percentage of occurrence in test words calculated	Frequency of each of the 15 processes calculated

Sound Preferences.   Another type of sound pattern that some clinicians have reported is called *sound preference*. In these situations, children seem to have a segment or two that they use for a large number of sounds or sound classes. Sometimes a particular sound is substituted for several or even all phonemes in a particular sound class (e.g., fricatives). Other children will substitute a single consonant for a variety of segments, such as [h] for /b, d, s, ʒ, z, dʒ, tʃ, ʃ, l, k, g, r/ (Weiner, 1981). It has been postulated that some children avoid the use of certain sounds in their productions and, instead, use those sounds they find easiest to produce.

Young children during the phonological acquisition stage simplify their productions as they learn the adult phonological system. The reasons that children simplify their productions likely include such factors as physiological and perceptual limitations/immaturities and a lack of linguistic knowledge. When such phonological simplifications (processes) persist in a child's productions, we use these patterns as a way to describe the child's phonological system and/or to identify the child's patterns of use. It is difficult to determine the precise reason for the persistence of a phonological process during normal sound acquisition.

Theoretical Considerations Regarding Phonological Processes.   An example demonstrating the inherent difficulty in arriving at an explanatory statement for a given phonological process was provided by Hoffman and Schuckers (1984). One explanation for the occurrence of a particular process might be that the child misperceives the adult word, for example, perceives [dɔg] as [dɔ]. A second explanation might be that the child's underlying word storage for *dog* is [dɔ]. A third possible explanation is that the child's perceptual system functions appropriately and the lexical match between what the child perceives and what he or she has stored is consistent with the adult standard, but he or she has a phonological production rule that calls for the deletion of word-final stops. A fourth possibility is that the child has a motor production problem; in this case the child may have the appropriate perception but does not possess the necessary motor skill to make the articulation gesture to produce the sound.

Shelton (1986) has identified three different theoretical interpretations of phonological processes/patterns in the speech-language pathology literature. One view is that phonological processes/patterns constitute a taxonomy or listing of speech sound error patterns, a catalog of descriptors that can be used to identify the simplifications or modifications used by children. This view makes no speculations or assumptions regarding the child's underlying representations (mental images or internal knowledge of the lexical items) in relation to the adult standard; it simply describes behavior at the observable or surface level. This atheoretical perspective posits nothing about the operation of processes, the nature of phonological structure, the relationship of surface forms and underlying representations, or even the relationship of production and perception.

A second view of phonological processes assumes that the child has underlying representations of lexical forms that are similar to those of the adult surface forms. This view, which comes from work in normal phonological development, assumes that the child is attempting to produce the adult form of the word and has an adultlike mental image of the lexical item. The surface forms produced by the child, however, reflect immature development. The child changes or simplifies the target production in some manner during the production of the word. It is these simplifications that are identified as errors in the individual's speech. The mismatches between the child's productions and his or her underlying representations (which are the same as the adult standard) are expressed as phonological processes/patterns.

The third theoretical position acknowledges the existence of underlying representations but makes no assumptions concerning their form. The clinician examines the child's surface forms (the child's articulatory productions) to determine the status or nature of the child's underlying representations. If a child uses a phoneme contrastively, it is assumed that he or she has the adult underlying form. If the child misarticulates a sound, and there is no evidence from phonological assessment or acoustical analysis that the sound is in the child's repertoire, it is not assumed the child has the adultlike underlying representation of the sound. For example, if a child says [dɔ] for [dɔg] but uses [g] in the diminutive *doggy* [dɔgi], one can assume that the child has the underlying form for [g] since /g/ is produced in the form [dɔgi]. On the other hand, if /g/ is not observed in any of the child's utterances, no assumption is made regarding the underlying form for /g/. Thus, this view of underlying structures differs from the second view, described above, in that it makes no assumptions concerning the underlying representations; the second assumes the child has the adult form.

Developmental Appropriateness

A fifth factor to consider in deciding if a client is a candidate for intervention is the age appropriateness of his or her phonological productions. If a child misarticulates sounds that are produced by 75 percent or 90 percent of children at that age (depending upon which criterion is selected), or if a child's performance on a normed speech sound test is one or more standard deviations below the mean, or if a child evidences phonological processes that typically are eliminated by other children of his/her age, the child is often identified as having a developmental delay or disorder.

Two methods traditionally have been employed to compare articulation performance and chronological age: (1) the number of correct responses on a speech sound articulation test are tabulated and then compared with normative data for a given age level on the same test (e.g., *Bankson-Bernthal Test of Phonology*, Bankson and Bernthal, 1990b); and (2) a comparison is made of the child's individual segmental productions with developmental norms for individual sounds (e.g., Prather, Hedrick, and Kern, 1975; Iowa-Nebraska norms, Smit, Hand, Freilinger, Bernthal, and Bird, 1990).

The comparison of a child's segmental productions with developmental norms for individual sounds is one way norms are frequently used. Although this appears to be a simple task, one must be cautious when assigning an age norm to a particular sound. Normative data are statistical averages that reflect overall patterns of mastery. One must remember that children learn sounds at different rates and in different sequences. Thus caution is required in the application of normative data for individual sounds produced by an individual child.

As discussed earlier, investigators have attached an age expectation to specific speech sounds by listing the age levels at which 75 percent and/or 90 percent of the children in a normative group have mastered each sound tested. Sander (1972) pointed out that such normative data are group standards which reflect upper age limits (i.e., 75 percent or 90 percent of children at a particular age produce the sound) rather than average performance or customary production (50 percent of children at a particular age produce the sound). Sander also argued that "variability among children in the ages at which they successfully produce specific sounds is so great as to discourage pinpoint statistics" (58).

Prather and colleagues (1975) reported speech sound acquisition norms for children from age 2 through 4 years on a test designed to elicit consonants in the prevocalic and postvocalic positions. With respect to the age levels at which 75 percent of the children had mastered specific sounds, these investigators reported earlier age levels than Templin (1957) although the sequence of acquisition was similar in both studies. They pointed out that the differences in findings could be due to their use of two-position versus Templin's three-position testing. A useful set of normative data for individual sound acquisition, which reflects an age range for sound development, is shown in Figure 5.3.

Smit and colleagues (1990) gathered three-position data from children in two midwestern states. Using a 75 percent criterion level, they reported that children acquire sounds at ages equal to or younger than ages reported by Templin except for /ŋ/ and /r/, for which the 75 percent criterion was later than that reported by Templin. They also found that clusters tended to reach the 75 percent criterion at the same age or later than singletons contained in the clusters. It is interesting to note, however, the overall similarity between the data of Smit and colleagues and those of Templin gathered 33 years earlier.

The clinician should keep in mind that in using the data from any large group study, individual subject data are obscured. Although the precise sequence and nature of phonological development varies from one person to another, in general, certain segments are mastered earlier than others, and this information is used in determining presence of phonological delay and the direction of treatment. For example, if 6-year-old Kirsten says all sounds usually produced by 75 percent of 3-year-old children, but is not yet using sounds commonly associated with 4-, 5-, and 6-year-olds, her phonological productions would be considered delayed. This developmental aspect of phonological acquisition makes age a useful factor in determining whether a child has a phonological delay.

A second commonly employed way of comparing phonology and chronological age is to compare a child's phonological performance with norms for a specific phonological measure (as opposed to individual segmental norms). In this procedure, the number of speech sound productions produced correctly on a specific test are compared with normative data for that instrument. In other words, the number of sounds that the child produces correctly are compared with normative data to determine whether a child's articulatory performance is typical for the child's age. This analysis is appropriate for children 8 years old and younger since correct production of speech sound segments is usually expected by age 8 in normal children. This procedure is the basis by which many states and school districts determine if children with phonological delay and disorders qualify for services. Tests such as the *Goldman-Fristoe Test of Articulation* (2000), the *Arizona Articulation Proficiency Scale* (Fudala and Reynolds, 1986), and the *Bankson-Bernthal Test of Phonology* (1990b) are examples of tests that report normative data.

The age appropriateness of certain phonological processes/patterns that may be present in a young child's speech is an additional normative factor taken into consideration in case selection. Several investigators have provided data that is relevant to young children's use of phonological processes. Preisser, Hodson, and Paden (1988), in a cross-sectional

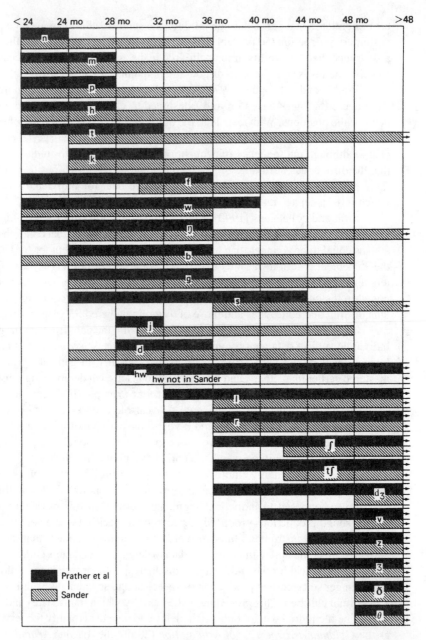

FIGURE 5.3 Normative articulation data. The left-hand margin of each bar represents the age at which 50 percent of the children in a normative study used the specified sound correctly. The right-hand margin shows the age at which 90 percent of the children used the sound correctly. Date reported in the lower bars are from Sander (1972). Date in the black bars are from the work of Hedrick, Prather, and Tobin (1975).

Adapted by permission from E.M. Prather, D.L. Hedrick, and C.A. Kern, "Articulation Development in Children Aged Two to Four Years," *Journal of Speech and Hearing Disorders*, *40* (1975): 179–191 (p. 186).

study, examined phonological processes used by young children. Between 24 and 29 months, the most commonly observed processes were cluster reduction, liquid deviation (which included deletions of a liquid in a consonant cluster, e.g., *black* → [bæk]), vowelization (e.g., *zipper*→ [zɪpo]), and gliding of liquids (e.g., *red* → [wɛd]). Next most common were patterns involving the strident feature.

Roberts, Burchinal, and Footo (1990) observed a group of children between 2;5 and 8 years in a quasilongitudinal study, that is, children were tested a varying number of times over the course of the study. They reported a marked decrease in the use of processes between the ages of 2;5 and 4 years. They also reported that at 2;5 years percentage of occurrence for the following processes was less than 20 percent: reduplication, assimilation, deletion of initial consonants, addition of a consonant, labialization shifts, methathesis, and backing. By age 4, only cluster reduction, liquid gliding, and deaffrication had a percentage of occurrence of 20 percent or more.

Stoel-Gammon and Dunn (1985) reviewed studies of process occurrence and identified those processes which typically are deleted by age 3 and those that persist after 3 years. Their summary is presented below:

Processes Disappearing by 3 Years	*Processes Persisting after 3 Years*
Unstressed syllable deletion	Cluster reduction
Final consonant deletion	Epenthesis
Consonant assimilation	Gliding
Reduplication	Vocalization
Velar fronting	Stopping
Prevocalic voicing	Depalatalization
	Final devoicing

Table 5.4 from Grunwell (1981) reflects "simplifying processes" used by young children in normal phonological development. The table is derived largely from data reported by Ingram (1976) and Anthony, Bogle, Ingram, and McIssac (1971) and is based on a relatively small number of subjects. The solid lines reflect typical ages at which particular processes are evidenced, and the broken lines reflect the approximate age at which the processes are modified or begin to disappear.

Bankson and Bernthal (1990b) reported data on the processes most frequently observed in a sample of over 1,000 children, 3 to 9 years of age, tested during the standardization of the *Bankson-Bernthal Test of Phonology (BBTOP)*. The BBTOP ultimately included the 10 processes that appeared most frequently in children's productions during standardization testing. The processes which persisted the longest in children's speech were gliding of liquids, stopping, cluster simplification, vocalization, and final consonant deletion. These data are almost identical to those reported by Khan and Lewis (1986, 2002) except they later found velar fronting as a process that also persisted in young children's speech.

Comparison of age and phonological development is widely practiced, and such data must be taken into consideration in intervention decisions. Justifiable criticism has been made of using such data as the single criterion for case selection (Turton, 1980). Criticism is based on the following factors: (1) Speech sound developmental norms typically reflect

TABLE 5.4 Chronology of Phonological Processes.

	2;0–2;6	2;6–3;0	3;0–3;6	3;6–4;0	4;0–4;6	4;6–5;0	5;0→
Unstressed Syllable Deletion	━━━	━━━	━━━	╌╌╌			
Final Consonant Deletion	━━━	╌╌╌					
Reduplication	╌╌						
Consonant Harmony	━━	╌╌					
Cluster Reduction (Initial)							
Obstruent—Approximant	━━━	━━━	╌╌╌				
/s/ + Consonant	━━━	━━━	╌╌				
Stopping /f/	╌╌╌	╌╌					
/v/		╌╌╌	╌╌				
/θ/ θ → [f]	━━	╌╌╌			╌╌╌	╌╌╌	╌╌╌
/ð/ /ð/ → [d] or [v]	━━━	━━━	━━━	━━━		╌╌╌	╌╌╌
/s/	━━	╌╌╌	╌╌				
/z/	━━━	╌╌╌	╌╌				
/ʃ/ Fronting '[s] type'	━━	╌╌╌	╌╌╌	╌╌╌	╌╌		
/tʃ, dʒ/ Fronting [ts, dz]	━━━	━━━	╌╌╌	╌╌╌	╌╌╌		
Fronting /k, g, ŋ/	━━	╌╌╌	╌╌				
Gliding r → [w]	━━━	╌╌╌	╌╌╌	╌╌╌	╌╌╌	╌╌╌	╌╌
Context-Sensitive Voicing	━━	╌╌╌	╌╌				

Source: Adapted by permission from P. Grunwell, "The Development of Phonology: A Descriptive Profile." *First Language, 3* (1981): 161-191. Used with permission.

upper age limits of customary consonant production (between 75 and 100 percent of children produce the sounds correctly) rather than average age estimates; (2) the norms are based on production in the initial, medial, and final positions of single words rather than spontaneous speech; (3) there is a great deal of variability across children; (4) norms frequently are based on a single production of a particular sound in one or two contexts; (5) norms represent a statement of average performance by age, but the resulting sequence of acquisition may not be applicable to a given individual; (6) although sounds generally appear to be acquired in a sequence, prior acquisition of certain sounds is not necessarily required for the learning of other sounds; and (7) the nature of the error may be a critical factor. For example, Stephens, Hoffman, and Daniloff (1986) reported that unlike most errors, lateralization of /s/ did not spontaneously improve with age. Our clinical experience is that lateralization of /s/ is a production which will likely self-correct with maturation. We would concur with the suggestion of Smit and colleagues (1990) that lateralized /s/ errors be treated earlier than other /s/ errors because unlike most speech sound errors they do not generally spontaneously correct with age.

Process norms can also be helpful in determining need for intervention. In this case, one is looking for processes/patterns or simplifications that are not typically used at a particular age. If processes/patterns persist beyond the expected age level, their presence is one of the factors that should be taken into consideration in case selection.

Case Selection Guidelines and Summary

The first question that must be answered through analysis of phonological sampling procedures is whether or not there is a phonological problem that warrants intervention. By reviewing the intelligibility of the speaker, the severity of the phonological problems that may be present, the developmental appropriateness of the child's phonological productions, and the error patterns, such a question can be answered.

As a general guideline for initiating intervention, a child, in order to be identifiable for services, should be one standard deviation or more (some state guidelines call for 1.5 to 2 standard deviations) below his or her age norm on a standardized measure of phonology. The clinician should recognize, however, that this is only a general guideline and that other considerations, such as, intelligibility, nature of the errors and error patterns, consistency of errors, speaker's perception of his or her problem, and other speech-language characteristics, may also be important in intervention decisions.

Children between ages 2.5 and 3 who are unintelligible are usually recommended for early intervention programs, which typically include parental education and assistance. Children age 3 years or older who evidence pronounced intelligibility and/or severity problems, or who evidence idiosyncratic phonological problems are candidates for intervention. Children age 8 and below whose phonological performance is at least one standard deviation below the mean for their age are also candidates for intervention. Most children 9 years or older are also recommended for intervention if they have consistently produced speech sound errors—often residual errors. Teenagers and adults who perceive that their phonological errors constitute a handicap should be considered for instruction. Likewise, children of any age should be considered for evaluation when they or their parents are concerned about their speech sound productions.

Target Behavior Selection

Once the need for intervention is established, sampling data are further reviewed to determine goals for intervention. The following paragraphs will delineate how the various components of the assessment battery are utilized to establish target behaviors for remediation.

Stimulability

As you will recall, stimulability testing consists of assessing client performance when the client is asked to imitate the adult form of speech sound errors in isolation, syllables, and words. Many clinicians have postulated that error sounds that can be produced through imitation are more rapidly corrected through intervention than sounds that cannot be imitated. McReynolds and Elbert (1978) reported that once a child could imitate a sound, generalization occurred to other contexts. Thus, imitation served as a predictor of generalization. Powell and colleagues (1991) also reported that stimulability explained many of the generalization patterns observed during treatment. They found that sounds that were stimulable were most likely to be added to the phonetic repertoire regardless of the sounds selected for treatment. Miccio and Elbert (1996) suggested that "teaching stimulability" may be a way to facilitate phonological acquisition and generalization by increasing the client's phonetic repertoire.

Intervention is usually initiated at the level of the most complex linguistic unit the client can imitate (i.e., isolation, syllable, word, phrase). Sounds from different sound classes are often chosen as exemplars, with stimulability data aiding in their selection. For example, if word-final stops, fricatives, and nasals are all deleted, the clinician might target one stimulable stop, fricative, and nasal as exemplars. Hodson (1989), in her cycles approach to remediation, suggested finding target sounds on which the child is stimulable when targeting processes.

Although there seems to be general agreement that more rapid generalization occurs for sounds which the child is stimulable on, some clinicians assign such sounds a lower priority for remediation. It has been reported that teaching sounds on which the child is not stimulable has the greatest potential to positively affect the child's overall phonological system although such sounds may be more difficult to teach (Powell et al., 1991). Thus, for children with multiple errors, greater gains in the overall phonological system may be made when intervention initially focuses on sounds not in the child's repertoire. This recommendation is in contrast to the notion that target selections should focus on sounds on which the client is stimulable since therapy will move rapidly and the child will enjoy faster success (Secord, 1989; Diedrich, 1983).

It has been postulated (Dinnsen and Elbert, 1984) that imitation of words by the child may reflect correct underlying representations (storage of the adult form). One might speculate then, that if a child is able to imitate a word, this performance may indicate that the child has acquired at a cognitive level the linguistic contrasts of the language necessary to produce a sound in at least some appropriate contrastive contexts. From this perspective, correct imitation is a reflection not only of phonetic or motor skill but also of the child's possession of the adult's (correct) underlying form of the error word. In a study of this issue, Lof (1994) concluded that stimulability testing reflects phonetic behavior only.

Frequency of Occurrence

Another factor used in target behavior selection is the frequency with which the sounds produced in error occur in the spoken language. Obviously, the greater the frequency of a sound in a language, the greater its potential effect on intelligibility. Thus, treatment will have the greatest impact on a client's overall intelligibility if frequently occurring segments produced in error are selected for treatment.

Table 5.5 lists the rank order and frequency of occurrence of the 24 most frequently used consonants in conversational American English (Shriberg and Kwiatkowski, 1983). These statistics are based on a collection of natural speech data from a variety of sources. Mines, Hanson, and Shoup (1978) noted a relatively high correlation among all frequency counts, based on both spoken and written expression. Seven consonants /n, t, s, r, d, m, z/ account for over half of all consonant occurrences in our language. The consonants /n, t, s, r, l, d, ð, k, m, w, z/ occur very frequently in connected speech and errors on these sounds will adversely affect intelligibility. Other data reported in the table show that almost two thirds of the consonants used are voiced, 29 percent are stops, 19 percent are sonorants, and 18 percent are nasals. Moreover, three of the six stops /t, d, k/, three of four sonorants /r, l, w/, and two of three nasals /n, m/ are among the 11 most frequently occurring consonants. Dental and alveolar consonants accounted for 61 percent of the productions and labial and labiodental sounds, 21 percent. In other words, over four-fifths of consonant occurrences are produced at the anterior area of the mouth.

Developmental Appropriateness

Earlier in this chapter we discussed, at length, the role of normative data in case selection. That discussion is also relevant to target selection. Traditionally clinicians have tended to select sounds for intervention that are earlier acquired and thus should already be in a client's repertoire. Research by Gierut, Morrisette, Hughes, and Rowland (1996) has suggested, however, that for children with multiple errors, treatment of later as opposed to earlier developing sounds results in greater overall improvement in a client's phonological system than does targeting early developing sounds. This finding is in keeping with other research (Dinnsen, Chin, Elbert, and Powell, 1990; Tyler and Figurski, 1994) which suggests that targeting sounds evidencing greater as opposed to lesser complexity is a more efficient way to proceed with phonological intervention. Data that does not support this assertion was reported by Rvachew and Nowak (2001). In a study of children with moderate or severe phonological delays, these investigators found that children who received treatment for phonemes that are early developing and associated with greater productive phonological knowledge showed greater progress toward acquisition of the target sounds than did children who received treatment for late-developing phonemes associated with little or no productive phonological knowledge. Further research appears warranted before a recommendation can be made regarding the efficacy of targeting early versus later developing sounds. In terms of processes/patterns, most clinicians would agree that targeting patterns that tend to be used early in acquisition (e.g., final consonant deletion) is better advised than targeting processes that tend to persist longer (e.g., gliding) during phonological acquisition because the early disappearing processes are more closely related to overall intelligibility. Age appropriateness is one factor to take into consideration in target selection, but it should be pointed out that other variables discussed in this section should also be reviewed when selecting targets for phonological remediation.

Contextual Analysis

As stated earlier, contextual testing is focused on the influence of surrounding sounds on error sounds. Contextual testing may identify facilitating phonetic contexts, which are

TABLE 5.5 Percentage of Occurrence of (Intended) English Consonants in Continuoius Speech.

Sound	Mean Rank	Mean %	Hoffman (1982)	Irwin and Wong (1983)[a]	Carterette and Jones (1974)	Mader (1954)	Shriberg and Kwiatkowski (1982)	Shriberg and Kwiatkowski (1983)	Mines et al. (1978)
n	1	12.01	11.22	9.84	13.63	13.14	11.7	13.04	11.49
t	2	11.83	12.43	14.05	7.91	11.74	13.7	13.08	9.88
s	3	6.90	6.78	6.66	6.94	6.50	7.1	6.43	7.88
r	4	6.68	7.06	5.99	8.20	7.83	5.2	5.84	6.61
d	5	6.41	4.26	6.89	6.31	10.25	5.8	5.33	5.70
m	6	5.93	5.20	5.52	7.49	4.63	5.6	7.97	5.11
z	7	5.36	8.69	4.88	4.58	3.70	3.0	3.97	4.70
ð	8	5.32	6.90	6.04	4.42	6.40	4.1	4.04	5.37
l	9	5.25	3.42	5.41	4.96	5.55	5.6	5.59	6.21
k	10	5.13	4.60	5.20	4.96	4.25	6.0	5.57	5.30
w	11	4.88	4.19	4.70	5.57	5.33	4.8	4.79	4.81
h	12	4.38	7.47	5.17	3.37	3.33	4.2	4.97	2.23
b	13	3.28	2.84	3.40	3.18	2.97	3.5	3.92	3.24
p	14	3.12	2.98	3.12	2.12	2.73	3.9	3.90	3.07
g	15	3.08	3.93	3.29	2.90	2.38	4.1	2.93	2.02
f	16	2.07	2.38	1.64	2.21	1.83	2.4	1.37	2.65
ŋ	17	1.58	0.94	1.86	1.05	1.61	2.5	1.24	1.85
j	18	1.56	1.22	1.49	1.41	0.77	2.2	1.94	1.87
v	19	1.52	1.03	1.46	1.64	1.91	1.2	0.42	2.97
ʃ	20	0.93	0.87	1.14	0.84	0.84	1.5	0.38	0.95
θ	21	0.89	0.59	0.84	1.03	0.93	0.9	0.76	1.19
dʒ	22	0.58	0.62	0.50	0.53	0.69	0.6	0.19	0.95
tʃ	23	0.55	0.34	0.31	0.51	0.55	0.7	0.56	0.85
ʒ	24	0.03	0.01	0.01	0	0.01	0	0	0.15

Source: L. Shriberg and J. Kwiatkowski, "Computer-Assisted Natural Process Analysis (NPA): Recent Issues and Data." In *Assessing and Treating Phonological Disorders: Current Approaches.* J. Locke (Ed.), *Seminars in Speech and Language, 4* (1983): 397. Used by permission.

[a]Data calculated from page 156. Table 8.4 to reflect only children aged 3, 4, and 6 years.

defined as surrounding sounds that have a positive influence on production of error sounds. Thus, contextual testing provides data on phonetic contexts in which an error sound may be produced correctly; this information may be helpful in treatment. Through the identification of such contexts, the clinician may find that a specific sound doesn't have to be taught, but rather should be isolated and stabilized in a specific context, since it is already in the client's repertoire. Both the client and clinician may save time and frustration that often accompany initial attempts to establish a speech sound by focusing first on a certain context in which a sound is produced correctly and then gradually shifting to other contexts. For example, if a child lisps on /s/ but a correct /s/ is observed in the /sk/ cluster in [bɪskɪt] (biscuit), one could have the client say *biscuit* slowly, emphasizing the medial cluster (i.e., sk), and hopefully hear a good /s/. The client could then prolong the /s/ before saying the /k/ (i.e., [bɪs ss kɪt]), and ultimately say the /s/ independent of the word context (i.e., /sss/). This production could then be used to progress to other contexts using the stabilized /s/ production. In general, when contexts can be found where target sounds are produced correctly, using such sound contexts can be used efficiently in remediation. The number of contexts in which a child can produce a sound correctly on a contextual test may provide some indication of the stability of the error. It seems logical that the less stable the error, the easier it may be to correct. However, some clinicians find that a stable error pattern is easier to focus on than is a more "elusive error." The clinician can utilize contexts in which a segment is produced correctly to reinforce correct production and facilitate generalization to other contexts. If a client's error tends to be inconsistent across different phonetic contexts, one might assume that the chances for improvement are better than if the error tends to persist across different phonetic contexts or situations.

Phonological Process Analysis

The comparison of a client's use of phonological processes/patterns with normative data regarding the use of phonological patterns or simplifications can be used in target selection. The processes or patterns used by a phonologically delayed child can be compared with those that might be expected in the speech of normally developing children. Patterns which are not normally present in children of a particular age are targeted for intervention. One caution, however, is that few data suggest that reduction in the use of phonological processes occurs in a prescribed order, although some processes tend to persist in older children and others tend to occur only in younger children. Moreover, no data suggest that the elimination or reduction of one process in a child's speech should occur before another process is targeted for treatment. There are, however, general trends that may be helpful in targeting processes for treatment, but a universally prescribed developmental order for process selection has not been established.

Hodson (1989) suggested that clinicians focus on teaching appropriate phonological patterns (rather than eliminate inappropriate patterns) and that stimulable sounds within those patterns be given priority for intervention. The following priority for targeting processes is based on suggestions from Hodson:

- Teaching word initial singleton consonants
- Teaching word final singleton consonants in CVC structures

- Evaluating syllable deletions in two- and three-syllable words
- Correcting errors related to velar sounds (e.g., velar fronting) and alveolar sounds
- Teaching /s/ clusters
- Evaluating liquids

Target Behavior Selection Guidelines

Few Errors

For children evidencing a small number of sound errors that are likely to be phonetic in nature, the clinician may wish to simultaneously work on all error productions. For example, if a child misarticulates /s/, /z/, /r/, and /l/, the clinician may target /s/ and /r/ for attention (assuming that the client will generalize from /s/ to /z/). If, however, a client is not able to handle multiple targets, one might wish to focus on a target that occurs most frequently in the language and/or affects intelligibility the most. Age of the client, attention span, and length and/or frequency of treatment sessions are variables to take into consideration in determining how many and which targets to focus on at any point in time.

Multiple Errors

For children with multiple phonological errors, target selection has some similarity to selection for clients with a small number of errors. However, some additional components and considerations exist. The first step for determining targets in clients with multiple errors is to determine the patterns or processes that are evident. Earlier we presented Hodson (1989), who suggested priorities for identifying target patterns for remediation (i.e., proceeding from initial and final consonant deletions to other processes, and ultimately liquid process errors).

When processes have been identified for intervention, one is then faced with selecting a specific sound to remediate, with the expectation that a selected target(s) or exemplar(s) will generalize to other sounds related to that target. For example, if final consonant deletion is identified as the first target process, one must then choose a sound, or perhaps two or more sounds, to work on in the word final position. Sound selection in this instance would be similar to the method identified above for choosing among sounds when there is a small number of errors (i.e., frequency of occurrence of a target, stimulability, developmental order).

In more recent years, these time-honored ways of selecting targets have been challenged because data has been provided (Gierut, 2001) that would suggest that other criteria for target sound selection may be more appropriate in terms of efficiency of treatment. More specifically, there are data to suggest that by targeting the following, a greater impact may be made on a child's overall sound system:

- Later developing as contrasted with early developing sounds
- Nonstimulable as contrasted with stimulable sounds
- Clusters as contrasted with singletons
- Difficult to produce as contrasted with easy to produce

Although many clinicians would suggest that these criteria for target selection should come into play after target processes have first been identified, some suggest that one could employ these criteria without reference to overall patterns present in a child's errors. However, the nature of sound collapses may also influence target sound selection. For example, if /w/ is used for /r/, /l/, /s/, /z/, /θ/, /ð/, /h/, one might attempt to initially target /s/ or /h/ to establish a contrast between /w/ and another sound in another sound class.

Other Factors to Consider in Case Selection— Intervention Decisions

Dialectal Considerations

As will be discussed in detail in Chapter 8, the linguistic culture of the speaker is a factor which must be considered when deciding on the need for speech-language intervention, particularly for those clients from ethnic or minority populations, where standard English may not be the norm. *Dialect*, as discussed in Chapter 8, refers to a consistent variation of a language, reflected in pronunciation, grammar, or vocabulary, that is used by a particular subgroup of the general population. Although many dialects are identified with a geographical area, those of greatest interest to clinicians are often dialects related to sociocultural or ethnic identification.

The phonological patterns of a particular dialect will differ from the general cultural norm, but these variations reflect only *differences* and not delays or deficiencies in comparison to the so-called standard version of the language. To view the phonological or syntactic patterns used by members of such subcultures as delayed, deviant, or substandard is totally inappropriate. As Williams (1972) put it years ago, "The relatively simple yet important point here is that language variation is a logical and expected phenomenon, hence, we should not look upon nonstandard dialects as *deficient* versions of a language" (111). This perspective has obvious clinical implications since persons whose speech and language patterns reflect a cultural dialect should not be considered for remediation unless their phonological patterns are outside the cultural norm for the region or ethnic group, or the individual wishes to learn a standard dialect.

Phonological differences may also occur in the speech of individuals within subcultures. The language patterns of inner-city African-Americans in New York City, for example, may be quite different from those in New Orleans. One cannot use normative data based on General American English (GAE) to judge the phonological status of individuals of some subcultures, and one should not assume that members of certain subcultures have homogeneous linguistic patterns, especially when geographic or ethnic factors are considered. Again, the reader is referred to Chapter 8 for further information on this topic.

Clinicians need to know about a child's linguistic and cultural background in order to make appropriate assessment-related decisions, including the need for intervention and instructional goals. Peña-Brooks and Hegde (2000) suggest that clinicians need to know:

1. The language and phonologic characteristics, properties, and rules of the linguistically-diverse child's primary language
2. How the primary language affects the learning of the second language

3. How to determine whether there are language or phonologic disorders in the child's first language, second language, or both

In the event that a speaker or the speaker's family wishes to modify their dialect or accent, the clinician may wish not only to use traditional sampling methods to describe the child's phonology, but also to employ measures specifically designed to assess the dialect and nonnative speaker's use of English phonology. Instructional decisions are then based on samples obtained and the variations that exist between Standard English and the person's dialect or accent.

Social-Vocational Expectations

Another factor to consider in the analysis and interpretation of a phonological sample is the attitude of the client or the client's parents toward the individual's phonological status. In cases where a treatment recommendation is questionable, the attitude of a client or family may be a factor in decisions for or against intervention. Extreme concern over an articulatory difference by the client or the client's parents may convince the clinician to enroll an individual for instruction. For example, the child who has a frontal lisp and also has a name that begins with /s/ may feel very strongly that the error is a source of embarrassment. Crowe-Hall (1991) and Kleffner (1952) found that fourth- and sixth-grade children reacted unfavorably to children who had even mild articulation disorders. There are many reports in the literature wherein elementary children have recounted negative experiences in speaking or reading situations when they produced only a few speech sounds in error. Even "minor distortions" can influence how one is perceived. Silverman (1976) reported that when a female speaker simulated a lateral lisp, listeners judged her more negatively on a personality characteristics inventory than when she spoke without a lisp.

The standard for acceptance of communication depends, to a large extent, on the speaking situation. People in public speaking situations may find that even minor distortions detract from their message. Some vocations, for example, radio and television broadcasters, may call for very precise articulation and pronunciations, and thus, some individuals may feel the need for intervention for what may be relatively minor phonetic distortions. We suggest that if an individual, regardless of age, feels handicapped by speech errors, treatment should usually be provided.

Computer-Assisted Phonological Analysis

Any discussion of phonological analysis and interpretation would be incomplete without calling attention to the fact that there are computer-based programs designed to assist with the analysis of phonological samples in clients who exhibit multiple errors. Masterson, Long, and Buder (1998) indicated that there are two primary reasons for using a computer-based analysis of a phonological sample: (1) it saves time, and (2) it provides greater detail of analysis than one typically produces with traditional paper and pencil (manual) analysis procedures. Computer phonological analysis (CPA) software involves inputting phonetic transcriptions from a computer keyboard and/or by selecting from predetermined stimuli, displaying this data on the screen, and ultimately printing results of an analysis. Analyses often include both relational and independent analyses of consonants and vowels, word position analysis, syllable shapes used, patterns among errors, and calculation of percentage of consonants correct. Each of the current programs has its own strengths and limitations, and undoubtedly future procedures will add new and helpful procedures for clinicians.

The Computerized Articulation and Phonology Evaluation System (CAPES) (Masterson and Bernhardt, 2002) is a good example of a system that was developed to elicit and analyze phonological productions. CAPES includes an online single-word (SW) elicitation task that is tailored to the client's phonological level. The SW task begins with a profile of 47 words (presented as picture files on the computer). The client's responses to those words are analyzed in order to select an additional set of words, the Individual Phonological Evaluation (IPE), for presentation. Four IPEs represent different phases of phonological development, from the earliest word structures and phonemes at Level 1 to complex multisyllabic words at Level 4. In addition to the SW elicitation task, CAPES allows the input of connected speech or user-constructed word lists or sentences. Video clips are available for elicitation of connected speech.

Client responses may be automatically recorded and digitized for later transcription or transcribed online with or without recording. To facilitate transcription, CAPES includes preselected transcriptions of the target form for each word in the SW task and a modest translation dictionary for the connected speech module. CAPES aids transcription of the words in the profile and IPEs 1 through 3 by providing a list of four predicted error responses (e.g., [tup] for *soup*). If the client produces one of these responses, the transcription is entered with a single click. When users need to enter transcriptions that are mismatches with the target, they access a click menu of IPA symbols. The IPA symbols allow phonological data from any language to be entered and analyzed in the connected speech module.

After transcriptions are entered, CAPES performs both independent and relational analyses. Reports for word shape, word length, stress pattern, consonants, and vowels may be accessed. Data regarding consonants and vowels may be viewed on the basis of individual segments, phonological sequences, phonological simplification processes, place/voice/manner features, and/or nonlinear features. Additionally, CAPES generates a list of potential treatment goals based on the results of the independent and relational analyses. Such goals are presented based on word shape, segment, or feature levels of organization.

In a study of time efficiency of procedures for phonological and grammatical analysis, comparing manual and computerized methods, Long (2001) reported that without exception, for both phonology and language, computerized analyses were completed faster and with equal or better accuracy than were manual analyses. Phonological analyses included the evaluation of variability, homonymy, word shapes, phonetic inventory, accuracy of production, and correspondence between target and production forms. Long further indicated that time needed for analyses, both computer and manual, was affected by the type of analysis, the type of sample, and the efficiency of individual participants.

A listing of some of the current CPA software programs is as follows:

Computer Analysis of Phonological Processes (CAPP). Hodson, B. (1985). Phonocomp, Box 46, Stonington, Ill. 62567.

Computerized Profiling (Version CP941.exe). Long, S.H., Fey, M.E., and Channell, R.W. (2002). Cleveland, OH: Case Western Reserve University.

Interactive System for Phonological Analysis (ISPA). Masterson, J., and Pagan, F. (1993). San Antonio, TX.: The Psychological Corporation.

Programs to Examine Phonetic and Phonological Evaluation Records (PEPPER). Shriberg, L. (1986). Hillsdale, NJ: Earlbaum.

Computerized Articulation and Phonology Evaluation System (CAPES). Masterson, J., and Bernhardt, B. (2002). San Antonio, TX: The Psychological Corporation.

Case Study

Assessment: Phonological Samples Obtained

Client

Kirk

Age

3.0 years

Reason for Referral

Parental referral due to Kirk's poor intelligibility when speaking

Case History/Speech and Hearing Mechanisms Status

The case history submitted by the parents and supplemented with the examination interview revealed normal motor and language development; however, speech sound development was delayed. Hearing screening indicated that hearing was within normal limits. A speech mechanism examination indicted normal structure and function.

Language.   Vocabulary, syntax, and pragmatics appeared normal based on case history, language sample obtained, and social interaction between Kirk and the examiner. Language skills, as measured by the *Peabody Picture Vocabulary Test* and the *Preschool Language Scale*, indicated language within normal limits. Poor intelligibility made it difficult to assess expressive morphosyntactic structures; however, a spontaneous speech sample obtained through storytelling evidenced four 6-word utterances, a seemingly rich vocabulary, and appropriate concepts for a 3-year-old child. Based on these data, Kirk's language skills were determined to be within normal limits.

Fluency and Voice.   Fluency was regarded as normal. However, a hoarse voice was noted. It was determined that vocal quality should be monitored over time by the parents and clinician to determine whether a problem was developing.

Phonological Samples Gathered

- **Conversation/Connected speech sample** of 180 words was obtained, with Kirk telling the story of "The Three Little Pigs." This story was used becaue Kirk was familiar with the story and words in the story were known to the examiner, thus facilitating phonological analysis.
- **Single word productions** were obtained through the *Bankson-Bernthal Test of Phonology* (BBTOP). All consonants and vowels produced by Kirk in the stimulus words were transcribed.
- **Stimulability testing** was done in isolation, syllables, and words for all target sounds produced in error.

Phonological Results and Analysis. The transcription of the connected speech sample and the single words from BBTOP were analyzed with the Proph phonological analysis component of the *Computerized Profiling* (Long, Fey, and Channell, 2002) program. Individual sound transcriptions were entered into the program and served as the basis for the analysis.

Phonological Analysis Outcomes. The percentage of consonants correct (PCC) was determined based on the connected speech sample. The PCC value was 34 percent, which translates to a rating of "severe" (i.e., level of handicap) for connected speech.

Segmental Analysis. Segmental analysis revealed numerous sound substitutions, particularly the use of /d/ in place of frictives, affricates, and some clusters. In addition there were inconsistent initial and final consonant deletions, including deletion of the initial /h/, /r/, and /l/. Other substitutions included /f/ for /s/ and some prevocalic voicing. These errors were evidenced in both single word productions and in running speech, though greater accuracy was reflected in single word productions. Table 5.6 reflects consonant singleton transcriptions from single word productions. Figures in the table indicate percent accuracy of production.

Stimulability Analysis. Kirk was instructed to "look at me, listen to what I say, and then you say it," followed by a model of the correct sound. Imitative testing (stimulability) was conducted for all sounds produced in error. Responses were solicited for sounds in isolation, syllables, and the initial position of words.

Kirk was stimulable for most error sounds in isolation, syllables, and initial word position. He did not imitate clusters that were in error. The following sounds were not stimulable: /ʃ/, /tʃ/, /z/, /dʒ/, /r/, and /ɚ/. The /s/ was stimulable only in isolation even though it was observed in the word-final position of some words during testing.

Pattern Analysis. A phonological process analysis was completed through the Proph program to determine error patterns that were evidenced in the single-word as well as connected speech sample of Kirk. This analysis revealed that the most prevalent process was stopping, with all fricatives and affricates impacted by this pattern (occurred in 85 percent of possible occasions in connected speech and with 44 percent occurrence in stimulus words from the BBTOP, particularly initial position). The most prevalent example of stopping was the use of /d/, which was substituted for initial /f/, /v/, /θ/, /ð/, /s/, /z/, /ʃ/, /tʃ/, /dʒ/,

TABLE 5.6 Consonant Singleton Productions in Single Word Productions Including Percent Accuracy of Production

Target	Error Productions			
	Error	Initial	Error	Final
p		100%		100%
b		100%		100%
m		100%		100%
w	ø	0%		
f	/d/	0%	/s/	0%
v	/d/	0%		100%
θ	/d/	0%	/t/	0%
ð	/d/	0%		
t		100%		100%
d		100%		100%
s	/d/	0%	/f/	50%
z	/d/	0%	/v/	0%
n		100%		100%
l	ø	0%	/o/	0%
ʃ	/d/	0%	/f/	0%
tʃ	/d/	0%		100%
dʒ	/d/	0%		
j	ø	0%		
r	ø	0%		
k		100%		100%
g		100%		100%
h	ø	0%		

and the clusters /sl/, /sn/, and /fl/. Kirk used frication (e.g., /s/, /f/, although inappropriately) when producing some single words. A diagram of his sound collapses for /d/ is as follows:

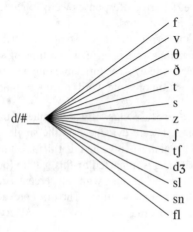

Clusters were simplified approximately 75 percent of the time in both isolated words and connected speech samples. Less frequently occurring patterns included **context sensitive voicing** (prevocalic voicing), and **initial consonant deletions**. Prevocalic voicing occurred in less than 25 percent of possible instances and initial consonants deletions less than 12 percent. Process analysis scoring on the BBTOP revealed similar error patterns.

Vowel Analysis.   The Proph program assesses vowel accuracy, and as might be expected for his age, Kirk's vowel productions were almost entirely accurate in both running speech and single word productions. Inconsistent misarticulations were observed on the vowels /ɛ/ and /ʊ/ in running speech.

Summary

These data reflect a 3-year-old boy with a speech sound disorder that, according to his PCC, BBTOP norms, and examiner subjective evaluation, is severe in nature. Although intelligibility was not formally measured, understanding his verbal productions was difficult even for family members. Most of Kirk's errors were sound substitutions, with some deletions in both initial and final word positions. Substitution errors were predominately the /d/ being substituted for fricatives and affricates. The presence of initial consonant deletions is developmentally an unusual process, but it is present only for the aspirate /h/ and liquids. Final consonant deletion is a process usually eliminated by age 3 and was observed only occasionally in Kirk's speech. Inconsistencies in all types of error productions were noted.

Sound errors appear to be both articulatory and phonological in nature. Articulatory errors are likely those errors for which Kirk was not easily stimulable. In other words, he did not demonstrate the motor skill to produce certain sounds via stimulability testing. This included the fricative /ʃ/, the affricates /tʃ/, and /dʒ/, prevocalic /r/, and the vowelized /ɝ/. Other errors seemed to involve both phonological and motor components. That is, several of the error consonants seemed to be difficult for Kirk to produce and likely will require motor practice before they are incorporated into appropriate sound contrasts. For /h/ and /k/, which were easily stimulated at the word level, it is likely that Kirk needs instruction in how these sounds are used contrastively in the language, or it may be necessary only to monitor these sounds to make sure they are acquired.

Assessment: Interpretation

Case Selection

Phonological intervention is warranted for Kirk. Factors that influenced this recommendation are as follows:

1. Normative data indicate that most normal developing 3-year-old children are approximately 75 percent intelligible. Although Kirk has just turned 3, we would nonetheless expect him to be more intelligible than he is. Intelligibility was not formally determined in our assessment battery, but observational data, as well as reports from

his family, indicate that much of Kirk's speech is unintelligible. This factor weighed heavily in our decision regarding Kirk's need for intervention.

2. With a PCC value in running speech of less than 40 percent, Kirk's phonological impairment is regarded as **severe** in nature. This rating relates to level of handicap reflected in his speech.

3. Phonological analysis evidences numerous substitution errors, some deletions, and several inappropriate phonological patterns. Positive indicators regarding Kirk's phonological status include the fact that he uses almost all vowels and some consonants correctly in his speech and is stimulable (with effort) for many of his error segments. His good vocabulary and the length of his utterances suggest that his linguistic deficits are confined to articulation and phonology, another positive indicator.

4. Intervention appears favorable because Kirk is stimulable for many of his error sounds, is highly verbal, and is not reluctant to speak for fear of negative consequences.

Target Sound Selection

Because Kirk has numerous misarticulations, and because these errors fall into patterns, target selection should begin with a review of these patterns. The error pattern that occurred most frequently was that of stopping, with several initial sounds, predominately fricatives and glides, collapsed into /d/. He also evidenced voicing of voiceless consonants in the initial position, gliding of liquids, and cluster reductions.

Although stopping is a process that persists in children sometimes past the age of 3, it is unusual for a child of this age not to be using more fricatives in speech. Most children are expected to use /f/ correctly by this age, and many are using the /s/ as well. Because the frication feature, including its correct usage, is diminished in Kirk's speech, reduction of stopping is the phonologic target of choice for initial therapy. The other two patterns evidenced in Kirk's speech (i.e., voicing, gliding), will be focused on later, largely because voicing does not have a great impact on intelligibility, and gliding occurred relatively infrequently and does not affect Kirk's intelligibility as much as stopping.

Intervention for Kirk is discussed in detail in Chapter 7. If one chooses to focus on one target sound, our suggestion for a priority focus is /f/. This is a highly visible sound and one that develops early, would address Kirk's stopping pattern, and frequently develops in final position prior to initial position. Kirk already uses the sound as a substitution for other fricatives in the final position; for example, he says /tif/ for /tiθ/ but /lis/ for /lif/. A second treatment target, likely one to work on simultaneously, is the correct use of /s/. The /s/ is in Kirk's repertoire; however, it is used inappropriately. Because Kirk is very young, one might choose to focus on only two sounds in the early sessions to avoid confusion among targets for the client. As progress is made, additional targets can be identified. Given Kirk's good attention span and good language skills, one might successfully focus on several error sounds in each lesson. If multiple targets are addressed, our suggestion would be to focus on collapses reflected in the /d/ replacement for numerous fricatives, clusters, and other stops. As stated, length of attention span, including ability to focus on multiple sounds and/or contrasts simultaneously, will influence the choice of intervention approach. This issue is addressed further in Chapter 7.

Summary

Kirk is a child who needs phonological intervention. Intelligibility, severity, and developmental level of his phonology support this decision. On the basis of his phonological samples, teaching frication to reduce stopping, producing sounds correctly in word-initial position, and further increasing Kirk's phonological repertoire are priority goals for initiating therapy.

QUESTIONS FOR CHAPTER 5

1. What are the purposes of phonological assessment?

2. Identify criteria for selecting a phonological assessment instrument.

3. Discuss the strengths and limitations of single-word testing and conversational sampling.

4. What is the nature and purpose of stimulability testing?

5. When might a clinician employ phonological perception testing as part of testing?

6. Discuss how the following factors may be utilized in case selection:

   - Intelligibility
   - Severity
   - Stimulability
   - Error patterns
   - Developmental appropriateness

7. Discuss how the following factors might influence target behavior selection:

   - Stimulability
   - Frequency of occurrence
   - Developmental appropriateness
   - Contextual analysis
   - Phonological process analysis

8. Differentiate between intelligibility and severity.

9. How do dialectal considerations influence intervention decisions?

REFERENCES

Aase, D., C. Hovre, K. Krause, S. Schelfhout, J. Smith, and L. Carpenter, *Contextual Test of Articulation*. Eau Clair, Wis.: Thinking Publications, 2000.

Anthony, A., D. Bogle, T. Ingram, and M. McIsaac, *Edinburgh Articulation Test*. Edinburgh: Churchill Livingston, 1971.

Ball, M. J., and F. Gibbon (Eds.), *Vowel Disorders*. Woburn, Mass.: Butterworth Heineman, 2001.

Bankson, N., and J. Bernthal, *Quick Screen of Phonology*. Chicago: Riverside Press, 1990a.

Bankson, N. W., and J. E. Bernthal, *Bankson-Bernthal Test of Phonology* (BBTOP). Austin, Tex.: PRO-ED, 1990b.

Bowen, C., Personal Communication, 2002.

Bzoch, K. R. (Ed.), *Communication Disorders Related to Cleft Lip and Palate* (4th ed.). Austin, Tex.: PRO-ED, 1997.

Carter, E., and M. Buck, "Prognostic testing for functional articulation disorders among children in the first grade." *Journal of Speech and Hearing Disorders, 23* (1958): 124–133.

Coplan, J., and J. Gleason, "Unclear speech: Recognition and significance of unintelligible speech in pre-school children." *Pediatrics, 82* (1988): 447–452.

Crowe-Hall, B. J., "Attitudes of fourth and sixth graders toward peers with mild articulation disorders." *Language, Speech, and Hearing Services in Schools, 22* (1991): 334–340.

Curtis, J., and J. Hardy, "A phonetic study of misarticulations of /r/." *Journal of Speech and Hearing Research, 2* (1959): 224–257.

Dawson, J. I., and P. J. Tattersall, *Structured Photographic Articulation Test—II.* DeKalb, Ill.: Janelle Publications, 2001.

Diedrich, W., "Stimulability and articulation disorders." In J. Locke (Ed.), *Assessing and Treating Phonological Disorders: Current Approaches. Seminars in Speech and Language, 4.* New York: Thieme-Stratton, 1983.

Dinnsen, D. A., S. B. Chin, M. Elbert, and T. Powell, "Some constraints on functionally disordered phonologies: Phonetic inventories and phonotactics." *Journal of Speech and Hearing Research, 33* (1990): 28–37.

Dinnsen, D., and M. Elbert, "On the relationship between phonology and learning." In M. Elbert, D. Dinnsen, and G. Weismer (Eds.), *Phonological Theory and the Misarticulating Child, ASHA Monographs, 22.* Rockville, Md.: ASHA, 1984.

Drumwright, A., *The Denver Articulation Examination.* Denver: Ladoca Project and Publishing Foundation, 1971.

Dubois, E., and J. Bernthal, "A comparison of three methods for obtaining articulatory responses." *Journal of Speech and Hearing Disorders, 43* (1978): 295–305.

Edwards, M., "Issues in phonological assessment." In J. Locke (Ed.), *Assessing and Treating Phonological Disorders: Current Approaches. Seminars in Speech and Language, 4.* New York: Thieme-Stratton, 1983.

Elbert, M., and L. V. McReynolds, "An experimental analysis of misarticulating children's generalization." *Journal of Speech and Hearing Research, 21* (1978): 136–149.

Farquhar, M. S., "Prognostic value of imitative and auditory discrimination tests." *Journal of Speech and Hearing Disorders, 26* (1961): 342–347.

Fluharty, N., *Fluharty Preschool Speech and Language Screening Test - Second Edition.* Austin, Tex.: PRO-ED, 2000.

Foster, D., K. Riley, and F. Parker, "Some problems in the clinical applications of phonological theory." *Journal of Speech and Hearing Disorders, 50* (1985): 294–297.

Fudala, J. B., and W. M. Reynolds, *Arizona Articulation Proficiency Scale* (2nd ed.). Los Angeles: Western Psychological Services, 1986.

Gallagher, R., and T. Shriner, "Contextual variables related to inconsistent /s/ and /z/ production in the spontaneous speech of children." *Journal of Speech and Hearing Research, 18* (1975): 623–633.

Gierut, J. A., "Complexity in phonological treatment: Clinical factors." *Language, Speech, and Hearing Services in Schools, 32* (2001): 229–241.

Gierut, J. A., M. L. Morrisette, M. T. Hughes, and S. Rowland, "Phonological treatment efficacy and developmental norms." *Language, Speech, and Hearing Services in Schools, 27* (1996): 215–230.

Goldman, R., and M. Fristoe, *Goldman-Fristoe Test of Articulation.* Circle Pines, Minn.: American Guidance Service, 1986, 2000.

Goldman, R., M. Fristoe, and R. Woodcock, *The Goldman-Fristoe-Woodcock Test of Auditory Discrimination.* Circle Pines, Minn.: American Guidance Service, 1970.

Gordon-Brannan, M., "Assessing intelligibility: children's expressive phonologies." In K. Butler, and B. Hodson (Eds.), *Topics in Language Disorders, 14* (1994): 17–25.

Grunwell, P., "The development of phonology: A descriptive profile." *First Language, 3* (1981): 161–191.

Harrington, J., I. Lux, and R. Higgins, "Identification of error types as related to stimuli in articulation tests." Paper presented at the annual convention of the American Speech-Language-Hearing Association. San Francisco, 1984.

Hodson, B., *Computer Analysis of Phonological Processes (CAPP).* Stonington, Ill.: Phonocomp, 1985.

Hodson, B., "Phonological remediation: A cycles approach." In N. Creaghead, P. Newman, and W. Secord (Eds.), *Assessment and Remediation of Articulatory and Phonological Disorders.* Columbus, Ohio: Charles E. Merrill, 1989.

Hodson, B. W., *Hodson Assessment of Phonological Process Patterns* (3rd ed.). Austin, Tex.: PRO-ED, 2003.

Hoffman, P. R., and G. H. Schuckers, "Articulation remediation treatment models." In R. G. Daniloff (Ed.), *Articulation Assessment and Treatment Issues.* San Diego: College-Hill Press, 1984.

Hoffman, P. R., G. Schuckers, and D. Ratusnik, "Contextual-coarticulatory inconsistency of /r/ misarticulations." *Journal of Speech and Hearing Research, 20* (1977): 631–643.

Ingram, D., *Phonological Disability in Children.* New York: American Elsevier, 1976, 1989.

Ingram, D., *Procedures for the Phonological Analysis of Children's Language.* Baltimore: University Park Press, 1981.

Ingram, D., and K. D. Ingram, "A whole-word approach to phonological analysis and intervention." *Language, Speech, and Hearing Services in Schools*, 32 (2001): 271–283.

Irwin, R. B., J. F. West, and M. A. Trombetta, "Effectiveness of speech therapy for second grade children with misarticulations: Predictive factors." *Exceptional Children*, 32 (1966): 471–479.

Kent, R., and F. Minifie, "Coarticulation in recent speech production models." *Journal of Phonetics*, 5 (1977): 115–133.

Kent, R. D., G. Miolo, and S. Bloedel, "Intelligibility of children's speech: A review of evaluation procedures." *American Journal of Speech-Language Pathology*, May (1994): 81–95.

Khan, L. M., *Basics of Phonological Analysis: A Programmed Learning Test*. San Diego, Calif.: College Hill, 1985.

Khan, L. M., and N. P. Lewis, *Khan-Lewis Phonological Analysis*. Circle Pines, Minn.: American Guidance Service, 1986, 2002.

Kisatsky, T., "The prognostic value of Carter-Buck tests in measuring articulation skills in selected kindergarten children." *Exceptional Children*, 34 (1967): 81–85.

Kleffner, F., "A comparison of the reactions of a group of fourth grade children to recorded examples of defective and nondefective articulation." Ph.D. thesis, University of Wisconsin, 1952.

Locke, J., "The inference of speech perception in the phonologically disordered child. Part II: Some clinically novel procedures, their use, some findings." *Journal of Speech and Hearing Disorders*, 45 (1980): 445–468.

Lof, G. L., "A study of phoneme perception and speech stimulability." Ph.D. thesis, University of Wisconsin—Madison, 1994.

Long, S., "About time: A comparison of computerized and manual procedures for grammatical and phonological analysis." *Clinical Linguistics and Phonetics*, 15 (2001): 399–426.

Long, S. H., M. E. Fey, and R. W. Channell, *Computerized Profiling (Version CP941.exe)*. Cleveland, Ohio: Case Western Reserve University, 2002.

Lowe, R. J., *Assessment Link Between Phonology and Articulation (ALPHA)*. Moline, Ill.: LinguiSystems, Inc., 1986.

Mason, R., and N. Wickwire, "Examining for orofacial variations." *Communiqué*, 8 (1978): 2–26.

Masterson, J., and B. Bernhardt, *Computerized Articulation and Phonology Evaluation System (CAPES)*. San Antonio, Tex.: The Psychological Corporation, 2002.

Masterson, J., S. Long, and E. Buder, "Instrumentation in clinical phonology." In J. Bernthal and N. Bankson (Eds.), *Articulation and Phonological Disorders* (4th ed.) (pp. 378–406). Needham Heights, Mass.: Allyn & Bacon, 1998.

Masterson, J., and F. Pagan, *Interactive System for Phonological Analysis (ISPA)*. San Antonio, Tex.: The Psychological Corporation, 1993.

McDonald, E., *A Deep Test of Articulation*. Pittsburgh: Stanwix House, 1964.

McReynolds, L.V., and M. Elbert, "An experimental analysis of misarticulating children's generalization." *Journal of Speech and Hearing Research*, 21 (1978): 136–150.

Miccio, A., and M. Elbert, "Enhancing stimulability: a treatment program." *Journal of Communication Disorders*, 29 (1996): 335–363.

Miccio, A. W., M. Elbert, and K. Forrest, "The relationship between stimulability and phonological acquisition in children with normally developing and disordered phonologies." *American Journal of Speech-Language Pathology*, 8 (1999): 347–363.

Mines, M., B. Hanson, and J. Shoup, "Frequency of occurrence of phonemes in conversational English." *Language and Speech*, 21 (1978): 221–241.

Morrison, J. A., and L. D. Shriberg "Articulation testing versus conversational speech sampling." *Journal of Speech and Hearing Research*, 35 (1992): 259–273.

Parker, F., "Distinctive features in speech pathology: Phonology of phonemics?" *Journal of Speech and Hearing Disorders*, 41 (1976): 23–39.

Paynter, W., and T. Bumpas, "Imitative and spontaneous articulatory assessment of three-year-old children." *Journal of Speech and Hearing Disorders*, 42 (1977): 119–125.

Peña-Brooks, A., and M. N. Hegde, *Assessment and Treatment of Articulation & Phonological Disorders in Children*. Austin, Tex.: PRO-ED, 2000.

Pigott, T., J. Barry, B. Hughes, D. Eastin, P. Titus, H. Stensil, K. Metcalf, and B. Porter, *Speech-Ease Screening Inventory (K–1)*, Austin, Tex.: PRO-ED, 1985.

Pollack, K., "The identification of vowel errors using transitional articulation or phonological process test stimuli." *Language, Speech, and Hearing Services in Schools*, 22 (1991): 39–50.

Powell, T. W., M. Elbert, and D. A. Dinnsen, "Stimulability as a factor in the phonologic generalization of misarticulating preschool children." *Journal of Speech and Hearing Research*, 34 (1991): 1318–1328.

Prather, E., D. Hedrick, and C. Kern, "Articulation development in children aged two to four years." *Journal of Speech and Hearing Disorders*, 40 (1975): 179–191.

Preisser, D. A., B. W. Hodson, and E. P. Paden, "Developmental phonology: 18–29 months." *Journal of Speech and Hearing Disorders*, 53 (1988): 125–130.

Roberts, J. E., M. Burchinal, and M. M. Footo, "Phonological process decline from 2½ to 8 years." *Journal of Communication Disorders*, 23 (1990): 205–217.

Rvachew, S., and M. Nowak, "The effect of target-selection strategy on phonological learning." *Journal of Speech, Language, and Hearing Research*, 44 (2001): 610–623.

Sander, E., "When are speech sounds learned?" *Journal of Speech and Hearing Disorders*, 37 (1972): 55–63.

Schmitt, L. S., B. H. Howard, and J. F. Schmitt, "Conversational speech sampling in the assessment of articulation proficiency." *Language, Speech, and Hearing Services in Schools*, 14 (1983): 210–214.

Secord, W., "The traditional approach to treatment." In N. Creaghead, P. Newman, and W. Secord (Eds.), *Assessment and Remediation of Articulatory and Phonological Disorders*. Columbus, Ohio: Charles E. Merrill, 1989.

Secord, W., and R. Shine, *Secord Contextual Articulation Tests (S-CAT)*. Sedona, Ariz.: Red Rock Educational Publications, 1997.

Shelton, R., Personal Communication, 1986.

Shriberg, L., *Programs to Examine Phonetic and Phonologic Evaluation Records (PEPPER)*. Hillsdale, N.J.: Earlbaum, 1986.

Shriberg, L., D. Austin, B. Lewis, J. McSweeney, and D. Wilson, "The percentage of consonants correct (PCC) metric: Extensions and reliability data." *Journal of Speech, Language, and Hearing Research*, 40 (1997): 708–722.

Shriberg, L., and J. Kwiatkowski, *Natural Process Analysis*. New York: John Wiley and Sons, 1980.

Shriberg, L. D., and J. Kwiatkowski, "Phonological disorders III: A procedure for assessing severity of involvement." *Journal of Speech and Hearing Disorders*, 47 (1982): 256–270.

Shriberg, L., and J. Kwiatkowski, "Computer-assisted natural process analysis (NPA): Recent issues and data." In J. Locke (Ed.), *Assessing and Treating Phonological Disorders: Current Approaches, Seminars in Speech and Language, 4*. New York: Thieme-Stratton, 1983.

Shriberg, L. D., J. Kwiatkowski, and K. Hoffman, "A procedure for phonetic transcription by consensus." *Journal of Speech and Hearing Research*, 27 (1984): 456–465.

Shriberg, L. D., and G. L. Lof, "Reliability studies in broad and narrow phonetic transcription." *Clinical Linguistics and Phonetics*, 5 (1991): 225–279.

Siegel, R., H. Winitz, and H. Conkey, "The influence of testing instruments in articulatory responses of children." *Journal of Speech and Hearing Disorders*, 28 (1963): 67–76.

Silverman, E., "Listeners' impressions of speakers with lateral lisps." *Journal of Speech and Hearing Disorders*, 41 (1976): 547–552.

Smit, A. B., and L. Hand, *Smit-Hand Articulation and Phonology Evaluation (SAAPE)*. Los Angeles, CA: Western Psychological Services, 1972, 1997.

Smit, A. B., L. Hand, J. J. Freilinger, J. E. Bernthal, and A. Bird, "The Iowa articulation norms project and its Nebraska replication." *Journal of Speech and Hearing Disorders*, 55 (1990): 779–798.

Smith, M. W., and S. Ainsworth, "The effect of three types of stimulation on articulatory responses of speech defective children." *Journal of Speech and Hearing Research*, 10 (1967): 333–338.

Snow, J., and R. Milisen, "The influences of oral versus pictorial representation upon articulation testing results." *Journal of Speech and Hearing Disorders*. Monograph Supplement, 4 (1954): 29–36.

Sommers, R. K., R. Leiss, M. Delp, A. Gerber, D. Fundrella, R. Smith, M. Revucky, D. Ellis, and V. Haley, "Factors related to the effectiveness of articulation therapy for kindergarten, first- and second-grade children." *Journal of Speech and Hearing Research*, 10 (1967): 428–437.

St. Louis, K., and D. Ruscello, *The Oral Speech Screening Examination*. Baltmore, Md.: University Park Press, 2000.

Stephens, M. I., P. Hoffman, and R. Daniloff, "Phonetic characteristics of delayed /s/ development." *Journal of Phonetics*, 14 (1986): 247–256.

Stoel-Gammon, C., "Normal and disordered phonology in two-year olds." In K. Butler (Ed.), *Early Intervention: Working with Infants and Toddlers* (pp. 110–121). Rockville, Md.: Aspen Publishers, 1994.

Stoel-Gammon, C., and C. Dunn, *Normal and Disordered Phonology in Children*. Baltimore: University Park Press, 1985.

Templin, M., "Spontaneous vs. imitated verbalization in testing pre-school children." *Journal of Speech and Hearing Disorders*, 12 (1947): 293–300.

Templin, M., *Certain Language Skills in Children*. Institute of Child Welfare Monograph Series, 26. Minneapolis: University of Minnesota, 1957.

Turton, L. J., "Development bases of articulation assessment." In W. D. Wolfe and D. J. Goulding (Eds.), *Articulation and Learning* (2nd ed.) (pp. 129–155). Springfield, Ill.: Charles C. Thomas, 1980.

Tyler, A. A., and G. R. Figurski, "Phonetic inventory changes after treating distinctions along an implicational hierarchy." *Clinical Linguistics and Phonetics*, 8 (1994): 91–107.

Walsh, H., "On certain practical inadequacies of distinctive feature systems." *Journal of Speech and Hearing Disorders*, 39 (1974): 32–43.

Weiner, F. F., "Systematic sound preference as a characteristic of phonological disability." *Journal of Speech and Hearing Disorders*, 46 (1981): 281–286.

Williams, F., *Language and Speech: Introductory Perspectives*. Englewood Cliffs, N.J.: Prentice Hall, 1972.

Wright, V., R. Shelton, and W. Arndt, "A task for evaluation of articulation change: III. Imitative task scores compared with scores for more spontaneous tasks." *Journal of Speech and Hearing Research, 12* (1969): 875–884.

Zehel, Z., R. Shelton, W. Arndt, V. Wright, and M. Elbert, "Item context and /s/ phone articulation results." *Journal of Speech and Hearing Research, 15* (1972): 852–860.

Zimmerman, I., V. Steiner, and R. Pond, *Preschool Language Scale*. Columbus, Ohio: Charles E. Merrill, 1992.

6

Remediation Procedures

NICHOLAS W. BANKSON
James Madison University

JOHN E. BERNTHAL
University of Nebraska—Lincoln

Basic Considerations

Introduction

The typical long-range objective of remediation for phonological disorders with a client not exhibiting significant cognitive/physical limitations is spontaneous use of speech sounds that reflect the adult standard of his or her linguistic community. Once a speech-language clinician has determined that an individual's phonology is disordered or otherwise warrants intervention, assessment data are used in the planning of management strategies to accomplish this instructional objective. As described in Chapter 5, phonological analyses are designed to assist the clinician in identifying appropriate target behaviors for instruction. After specific goals and objectives for intervention have been determined, the clinician is then faced with the task of determining the type of treatment approach that is best suited for an individual client. Before discussing specifics of particular treatment approaches in the next chapter, we focus in this chapter on some basic underlying concepts that must be taken into consideration when developing a treatment plan. Although the focus of the chapter is on disordered phonology, concepts and principles described may also be useful in terms of instruction related to other speech/language disorders as well as accent/dialect modification (speech sound differences).

Framework for Conducting Therapy

Before clinical speech instruction is initiated, regardless of the disorder area being treated, certain administrative or organizational factors must be considered as part of developing the framework from which specific treatment methodologies will emerge. In this section we review several overarching variables to be considered as a first step in treatment planning.

Temporal Sequencing of Instructional Components

Once intervention objectives have been determined, the clinician formulates a treatment plan that spells out activities that will be used in accord with the moment-to-moment temporal sequence of instructional components. The typical sequence of clinical speech instruction components is:

Antecedent events (AE)	Delineation of stimulus events designed to elicit particular responses (e.g., auditory/visual modeling or pictures presented by the clinician, followed by a request for the client to imitate the model or name a picture)
Responses (R)	Production of a target behavior (often a particular sound in isolation or in a given linguistic and/or social context)
Consequent events (CE)	Reinforcement or feedback that follows the response (the clinician says "good" if a response is accurate, or may say "try again" if inaccurate: tokens to reinforce correct responses)

Antecedent events are the stimulus events presented during or just prior to a response. Such events typically consist of a verbal model, a picture, printed material, or verbal instructions designed to elicit particular verbal responses. For example, if a client is working on the /s/ phoneme at the word level, the clinician may show the child a picture of soap, and ask the child, "What do we wash with?" The child may be further asked to "say the word three times," or to "put it in a sentence." The type of antecedent events will vary depending on whether the clinician is seeking to establish a motor behavior in the client or is trying to help the client use a motor behavior in accord with the phonological rules of the language.

Responses are the behaviors the clinician has targeted for the client. These may range from approximations of the desired behavior (e.g., movement of the tongue backward for production of /k/), to production of the correct behavior (e.g., /k/ in connected speech). The clinician is concerned with the functional relationship between an antecedent event and a response or, in other words, the likelihood that a given stimulus will elicit the desired response. Movement to the next level of instruction is often contingent upon a certain number of correct responses. It is important in phonologic training that clients have the opportunity to produce many utterances in the course of a therapy session. A high rate of utterances provides the opportunity for both the clinician's external monitoring and the client's automatization of the response. It is usual that responses are stabilized on one level of complexity before proceeding the next level (e.g., sounds are often easier to produce in syllables than in words; word production is easier than it is in phrases).

The third aspect of the temporal sequence for instruction is **consequent events** (CE). Consequent events are events that occur following a particular response, and usually are labeled reinforcement or punishment. Whether or not a response is learned (and how quickly it is learned) is closely related to what happens following the occurrence of a behavior or response. The most frequently used consequent event in clinical speech instruction is positive **reinforcement**. Tangible consequents such as tokens, points, chips, and informal reinforcers such as a smile or verbal feedback are also used. Consequent events intended to reinforce should immediately follow the correct or desired behavior and should only be used when the desired or correct response is produced. Reinforcement is defined by an increase in a behavior following the presentation of consequent events. Using reinforcement after an incorrect behavior sends the "wrong message" to the speaker, reinforces an incorrect response, and does not facilitate learning of correct responses. Formal use of "punishment" as a consequence seldom occurs in phonological treatment.

Instructional steps are organized so that a sequential series of antecedent events, responses, and consequent events are followed as one moves through therapy. See Table 6.1 for an example.

Goal Attack Strategies

An early treatment decision relates to the number of treatment goals targeted in a given session. Fey (1986) described three "goal attack strategies" applicable to children with phonological disorders. The first strategy is called a *vertically structured treatment program*, in which one or two goals or targets are trained to some performance criterion before proceeding to another target. Treatment sessions of this type involve a high response rate for a single target, involving lots of repetition of that target. The traditional approach to treatment of phonological disorders, to be described in detail later in this book, is an example of a vertically structured program. In this approach, one or two phonemes are targeted for treatment and are worked on until they are produced in conversation before training is initiated on other target sounds. For a client who exhibits five different phonologic processes, the clinician may target one process and focus treatment on one or two sounds related to

TABLE 6.1   Sequential Series of Antecedent Events, Responses, and Consequent Events

Step	Anecedent Event	Response	Consequent Event
1	Clinician: Put your tongue behind your teeth, have the tip of your tongue lightly touch the roof of your mouth as if you were saying /t/, and blow air. Say /s/.	/t/	Clinician: No, I heard /t/.
2	Clinician: Keep your tongue top a little bit down from the roof of your mouth and blow air. Say /s/.	/s/	Clinician: Good! Perfect!
3	Now say /s/ 3 times.	/s/, /s/, /s/	Great!
4	Now say /sa/.	/sa/	Super!

that process/pattern until some criterion level is reached before proceeding to the next target process and other sounds. Elbert and Gierut (1986) termed this vertical type of strategy *training deep*. The assumptions behind the vertical strategy are that (1) mass practice on a restricted number of target sounds with a limited number of training items will facilitate generalization to other nontrained items; and (2) some clients are best served by focusing on one goal or target rather than many.

A second instructional strategy is a *horizontally structured treatment program* (Fey, 1986; Williams, 2000), or what Elbert and Gierut (1986) have called *training broad*. Using this strategy, the clinician addresses multiple goals in each session. Thus, more than one goal may be incorporated into each session, and goals may change across sessions. By working on several sounds in the same session, the client will presumably learn commonalities or relationships among sound productions and treatment will be more efficient. In other words, the client receives less training about more aspects of the sound system than in the vertical approach. The concept behind training broad is that limited practice, with a range of exemplars and sound contrasts, is an efficient way to modify a child's phonological system. The goal is to expose the child to a wide range of target sound productions so that this broad-based training will facilitate simultaneous acquisition of several treatment targets.

A third strategy (Fey, 1986), which combines aspects of the vertical and horizontal approaches, is a *cyclically structured treatment program* (Hodson and Paden, 1991). In this approach a single phonemic target (related to a particular phonological pattern) is addressed for a single session or week. The following session or week another goal is addressed. The movement from goal to goal is essentially a horizontal approach to treatment, while the focus on a single sound for a session or week may be viewed as vertical. Historically, the most common strategy employed in remediation was the vertical approach, but many clinicians now favor the horizontal or cyclical approach, especially once clients have a sound in their repertoire (i.e., they can produce a sound at the motor level with some consistency). Our preference with children who produce multiple errors is the cyclical approach, although all three approaches have been shown to improve phonological productions. For clients who evidence a small number of errors, such as misarticulate /r/, /s/, /l/, or /θ/ (residual errors), a vertical approach is preferable.

Scheduling of Instruction

Another basic consideration in planning for phonological intervention relates to the scheduling of treatment sessions. Relatively little is known about the influence that scheduling of instruction has upon remediation efficacy, and sufficient research has not been reported to determine which scheduling arrangements are most desirable. In addition, it is often not practical to schedule treatment sessions on an "ideal" basis. Scheduling of treatment may be related to age of the client, attention span of the client, severity of the disorder, and practical realities such as availability of instructional services, size of a clinician's caseload, and treatment models employed by a school system (e.g., pull-out versus classroom-based instruction). Investigators who have studied scheduling have generally focused on the efficacy of intermittent scheduling versus block scheduling of treatment sessions. *Intermittent scheduling* usually refers to two or three sessions each week over an extended period of time (such as eight months), while *block scheduling* refers to daily sessions for a shorter temporal span (such as an eight-week block). Several investigators have compared dismissal rates associated with intermittent and block scheduling, primarily for public school students with articulation disorders (Van Hattum, 1969). Based on these studies, Van Hattum reported that block scheduling was a more efficient way to achieve articulatory/ phonological progress than was intermittent scheduling. Unfortunately, however, variables such as articulation disorder severity, stimulability, and treatment methodology employed were not well enough controlled to make definitive clinical recommendations from these investigations.

Bowen and Cupples (1999) described a scheduling protocol where children were seen once weekly for approximately 10-week blocks, followed by approximately 10 weeks without treatment. They reported positive results with this treatment schedule. It should be pointed out, however, that their treatment included multifaceted components including parent education. The specific influence of the break in treatment schedule on treatment outcome is unknown; however, this study reflects a contemporary approach that utilizes a form of block scheduling.

Although control experiments on scheduling are lacking, suggestions for scheduling of phonological intervention seem appropriate:

1. Scheduling of intervention four to five times per week for 8 to 10 weeks may result in slightly higher dismissal rates than intermittent scheduling for a longer period of time, the greater gains being made early in the treatment process.
2. Intensive scheduling on only a short-term basis does not appear to be as appropriate with clients who have severe articulation/phonological disorders and need ongoing services.
3. Scheduling a child for three 20-minute sessions appears to yield better results than one 60-minute session.

Pull-Out Versus Classroom-Based Instruction

Basic considerations related to phonological intervention relate to the place and format whereby services will be delivered. One issue is the matter of whether treatment will be provided through a *pull-out model* (the client is instructed in a treatment room) or *inclusion model* (the client is instructed in a classroom setting), or a combination of the two. Historically, the pull-out model was the choice for articulation/phonological treatment. In recent years, an increased emphasis has been placed on integrating speech and language services within the classroom. The opportunity to incorporate a child's phonological instruction with the academic curriculum and communication events associated with a child's daily school routine is the optimal way to enhance the efficiency and effectiveness of therapy. Furthermore, classroom inclusion capitalizes on the opportunity for collaboration among regular educators, special education educators, speech-language pathologists, and other professionals within a child's educational environment.

Masterson (1993) suggested that classroom-based approaches for school-age children allow the clinician to draw on textbooks, homework, and classroom discourse to establish instructional goals, target words, and instructional procedures. For preschoolers, classroom activities such as crafts, snacks, and toileting are similarly helpful activities for language and phonological instruction. In addition, for preschool and early primary grade children, classroom-based phonological awareness activities may provide the clinicians with the opportunity to extend services to all children in a classroom as they collaborate with teachers. Masterson (1993) further indicated that classroom-based approaches may be most useful for treating conceptual- or linguistic-based errors, as opposed to errors that require motor-based habilitation. Instruction in the context of the classroom setting is typically less direct than that involved in a pull-out model and requires collaborative efforts between the clinician and the classroom teacher. Classroom instruction is particularly appropriate when a client is in the generalization, or "carryover," phase of instruction, in which academic material and other classroom activities allow for an emphasis on communication skills and intent. It is likely that both of these models (i.e., pull-out; classroom inclusion) may be appropriate for a given client during the course of intervention, depending on where they are on the treatment continuum.

Clinicians must determine whether clients are treated individually or in a small group. Although group instruction is sometimes conducted because of large caseloads, reports have indicated that group instruction may well be as effective as individual instruction in remediating articulation disorders (Sommers, Furlong, Rhodes, Fichter, Bowser, Copetas, and Saunders, 1964; Sommers, Schaeffer, Leiss, Gerber, Bray, Fundrella, Olson, and Tomkins, 1966).

Sommers and colleagues (1964) reported that 50-minute group instruction based on the pull-out model resulted in as much articulatory change as 30-minute individual instruction when both group and individual sessions were conducted four times per week for 4 weeks. In a subsequent study (Sommers et al., 1966), similar results were obtained from group sessions held 45 minutes each week and individual instruction sessions held 30 minutes each week over a period of 8½ months. These investigators concluded that group and individual sessions were equally effective and that the results were not influenced by the grade level (fourth to sixth grade versus second grade) or the severity of the phonologic disorder. Phonologic groups usually contain three or four clients of about the same age who work on similar target behaviors. Unfortunately, such group sessions frequently have a tendency to become regimented so that all individuals work on the same activity, the same target behavior, and the same level of behavior; they are even given the same homework assignments.

It should be pointed out that *group instruction* should be different from *individual instruction in a group*. When assigned a group of clients, the clinician may simply work with each client individually while remaining group members observe. Group instruction can and should be structured so that individuals in the group can benefit from interaction with other members and from activities that involve the entire group. For example, individuals can monitor and reinforce each other's productions and can serve both as correct models for each other and as listeners to see whether the communication intent of the message was met.

It is our suggestion that a combination of group and individual sessions may be advantageous for most individuals with phonologic problems. Furthermore, instructional groups should usually be limited to three or four individuals whose ages do not exceed a three-year range. Some would suggest that when children are learning the motor skills involved in production of a given sound, individual instruction is perhaps the best environment, if only for relatively short sessions or a part of a session. Once a sound is in the child's repertoire, group activities may be incorporated into the instructional plans. Having the flexibility to make such shifts sometimes, however, proves difficult in terms of classroom demands or a child's schedule.

Intervention Style

A final consideration before we begin our discussion of specific therapy approaches is intervention style. In addition to selecting target behaviors and training stimuli to be used in treatment, the clinician must also consider the management mode or style most appropriate for a given client. A key issue here is the amount of structure that may be prescribed for or tolerated by a given client.

Shriberg and Kwiatkowski (1982) described the structure of treatment as a continuum ranging from drill (highly structured therapy) to play (little structure to therapy), with combinations of these *two end points as in-between stages* on the continuum. These authors described the following four modes of management:

1. *Drill.* This type of therapy relies heavily on clinician presentation or some form of antecedent instructional events, followed by client responses. The client has little control over the rate and presentation of training stimuli.
2. *Drill play.* This type of therapy is distinguished from drill by the inclusion of an antecedent motivational event (e.g., activity involving a spinner; card games).
3. *Structured play.* This type of instruction is structurally similar to drill play. However, training stimuli are presented as play activities. In this mode, the clinician moves from formal instruction to playlike activities, especially when the child becomes unresponsive to more formal instruction.
4. *Play.* The child perceives what he or she is doing as play. However, the clinician arranges activities so that target responses will occur as a natural component of the activity. Clinicians may also use modeling, self-talk, and other techniques to elicit responses from a child.

Shriberg and Kwiatkowski (1982) conducted several studies with young children with phonological disorders to compare the relative effects of these four treatment modes. Their data indicated that drill and drill play modes were more effective and efficient than structured play and play modes. In addition, drill play was as effective and efficient as drill.

Clinicians' evaluation of the four modes indicated that they felt drill play was most effective and efficient for their clients, and they personally preferred it. They also urged that three factors be considered when making a choice of management mode: (1) a general knowledge of the child's personality, (2) the intended target response, and (3) the stage of therapy (Shriberg and Kwiatkowski, 1982).

It should be kept in mind that details regarding the organization of intervention sessions focused on phonological impairments are impacted by the presence of additional communication impairments, particularly language disorders. Because language and phonological disorders often both occur in young children, decisions discussed above related to planning therapy are influenced by the severity of disorders in each of these areas, and their priority for treatment. Instruction for children with phonological and other language impairments is discussed in Chapter 7.

Summary

Before deciding on a specific treatment methodology, the clinician must make several administrative decisions that interact significantly with treatment approaches and, potentially, clients' progress. These include the following:

1. What is the severity of the problem, and how many targets will you select to be incorporated into treatment planning?
2. Which targets need to be focused on at a motor level and which may be approached from a rule or phonological basis?
3. How many targets will I work on in a given session, and how long will I stay with a target before I move on to another?
4. How frequently will therapy sessions be held, and how long will each session last?
5. Will instruction be individual or in a small group? If it is conducted in a school environment, will it be pull-out, classroom based, or a combination of the two? Is drill and practice the best approach, or play, or a combination of the two?
6. For children with both phonological and language impairments, how should intervention be structured (e.g., an integrated approach; target each area separately)?

Making Progress in Therapy: Generalization

Once target behaviors are in a client's repertoire and can be produced on demand, the next task is to facilitate generalization to other linguistic contexts and nonclinical settings. Generalization is a process that is facilitated rather than taught, and it is relevant to correction of all phonologic errors whether they be viewed as motor and/or linguistic in nature. Generalization is a critical and all-important step in the learning process for all children who receive treatment for phonologic disorders. Our discussion of generalization includes an introduction to the concept, followed by a review of (1) across-position generalization, (2) across-context generalization, (3) across-linguistic unit generalization, (4) across-sound and feature generalization, and (5) across-situation generalization.

Generalization has been defined by Stokes and Baer (1977) as

> The occurrence of relevant behavior under different non-training conditions (i.e., across subjects, settings, people, behavior, and/or time) without the scheduling of the same events in those conditions as had been scheduled in the training conditions. Thus, generalization may be claimed when no extra training manipulations are needed for extra training changes (350).

In other words, generalization (sometimes called *transfer*) is the principle that learning one behavior in a particular environment often carries over to other similar behaviors, environments, or untrained contexts. For example, if one learns to drive in a Ford Taurus, there is a high probability that one can also drive a Honda Accord. Generalization of training occurs from the driving apparatus in the Taurus to the driving apparatus in the Honda. In terms of articulation remediation, if a client learns to produce /f/ in the word *fish*, [f] production will probably generalize to other words that contain /f/, such as *fun*. If generalization did not occur, it would be necessary to teach a sound in every word and context—an impossible task. The clinician must rely on a client's ability to generalize in order to effect a change in phonologic use. Generalization, however, does not occur automatically, nor do all persons have the same aptitude for it. People vary in their ability to achieve generalization, but certain activities can increase the likelihood of generalization.

One type of generalization is **stimulus generalization**, which occurs when a learned response to a particular stimulus is evoked by similar stimuli. The importance of reinforcement in such generalization cannot be overemphasized. Behaviors that have been reinforced in the presence of a particular stimulus may be said to have generalized when they occur in the presence of novel but similar stimuli, even though the response was not reinforced. Consider this example: A client who utilizes the process of "velar fronting" (/t/ for /k/ substitution) has been taught to produce /k/ correctly at the word level in response to the auditory stimulus, "Say kangaroo." The client is later shown a picture of a kangaroo and asked to name it, but no model is provided. If the client says "kangaroo" with [kʰ] produced correctly in response to the picture (i.e., the model is no longer necessary for a correct production), stimulus generalization has occurred.

Response generalization is another type of generalization that is especially relevant to speech sound remediation. This is the process in which responses that have been taught carry over to other behaviors that are not taught. An example of response generalization is as follows: A client with /s/ and /z/ errors is taught to say [s] in response to an auditory model of [s]. He or she is then presented with an auditory model [z] and asked to imitate it. If the client emits a correct [z], response generalization has occurred. Such generalization is well documented in the literature, including an early study by Elbert, Shelton, and Arndt (1967) in which children with /s/, /z/, and /r/ errors were taught to say [s] correctly. Generalization was evident by correction of the untrained /z/, which has many features in common with /s/. However, no generalization to the untrained [r] was noted. Obviously, sounds in the same sound class and having similar features with the target sound are those where response generalization is most likely to occur.

Several other types of generalization may also occur during phonologic remediation, including generalization from one position to another, from one context to another, to increasingly complex linguistic levels, to nontrained words, to other sounds and features, and to various speaking environments and situations. Clinicians often attempt to facilitate generalization by sequencing instructional steps from simple to more complex behaviors. By proceeding in small, progressive steps, the clinician seeks to gradually extend the behavior developed during the establishment period to other contexts and situations.

The amount of training required for the different types of generalization has not been established and seems to vary considerably across subjects. Elbert and McReynolds (1978) have reported data from five children indicating that from 5 to 26 sessions were required before across-word generalization occurred. They speculated that the error patterns exhibited by children affected both the time required and the extent of transfer that occurs.

For those clients who begin remediation with an established target behavior in their repertoire, generalization may be the primary task of instruction. Following is a discussion of the various types of generalization that are expected in the articulation remediation process.

Across Word-Position/Contextual Generalization

Generalization of correct sound productions across word-positions is well documented (Elbert and McReynolds, 1975, 1978; Powell and McReynolds, 1969). This term refers to generalization from a word-position that is taught (initial, medial, or final) to a word-position that is not taught. By teaching a sound in a particular position (e.g., initial position), generalization may occur to a second position (e.g., final position). Speech-language pathologists have traditionally taught target sounds first in the initial position of words, followed by either the final or medial position. One rationale for beginning with the initial position is that, for most children, many sounds are first acquired in the prevocalic position (the most notable exception is certain fricatives that appear first in word-final position).

In the process of investigating a particular approach to articulation remediation (paired-stimuli), Weston and Irwin (1971) examined position generalization. They observed in children with pre- and postvocalic substitutions that when a sound was taught in the prevocalic position, generalization usually occurred to the postvocalic position. Similarly, they observed that sounds taught in the postvocalic position usually generalized to the prevocalic position.

Ruscello (1975) studied the influence of training on generalization across word-positions. Two groups, each containing three subjects, were presented training programs that differed with respect to the number of word-positions practiced in each session. Ruscello reported significantly more generalization across training sessions for those subjects who practiced a target sound in the initial, medial, and final word-positions than the group who practiced a target sound only in the word-initial position. Weaver-Spurlock and Brasseur (1988) also reported that simultaneous training of /s/ in the initial, medial, and final positions of familiar words was an effective training strategy for across-position generalization to nontrained words.

Olswang and Bain (1985) reported different amounts of position generalization for /s/ and /l/ in two subjects. For both subjects, improvement in initial /l/ had little influence on final /l/. In other words, improvement on initial /l/ did not seem to facilitate improvement of final /l/. By contrast, when /s/ was trained in one word-position in one subject, it seemed to facilitate production of the sound to other positions. They attributed the differences in position generalization between /l/ and /s/ to the greater allophonic variation between initial and final /l/ (i.e., initial and final /l/ are produced differently) compared to that of initial and final /s/. Wolfe, Blocker, and Prater (1988) reported that generalization of sounds in the medial word position may be related to whether the word reflects a sound in the traditional medial position (e.g., /k/ in *bacon*), or is related to inflection (e.g., /k/ in *picking*). In their study, greater generalization occurred with medial inflection, which they attributed to factors of coarticulation, perceptual salience, and representational integrity of the word.

It can be inferred from the available data that generalization from initial to final position is just as likely to occur as generalization from final to initial. A preferred word-position that would maximally facilitate position generalization has not been established. Thus, the word-position in which a target sound is trained does not seem to be a factor in position generalization. In terms of clinical management, unless the pattern of errors suggests a particular word-position for initial training (such as final consonant deletion), it is recommended that the clinician train the word-position that the client finds easiest to produce, check for generalization to other positions, and then proceed to train the other word-positions if generalization has not already occurred. Except for selected fricative sounds (those that develop earliest in the final position), the easiest position to teach is the initial position. However, contextual testing may result in the identification of singleton or cluster contexts that are facilitating for an individual child.

Technically, position generalization may be viewed as a type of contextual generalization. The term *contextual generalization*, however, also refers to phonetic context transfer—for example, generalization from /s/ in *ask* to /s/ in *biscuit* or to /s/ in *fist*. This type of generalization where a production transfers to other words without direct treatment is an example of response generalization as described above. When preliminary testing has indicated specific contexts in which an error sound may be produced correctly, clinicians will frequently attempt to stabilize such productions—that is, see that a target sound can be consistently produced correctly in that context—and then provide instruction designed to facilitate generalization of the correct sound to other contexts. As with all types of generalization, the client must exhibit transfer to untrained contexts at some point for the remediation process to be complete. In a study of phoneme generalization, Elbert and McReynolds (1978) reported that although facilitative phonetic contexts have been posited as a factor in generalization, their data did not support the idea that certain contexts facilitate generalization across subjects. Instead, they found a great deal of variability in facilitative contexts across subjects. The authors also reported that once a child imitated the sound, generalization occurred to other contexts. They concluded that the client's position of the sound in his or her productive repertoire had more to do with generalization than did contextual factors.

Elbert, Powell, and Swartzlander (1991) examined the number of minimal word-pair exemplars necessary for phonologically impaired children to meet a generalization criterion. They reported that for their subjects (primarily preschool children), generalization occurred using a small number of word-pair exemplars (five or less for 80 percent of the children) but there was substantial variability across subjects. The occurrence of response generalization subsequent to teaching a small number of exemplars is consistent with findings from previous treatment reports (Elbert and McReynolds, 1978; Weiner, 1981).

Across-Linguistic Unit Generalization

A second type of generalization involves shifting correct sound productions from one level of linguistic complexity to another (e.g., from syllables to words). For some clients, the first goal in this process is to transfer production of isolated sounds to syllables and words; others begin at the syllable or word level and generalize target sound productions to phrases and sentences.

Van Riper and Erickson (1996) recommended that the transfer sequence be initiated with sounds in isolation, followed by syllables, words, and finally sentences. This hierarchy of production complexity is the usual treatment sequence in traditional therapy. Instruction at the transfer phase of the instructional continuum begins at the highest level of linguistic complexity at which a client can produce a target behavior on demand. Instruction progresses from that point to the next level of complexity. When sounds are taught in isolation, the effects of coarticulation are absent, and therefore the potential for generalization to syllables and words may be diminished. This notion received some support from a study reported by McReynolds (1972), in which the transfer of /s/ productions to words was probed after each of four sequential teaching steps: (1) /s/ in isolation, (2) /sa/, (3) /as/, and (4) /asa/. Although no transfer to words was observed following training on /s/ in isolation, over 50 percent transfer to words was observed following training on /sa/. It should be recognized, however, that the training of /s/ in isolation prior to syllables may have had a learning effect and influenced the generalization observed following syllable instruction. Some clinicians prefer initially to teach sounds in isolation or in syllables rather than in words in order to decrease interference from previous learning.

Van Riper and Erickson (1996) and Winitz (1975) recommended that sounds be taught in nonsense syllables or nonsense (nonce) words before they are practiced in meaningful words, thereby reducing the interference of previously learned error productions of the target sound. This view is in contrast with the language-based perspective that phonologic contrasts should be established at the word level because *meaningful* contrasts are a key to acquisition. Powell and McReynolds (1969) studied generalization in four subjects who misarticulated /s/. They reported that when two of the subjects were taught consonant productions in nonsense syllables, transfer of the target sound to words occurred without additional training. The other two subjects had to be provided instruction for generalization from nonsense syllables to words to occur.

Elbert, Dinnsen, Swartzlander, and Chin (1990) reported that when preschool children were taught target sounds within a minimal pair contrast training paradigm, generalization occurred to other single-word productions as well as to conversational speech. Based on a three-month posttreatment probe, they reported that subjects continued to generalize to other nontrained productions.

In summary, it appears that some clients generalize from one linguistic unit to another without specific training; others require specific instructional activities for transfer from one linguistic unit to another. The process of generalization across linguistic units varies across individuals as do all types of generalization.

Across-Sound and Across-Feature Generalization

A third type of generalization is observed when correct production of a target sound generalizes from one sound to another. Generalization most often occurs within sound classes and/or between sounds that are phonetically similar (e.g., /k/ to /g/; /s/ to /z/ and /ʃ/). Clinicians have long observed that training on one sound in a cognate pair frequently results in generalization to the second sound (e.g., Elbert et al., 1967). McNutt (1994), in a study of bilingual children, reported that correction of /s/ in English generalized to correction of a defective /s/ in French.

Generalization of correct production from one sound to another is expected when remediation targets are selected on the basis of place, manner, and voicing analysis, distinctive feature analysis, or phonologic process/pattern analysis. Often in these approaches, target behaviors are selected that reflect features or processes/patterns common to several error productions. This is done on the assumption that generalization will occur from exemplars to other error sounds within the same sound class or, in some instances, across sound classes. For example, an underlying assumption of distinctive feature analysis and remediation is that features generalize from one sound production to another production containing the same features. This type of generalization can be seen in the client who initially did not correctly produce any sounds containing [+ stridency], yet after learning to produce /s/, was able to correctly articulate /ʃ/ and /z/, which also contain the feature [+ stridency].

A client can learn a feature and transfer the feature without necessarily correcting a sound. For example, a client who substitutes stops for fricatives may learn to produce /f/ and overgeneralize its use to several fricative sounds. Although the client no longer substitutes stops for fricatives, he or she now substitutes /f/ for other fricatives (e.g., [sʌn] → [fʌn]; [ʃou] → [fou]. While the same number of phonemes is in error, the fact that the client has incorporated a new sound class into his or her repertoire represents enhancement of the child's phonological system (Williams, 1993).

McReynolds and Bennett (1972) studied three subjects who received training to facilitate feature generalization. Instruction for each subject focused on a specified sound that was selected to reflect a particular feature. Specifically, one subject was taught an exemplar containing the [+ stridency] feature, another the [+ voicing] feature, and the third the [+ continuancy] feature. Feature generalization to other error sounds was assessed through deep testing of nontrained phonemes. Results for the three subjects indicated that the feature generalized to several sounds even though training was limited to a single sound exemplar.

Frequently, the establishment of feature contrasts is part of the effort to reduce and eliminate process usage; thus, feature teaching and process reduction approaches are inextricably intertwined. The notion of feature and sound generalization, like other types of generalization, is critical to the remediation process.

During the 1990s, several studies of children with multiple phonological errors were conducted wherein data was collected regarding the impact on generalization of various types of treatment targets. Results of these studies are relevant to our discussion of across-sound and across-feature generalization.

In a study related to teaching stimulable versus nonstimulable sounds, Powell, Elbert, and Dinnsen (1991) reported that teaching a nonstimulable sound prompted change in the target sound and other errored stimulable sounds. However, teaching a stimulable sound did not necessarily lead to changes in untreated stimulable or nonstimulable sounds. The implication of this study is that treatment of nonstimulable sounds may lead to increased generalization and thus have a more widespread impact on the child's overall sound system.

Gierut, Morrisette, Hughes, and Rowland (1996) examined generalization associated with teaching early developing sounds versus later developing sounds. They reported that children taught later developing sounds evidenced change in the treated sound, with generalization occurring both within and across sound classes. For those taught early developing sounds, improvements were noted on the target sound within class sounds, but not across class sounds.

Studies of generalization associated with teaching sounds evidencing "least" versus "most" knowledge of sounds in the sound system (Dinnsen and Elbert, 1984; Gierut, Elbert, and Dinnsen, 1987) have indicated that treatment focused on least knowledge resulted in extensive systemwide generalization, wherein treatment of most knowledge contributed to focused but limited change in a child's overall sound system. Studies comparing generalization associated with teaching phonetically more complex sounds to those less phonetically complex sounds (Dinnsen, Chin, Elbert, and Powell, 1990; Tyler and Figurski, 1994) have evidenced that more extensive changes were obtained when treatment was focused on more complex phonetic distinctions between error sounds as compared to simpler distinctions between sounds.

As a follow-up to the studies reported in the paragraphs above, Rvachew and Nowak (2001) studied the amount of phonological generalization associated with treatment targets that reflected early developing and greater phonological knowledge, as contrasted with later developing and little or no productive phonological knowledge. In contrast to previous findings, these investigators reported that greater treatment efficiency was associated with phoneme targets that reflected early developing and greater productive phonological knowledge. Further investigation is necessary before definitive statements may be made with regard to the issue of targeting early versus later acquired sounds, and more versus less phonological knowledge.

Powell and Elbert (1984) investigated the generalization patterns of two groups of children with misarticulations. Specifically, they wanted to see if the group receiving instruction on earlier developing consonant clusters (stop + liquid) would exhibit generalization patterns different from those of the group receiving instruction on later-developing consonant clusters (fricative + liquid). The authors reported that no clear overall pattern was observed; instead, the six subjects exhibited individual generalization patterns. All subjects evidenced some generalization to both the trained and untrained consonant clusters. The most interesting finding was that generalization to both cluster categories occurred on the final probe measure in five of six subjects regardless of the treatment received. Powell and Elbert (1984) attributed generalization across sound and classes in part to good pretreatment stimulability skills.

Weiner (1981) also reported across-sound generalization in teaching final consonants in children who deleted final consonants. He trained subjects to produce word-final stops and reported generalization to word-final fricatives.

Across-Situations Generalization

The fourth and final type of generalization to be discussed in this chapter, called *situational generalization*, involves transfer of behaviors taught in the clinical setting to other situations and locations, such as school, work, or home. This type of generalization is critical to the remediation process because it represents the terminal objective of instruction (i.e., correct phonologic productions in conversational speech in nonclinical settings). Such generalization has also been called *carryover* in the speech-language pathology literature.

Most clinicians focus on activities to facilitate situational transfer during the final stages of remediation. Some, including the authors, have argued that clinicians should incorporate these activities into early stages of instruction. For example, once a client can produce single words correctly, efforts should be made to incorporate these words into nonclinical settings. A major advantage of providing phonological instruction in the classroom setting (inclusion model) is the opportunity to incorporate treatment targets into a child's natural communicative environment. For example, if a child's science lesson incorporates a word containing a target sound (such as /s/) the teacher or clinician can provide the opportunity for the child to utilize his/her new speech sound in words like *sun, solar, ice, estimate, season, summer*, and so on. Although much emphasis is placed on facilitating situational generalization, little experimental data are available to provide specific guidance to the clinician.

Studies by Costello and Bosler (1976), Olswang and Bain (1985), and Bankson and Byrne (1972) have shown that situational generalization is facilitated through treatment, but the extent of such transfer varies greatly from one individual to another. Costello and Bosler (1976) investigated whether certain clinical situations were more likely to evidence generalization than others. They recorded the transfer that occurred from training in the home environment to probes obtained in the following four settings:

1. A mother administered the probe while sitting across from her child at a table in a treatment room of the speech clinic.
2. An experimenter (who was only vaguely familiar to the child) administered the probe while sitting across from the child at the same table in the same room as setting 1.
3. The same experimenter administered the probe while she and the child were seated at separate desks facing each other in a large classroom outside the speech clinic.
4. A second experimenter (unknown to the child prior to the study) administered a probe while she and the child were alone and seated in comfortable chairs in the informal atmosphere of the clinic waiting room.

Although all three subjects generalized from therapy to one or more of the above testing settings, there was no evidence that one setting was more likely to evidence generalization than another. It may be that generalization variables differ so much from person to person that it is impossible to predict which environments are most likely to facilitate situational transfer.

Olswang and Bain (1985) monitored situational generalization for three 4-year-old children in two different settings during speech sound remediation. They examined connected speech samples recorded in conversational activities in a clinic treatment room and connected speech samples audio recorded by parents during conversational activities at home. They reported similar rates and amounts of generalization of target sounds for both settings.

Bankson and Byrne (1972) reported that four out of five subjects generalized correct sound production in words from a motor-based remediation procedure to conversational samples gathered both in the training setting (school) and the home environment. Although the amount of generalization seen in the home and school training probes varied from day to day for each subject, the daily fluctuations were consistent between settings for each subject. The overall extent to which generalization occurred varied greatly across individuals and from day to day.

One strategy that has been suggested to facilitate situational generalization is the use of self-monitoring (self-evaluation). Self-monitoring techniques have included hand raising (Engel and Groth, 1976), charting (Diedrich, 1971; Koegel, Koegel, and Ingham, 1986), and counting of correct productions, both within and outside the clinic (Koegel, Koegel, Van Voy, and Ingham, 1988). Bennett, Bennett, and James (1996) suggested the following steps to facilitate self-monitoring:

1. External monitoring and verbal feedback
2. External monitoring with cues provided for revision (e.g., raise hand)
3. Self-revision by client when errors occur

4. Anticipating when errors may occur
5. Automatic usage of correct production

Koegel and colleagues (1988) examined generalization of /s/ and /z/ in seven children. They reported that when children self-monitored their conversational productions in the clinic, no generalization of the correct target production outside the clinic occurred. However, when children were required to monitor their conversational speech outside the clinic, "rapid and widespread generalization" occurred across subjects, although at slightly different rates. They reported high levels of generalization for all subjects. In contrast, when Gray and Shelton (1992) field tested the self-monitoring strategy of Koegel and colleagues (1988), the results did not replicate the positive generalization treatment effect reported by the latter.

Shriberg and Kwiatkowski (1987), in a retrospective study of efficacy of intervention strategies, identified self-monitoring procedures as a potentially effective component to facilitate generalization to continuous speech. In a subsequent experimental study, Shriberg and Kwiatkowski (1990) reported that seven of the eight preschool subjects generalized from such self-monitoring instruction to spontaneous speech. They concluded, however, that while self-monitoring facilitated generalization, it varied in terms of type, extent, and point of onset.

Despite a paucity of data on situational generalization, available evidence indicates that, as with other forms of generalization, the extent to which it occurs in different settings varies greatly among individuals. There is also the suggestion that situational generalization may be influenced by age and how well developed the child's phonologic system is (Elbert et al., 1990).

Several investigators have suggested that productive phonologic knowledge (accuracy and consistency of sound production) influences children's generalization learning (Dinnsen and Elbert, 1984; Elbert and Gierut, 1986; Gierut et al., 1987; Gierut, 1989). They have inferred that phonologic knowledge accounts for some of the individual differences that occur in generalization. Gierut et al. (1987) reported that greater generalization occurred in sounds where children exhibited more knowledge (correct productions in a wide array of contexts) as opposed to less knowledge (correct productions in fewer contexts; more positional constraints), but the greatest generalization occurred on those sounds for which training was provided. They also reported that when intervention was directed toward sounds where the child evidenced the least phonologic knowledge, generalization learning occurred across the child's phonologic system. These investigators recommended that clinicians choose sounds for treatment that reflect the least phonologic knowledge (inventory constraints). Even though training on sounds in which children showed most knowledge facilitated greater generalization within a sound class, training on sounds for which children exhibited least knowledge resulted in more broad-based generalization. Gierut and colleagues (1987) inferred from these findings that training on sounds in which children displayed least knowledge (e.g., no correct production of a sound) resulted in more system-wide changes and reorganization of the child's phonologic system than did training on sounds in which children showed most knowledge (e.g., inconsistent productions).

Williams (1991) examined generalization of nine children on /s/ and /r/ sounds for which they exhibited least phonologic knowledge as reflected by inventory constraints (i.e., the children did not produce /s/ and /r/ on a conversational sample or on a 306-item probe test). The misarticulated [s] and [r] were trained in consonant clusters. Williams reported three different generalization and learning patterns across the subjects and hypothesized that differences in generalization reflected different levels of phonological knowledge, even though all error targets were classified in the least phonologic knowledge category (sound is not in child's repertoire). Williams questioned if Gierut and colleagues' (1987) category of least knowledge was too broad to capture subtle differences in children's knowledge and recommended acoustical measurements to supplement transcription to further differentiate the amount of phonologic knowledge demonstrated for sounds in the least knowledge category of this system. This observation is consistent with recommendations from Weismer, Dinnsen, and Elbert (1981); Smit and Bernthal (1983); and Tyler, Edwards, and Saxman (1990).

Parental Assistance with Generalization

Clinicians have long recognized that the generalization process in phonologic remediation might be facilitated if individuals from the client's environment could be drawn into the generalization phase of the treatment process. The assumption has been that persons significant to the client, including parents, spouse, teachers, or peers could engage in activities designed to extend what the clinician was doing in the clinical setting. Several programs include instructional activities designed for parents to use with their children at home (Bowen and Cupples, 1999; Mowrer, Baker, and Schutz, 1968; Gray, 1974). Sommers (1962) and Sommers and colleagues (1964) studied several variables related to articulation instruction. Greater improvement between pre- and post-test scores was reported for children whose mothers were trained to assist with instruction than for a control group of children whose mothers had not received training. Carrier (1970) reported a study comparing a group of ten children 4 to 7 years old who participated in an articulation training program administered by their mothers and a similar control group who received minimal assistance from their mothers. The experimental group obtained significantly higher scores on four phonologic measures than the control group. Other investigations in which parents provided directed articulation instruction for their children (Shelton, Johnson, and Arndt, 1972; Shelton, Johnson, Willis, and Arndt, 1975) reported that parents can be utilized to enhance phonological intervention.

The clinician must be sensitive to the role parents or other nonprofessionals can assume in the treatment process and must keep several things in mind. For example, parents can: (1) provide good auditory models of target words, (2) have their children practice target words that the child can easily produce correctly, and (3) reinforce correct productions. First, if parents are to judge the accuracy of sound productions, they must be able to discriminate the sounds correctly. Second, the clinician must demonstrate to the parents the procedures to be used in the program; then the parents must demonstrate to the clinician the same procedures to ensure that they can carry them out. Third, the clinician must recognize that parents have only a limited amount of time; consequently, programs should be designed for short periods. Fourth, written instructions of the specific tasks should be provided to the caregivers/parents. Finally, clinicians should keep in mind that parents probably function better as monitors of productions than as teachers. Often parents lack the patience and objectivity necessary to teach their own children. However, if parents or other individuals in the child's environment have the desire, skill, time, and patience to work with their children, the clinician may have a helpful facilitator of the generalization process.

Generalization Guidelines

1. For most rapid context and situational generalization, begin instruction with target behaviors (sounds) that are stimulable or in the client's repertoire.
2. For children with multiple errors, there are data to support each of the following as ways to facilitate generalization:
   A. Nonstimulable sounds are treated before stimulable sounds.
   B. More phonetically complex sounds are treated before those less complex.
   C. Late developing sounds are treated before early developing sounds.
   D. Sounds evidencing least knowledge are treated before those evidencing most knowledge.
   E. Early developing sounds that also reflect greater productive knowledge are treated before later developing sounds with less productive knowledge.
3. Because word productions form the basis of position generalization, productions at this level should be incorporated into the instructional sequence as soon as possible. When teaching a sound, utilize words and syllable shapes within the child's lexicon.
4. The more features that sounds have in common, the more likely that generalization will occur from one to another. For example, teaching [ɝ] usually results in generalization to the unstressed [ɚ] and the consonantal [r]; teaching one member of a cognate sound-pair, such as [s], usually results in the client's correction of the cognate [z].
5. Teaching a distinctive feature in the context of one sound, such as frication in [f], may result in generalization of that feature to other untreated sounds, such as [z].
6. Data are lacking to support a particular order for teaching sounds in various word-positions to facilitate generalization. Beginning with the word-position that is easiest for the client is an often used starting point.
7. When selecting sounds to target phonologic patterns, select target sounds from across sound classes in which the pattern occurs to increase the likelihood of generalization across the phonological system.
8. Nonsense syllables may facilitate production of sounds in syllable contexts during establishment of sound production because nonsense syllables pose less interference with previously learned behaviors than do words.
9. Meaningful words may generalize more rapidly than nonsense syllables because they reflect phonemic contrasts and may be reinforced in the environment.
10. Activities to facilitate situational generalization are advised as soon as the client can say a sound in words, rather than waiting until sounds are produced at the sentence level. In the case of preschool children, generalization frequently takes place without a plan to facilitate situational generalization in treatment.
11. Parents and others in the child's environment can be used effectively to facilitate phonologic change in children.

Dismissal from Instruction

The final phase of phonologic instruction occurs when the client habituates new target behaviors and otherwise assumes responsibility for self-monitoring of target phonologic productions. This phase of therapy is an extension of the generalization phase.

During the final phase of therapy, sometimes referred to as the *maintenance phase*, clients decrease their contact with the clinician. Shelton (1978) labeled the terminal objective of articulation remediation as **automatization** and described it as automatic usage of standard articulation patterns in spontaneous speech. The term *automatization* implies that phonologic productions can be viewed as motor behavior that develops into an automatic response. When phonologic errors are linguistic in nature, maintenance may be viewed as the mastery of phonologic rules or phonemic contrasts. In reality, both the motor production and phonologic rules become part of a person's everyday productive behavioral responses by this point in treatment. The maintenance phase may be considered complete once the client can consistently use target behaviors in spontaneous speech.

To determine the extent to which a client has maintained target behaviors, the clinician must assess a client's behavior during the conversational speech. Diedrich (1971) suggested that three-minute "Talk" samples are a good way to monitor correct and incorrect speech productions during conversation.

During maintenance, the client usually receives intermittent reinforcement for the new speech patterns because this type of schedule results in behavior that is most resistant to extinction. Clients are also required to monitor their own articulation productions during maintenance. Having the client keep track of target productions during specified periods of the day is a procedure that can be used to self-monitor target production.

Information from the learning literature offers insights into the maintenance or retention of newly acquired phonologic patterns. **Retention**, in the context of phonologic remediation, refers to the continued and persistent use of responses learned during instruction. Once an individual learns a new phonologic pattern or response, he or she must continue to use (retain) the response. In clinical literature, retention is sometimes discussed in terms of intersession retention and sometimes in terms of habitual retention. *Intersession retention* refers to the ability to produce recently taught responses correctly. Speech clinicians frequently observe "between-session forgetting" in many clients. This is an instance where the decision above concerning parental assistance with therapy is useful. Short practice sessions for an hour between therapy sessions may improve intersession retention. *Habitual retention* is the persistent and continued use of the response after instruction has been terminated. The term *maintenance* is frequently used to refer to this phenomenon. Speech clinicians occasionally dismiss clients from instruction only to have them return for additional therapy some months later. Such individuals obviously did not habituate or retain their newly learned responses. Mowrer (1977) pointed out that lack of intersession retention is a particular problem with mentally retarded children.

Sommers (1969) reported that articulation errors are susceptible to regression. In a follow-up study of 177 elementary school children who had been dismissed from articulation instruction during a six-month period, he found that approximately one-third had regressed. Based on conversational samples of target sound productions, 59 percent of those who had worked on /s/ and /z/ had regressed, but only 6 percent of those who had worked on /r/ had regressed. He did not report dismissal criteria or the level of performance prior to dismissal.

In contrast, Elbert and colleagues (1990) reported that for preschool children, learning continued to improve on both single-word and conversational speech samples obtained three months post-treatment. These data support the idea that young children are actively involved and continue to learn the phonologic system even after treatment was terminated. It appears that phonologic errors in preschool children are less habituated than in older school-age children and easier to correct.

Winitz (1969) proposed that interference, which results in competition between the error sound and the newly acquired sound, may explain why individuals forget articulatory responses. Winitz pointed out that the years of motor production practice using an incorrect articulatory gesture, such as /t/ for /tʃ/, will interfere with the individual's ability to produce a newly learned /tʃ/. Similarly, speech clinicians frequently observe individuals who, during the early stages of /s/ instruction, insert a /θ/ following a newly learned /s/ in a word context (e.g., [sθup]).

Mowrer (1982) pointed out several factors that have been shown to influence the degree to which information will be retained, whether in the child who is dismissed from therapy but returns for lack of long-term maintenance or in the child who seems to have forgotten previous learning between sessions. First, the meaningfulness of the material used to teach the new responses may affect retention, although there is little empirical evidence in the articulation learning literature on this point. In general, as the meaningfulness of the material increases, the rate of forgetting tends to decrease, and thus the use of meaningful material is recommended during remediation. Thus, names of friends, family members, pets, familiar objects, and classroom vocabulary are appropriate choices. Although meaningfulness of material may be an important aid to long-term retention, the clinician may find, as stated earlier, that nonmeaningful material (e.g., nonsense syllables) may be useful during earlier phases of instruction (i.e., establishment). Leonard (1973) reported that when /s/ had been established in meaningful words, fewer training trials were required to transfer to other words than when nonsense items were utilized. But this finding on generalization must be distinguished from the finding presented earlier in our discussion of interference—that acquisition or establishment of new responses can be accomplished in fewer trials with nonsense items than with meaningful items.

A second factor believed to affect retention is the degree or extent to which something has been learned. In general, the greater the number of trials during the learning process, the greater the retention. Retention improves when some overlearning of verbal material takes place. To avoid unnecessary practice, it is important to determine the minimum amount of learning needed to provide a satisfactory level of retention. The optimum point for stopping instruction occurs when additional training does not produce sufficient change in performance to merit additional practice; however, there is little data to guide the clinician about where this point may be.

A third factor affecting retention is the frequency of instruction or the distribution of practice. Retention is superior when tasks are practiced during several short sessions (distributed practice) than during fewer, longer sessions (massed practice). On the basis of this fact, frequent, short practice sessions are recommended. In his review of this topic, Mowrer (1982) concluded: "On the basis of controlled learning experiments in psychology alone, it could be recommended that clinicians could increase retention by providing frequent instruction; but bear in mind that no data are available from speech research that confirms this recommendation . . . the important factor in terms of frequency of instruction is not how much instruction . . . but the total number of instruction periods" (259).

A fourth factor shown to affect retention is the individual's motivational state. The more motivated a person, the greater the retention of the material that has been learned. Little, if any, experimental work reported in the phonologic literature has attempted to examine motivational state during speech instruction.

Dismissal Criteria

The maintenance phase provides a period for monitoring retention, and it is during this period that dismissal decisions are made. Limited data on dismissal criteria have been reported, and thus evidence is lacking to support a single dismissal criterion. Elbert (1967) suggested dismissal might be based on two questions: (1) Has the maximum change in this individual's speech behavior been attained? (2) Can this individual maintain this level of speech behavior and continue to improve without additional speech instruction? Whatever criteria are used for dismissal, they should be based upon periodic samples of phonologic behavior over time. The maintenance phase provides the final opportunity for the clinician to monitor, reinforce, and encourage the client to assume responsibility for habituation of the new speech patterns.

Diedrich and Bangert (1976) reported data on articulatory retention and dismissal from treatment. Some of the children studied were dismissed after reaching a 75 percent criterion level for correct /s/ and /r/ productions, as measured on a 30-item probe word test plus a three-minute sample of conversational speech. Four months later, 19 percent of the subjects had regressed below the 75 percent criterion level. No greater retention was found, however, among those children who remained in treatment until achieving higher than 75 percent criterion level on the probe measure. Diedrich and Bangert concluded that most speech clinicians tend to retain children with /s/ and /r/ errors in articulation instruction longer than necessary.

Maintenance and Dismissal Guidelines

1. Dismissal criteria may vary depending on the nature of the client's problem and the client's age. Preschool children with multiple errors generally require less stringent dismissal criteria than older children because they have been reported to continue to improve phonological productions without instruction once they begin to incorporate a new sound(s) into their repertoire. School age and older clients who evidence residual errors /r/, /s/, and /l/ may require more stringent dismissal criteria in order to retain the new behavior.
2. During the maintenance phase, clients assume increased responsibility for self-monitoring their production and maintaining accurate production.
3. The reinforcement schedule should continue to be intermittent during maintenance, as is the situation during the latter stages of generalization.

4. It has been suggested that clinicians may tend to keep many clients enrolled for phonologic remediation longer than is necessary. In other words, the cost-benefit ratio for intervention may significantly decline after a certain point is reached in treatment.

QUESTIONS FOR CHAPTER 6

1. When in the treatment process would it be appropriate to use continuous versus intermittent reinforcement?

2. What are critical considerations in selecting consequent events?

3. Describe vertical, horizontal, and cyclical structured treatment programs.

4. Describe and give examples of three types of phonological generalization.

5. Present five expectations relative to phonological generalization.

REFERENCES

Bankson, N. W., and M. C. Byrne, "The effect of a timed correct sound production task on carryover." *Journal of Speech and Hearing Research*, 15 (1972): 160–168.

Bennett, B., C. Bennett, and C. James, "Phonological development from concept to classroom." Paper presented at the Speech-Language-Hearing Association of Virginia Annual Conference, Roanoke, Virginia, 1996.

Bowen, C., and L. Cupples, "Parents and children together (PACT): A collaborative approach to phonological therapy." *International Journal of Language and Communication Disorders*, 34 (1999): 35–55.

Carrier, J. K., "A program of articulation therapy administered by mothers." *Journal of Speech and Hearing Disorders*, 33 (1970): 344–353.

Costello, J., and C. Bosler, "Generalization and articulation instruction." *Journal of Speech and Hearing Disorders*, 41 (1976): 359–373.

Diedrich, W. M., "Procedures for counting and charting a target phoneme." *Language, Speech, and Hearing Services in Schools*, 2 (1971): 18–32.

Diedrich, W. M., and J. Bangert, "Training and speech clinicians in recording and analysis of articulatory behavior." Washington, D.C.: U.S. Office of Education Grant No. OEG-0-70-1689 and OEG-0-71-1689, 1976.

Dinnsen, D. A., S. B. Chin, M. Elbert, and T. W. Powell, "Some constraints on functionally disordered phonologies: Phonetic inventories and phonotactics." *Journal of Speech and Hearing Research*, 33 (1990): 28–37.

Dinnsen, D., and M. Elbert, "On the relationship between phonology and learning." In M. Elbert, D. A. Dinnsen, and G. Weismer (Eds.), *Phonological Theory and the Misarticulating Child*, ASHA Monographs (No. 22, pp. 59–68). Rockville, Md.: American Speech-Language-Hearing Association, 1984.

Elbert, M., "Dismissal Criteria from Therapy." Unpublished Manuscript, 1967.

Elbert, M., D. A. Dinnsen, P. Swartzlander, and S. B. Chin, "Generalization to conversational speech." *Journal of Speech and Hearing Disorders*, 55 (1990): 694–699.

Elbert, M., and J. Gierut, *Handbook of Clinical Phonology Approaches to Assessment and Treatment.* San Diego, Calif.: College-Hill Press, 1986.

Elbert, M., and L. V. McReynolds, "Transfer of /r/ across contexts." *Journal of Speech and Hearing Disorders*, 40 (1975): 380–387.

Elbert, M., and L. V. McReynolds, "An experimental analysis of misarticulating children's generalization." *Journal of Speech and Hearing Research*, 21 (1978): 136–149.

Elbert, M., T. W. Powell, and P. Swartzlander, "Toward a technology of generalization: How many exemplars are sufficient?" *Journal of Speech and Hearing Research*, 34 (1991): 81–87.

Elbert, M., R. L. Shelton, and W. B. Arndt, "A task for education of articulation change." *Journal of Speech and Hearing Research*, 10 (1967): 281–288.

Engel, D. C., and L. R. Groth, "Case studies of the effect on carry-over of reinforcing postarticulation responses based on feedback." *Language, Speech, and Hearing Services in Schools*, 7 (1976): 93–101.

Fey, M. E., *Language Intervention with Young Children*. San Diego, Calif.: College Hill Press/Little Brown, 1986.

Gierut, J., "Maximal opposition approach to phonological treatment." *Journal of Speech and Hearing Disorders*, 54 (1989): 9–19.

Gierut, J. A., M. Elbert, and D. A. Dinnsen, "A functional analysis of phonological knowledge and generalization learning in misarticulating children." *Journal of Speech and Hearing Research*, 30 (1987): 462–479.

Gierut, J. A., M. L. Morrisette, M. T. Hughes, and S. Rowland, "Phonological treatment efficacy and developmental norms." *Language, Speech, and Hearing Services in Schools*, 27 (1996): 215–230.

Gray, B., "A field study on programmed articulation therapy." *Language, Speech, and Hearing Services in Schools*, 5 (1974): 119–131.

Gray, S. I., and R. L. Shelton, "Self-monitoring effects on articulation carryover in school-age children." *Language, Speech, and Hearing Services in Schools*, 23 (1992): 334–342.

Hodson, B., and E. Paden, *Targeting Intelligible Speech: A Phonological Approach to Remediation*, 2nd ed. Austin, Tex.: PRO-ED, 1991.

Koegel, L. K., R. L. Koegel, and J. C. Ingham, "Programming rapid generalization of correct articulation through self-monitoring procedures." *Journal of Speech and Hearing Disorders*, 51 (1986): 24–32.

Koegel, R., L. Koegel, K. Van Voy, and J. Ingham, "Within-clinic versus outside-of-clinic self-monitoring of articulation to promote generalization." *Journal of Speech and Hearing Disorders*, 53 (1988): 392–399.

Leonard, L., "The nature of deviant articulation." *Journal of Speech and Hearing Disorders*, 38 (1973): 156–161.

Masterson, J., "Classroom-based phonological intervention." *American Journal of Speech-Language Pathology: A Journal of Clinical Practice*, 2 (1993): 5–9.

McNutt, J., "Generalization of /s/ from English to French as a result of phonological remediation." *Journal of Speech-Language Pathology and Audiology/Revue d'orthophonic et d'audiologie*, 18 (1994): 109–114.

McReynolds, L. V., "Articulation generalization during articulation training." *Language and Speech*, 15 (1972): 149-155.

McReynolds, L. V., and S. Bennett, "Distinctive feature generalization in articulation training." *Journal of Speech and Hearing Disorders*, 37 (1972): 462–470.

Mowrer, D. E., *Methods of Modifying Speech Behaviors*. Columbus, Ohio: Charles E. Merrill, 1977.

Mowrer, D. E., *Methods of Modifying Speech Behaviors*, 2nd ed. Columbus, Ohio: Charles E. Merrill, 1982.

Mowrer, D. E., R. Baker, and R. Schutz, *S-Programmed Articulation Control Kit*. Tempe, Ariz.: Educational Psychological Research Associates, 1968.

Olswang, L. B., and B. A. Bain, "The natural occurrence of generalization articulation treatment." *Journal of Communication Disorders*, 18 (1985): 109–129.

Powell, T., and M. Elbert, "Generalization following the remediation of early-and later-developing consonant clusters." *Journal of Speech and Hearing Disorders*, 49 (1984): 211–218.

Powell, T., M. Elbert, and D. Dinnsen, "Stimulability as a factor in the phonological generalization of misarticulating preschool children." *Journal of Speech and Hearing Research*, 34 (1991): 1318–1328.

Powell, T., and L. McReynolds, "A procedure for testing position generalization from articulation training." *Journal of Speech and Hearing Research*, 12 (1969): 625–645.

Ruscello, D. M., "The importance of word position in articulation therapy." *Language, Speech, and Hearing Services in Schools*, 6 (1975): 190–196.

Rvachewi, S., and M. Nowak, "The effect of target-selection strategy on phonological learning." *Journal of Speech, Language, and Hearing Research*, 44 (2001): 610–623.

Shelton, R., "Disorders of articulation." In P. Skinner, and R. Shelton (Eds.), *Speech, Language, and Hearing*. Reading, Mass.: Addison-Wesley, 1978.

Shelton, R. L., A. F. Johnson, and W. B. Arndt, "Monitoring and reinforcement by parents as a means of automating articulatory responses." *Perceptual and Motor Skills*, 35 (1972): 759–767.

Shelton, R. L., A. F. Johnson, V. Willis, and W. B. Arndt, "Monitoring and reinforcement by parents as a means of automating articulatory responses: II. Study of preschool children." *Perceptual and Motor Skills*, 40 (1975): 599–610.

Shriberg, L. D., and J. Kwiatkowski, "Phonological disorders III: A procedure for assessing severity of involvement." *Journal of Speech and Hearing Disorders*, 47 (1982): 256–270.

Shriberg, L. D., and J. Kwiatkowski, "A retrospective study of spontaneous generalization in speech-delayed children." *Language, Speech and Hearing Services in Schools*, 18 (1987): 144–157.

Shriberg, L. D., and J. Kwiatkowski, "Self-monitoring and generalization in preschool speech-delayed children." *Language, Speech and Hearing Services in Schools*, 21 (1990): 157–170.

Smit, A. B., and J. Bernthal, "Voicing contrasts and their phonological implications in the speech of articulation-disordered children." *Journal of Speech and Hearing Research*, 26 (1983): 19–28.

Sommers, R. K., "Factors in the effectiveness of mothers

trained to aid in speech correction." *Journal of Speech and Hearing Disorders, 27* (1962): 178–186.

Sommers, R. K., "The therapy program." In R. Van Hattum (Ed.), *Clinical Speech in the Schools.* Springfield, Ill.: Charles C. Thomas, 1969.

Sommers, R. K., A. K. Furlong, F. H. Rhodes, G. R. Fichter, D. C. Bowser, F. H. Copetas, and Z. G. Saunders, "Effects of maternal attitudes upon improvement in articulation when mothers are trained to assist in speech correction." *Journal of Speech and Hearing Disorders, 29* (1964): 126–132.

Sommers, R. K., M. H. Schaeffer, R. H. Leiss, A. J. Gerber, M. A. Bray, D. Fundrella, J. K. Olson, and E. R. Tomkins, "The effectiveness of group and individual therapy." *Journal of Speech and Hearing Research, 9* (1966): 219–225.

Stokes, T. F., and D. M. Baer, "An implicit technology of generalization." *Journal of Applied Behavior Analysis, 10* (1977): 349–367.

Tyler, A., M. Edwards, and J. Saxman, "Acoustic validation of phonological knowledge and its relationship to treatment." *Journal of Speech and Hearing Disorders, 55* (1990): 251–261.

Tyler, A. A., and G. R. Figurski, "Phonetic inventory changes after treating distinctions along an implicational hierarchy." *Clinical Linguistics and Phonetics, 8* (1994): 91–107.

Van Hattum, R. J., "Program scheduling." In R. Van Hattum (Ed.), *Clinical Speech in the Schools.* Springfield, Ill: Charles C. Thomas, 1969.

Van Riper, C., and R. Erickson, *Speech Correction: An Introduction to Speech Pathology and Audiology,* 9th ed. Englewood Cliffs, N.J.: Prentice-Hall, Inc., 1996.

Weaver-Spurlock, S., and J. Brasseur, "Position training on the generalization training of [s]." *Language, Speech, and Hearing Services in Schools, 19* (1988): 259–271.

Weiner, F., "Treatment of phonological disability using the method of meaningful minimal contrast: Two case studies." *Journal of Speech and Hearing Disorders, 46* (1981): 97–103.

Weismer, G., D. Dinnsen, and M. Elbert, "A study of the voicing distinction associated with omitted, word-final stops." *Journal of Speech and Hearing Disorders, 46* (1981): 91–103.

Weston, A. J., and J. V. Irwin, "Use of paired-stimuli in modification of articulation." *Perceptual and Motor Skills, 32* (1971): 947–957.

Williams, A. L., "Generalization patterns associated with training least phonological knowledge." *Journal of Speech and Hearing Research, 34* (1991): 722–733.

Williams, A. L., "Phonological reorganization: A qualitative measure of phonological improvement." *American Journal of Speech-Language Pathology, 2* (1993): 44–51.

Williams, A. L., "Multiple oppositions: Theoretical foundations for an alternative approach. *American Journal of Speech-Language Pathology, 9* (2000): 282–288.

Winitz, H., *Articulatory Acquisition and Behavior.* Englewood Cliffs, N.J.: Prentice-Hall, 1969.

Winitz, H., *From Syllable to Conversation.* Baltimore, Md.: University Park Press, 1975.

Wolfe, V. I., S. D. Blocker, and N. J. Prater, "Articulatory generalization in two word-medial and ambisyllabic contexts." *Language, Speech, and Hearing Services in Schools, 19* (1988): 251–258.

7

Treatment Approaches

NICHOLAS W. BANKSON
James Madison University

JOHN E. BERNTHAL
University of Nebraska—Lincoln

Introduction

In Chapter 6 we discussed concepts and principles that underlie phonological remediation. These principles and considerations are applicable to all of the treatment approaches that will be discussed in this chapter.

Historically, speech-language pathologists approached the correction of speech sound errors from the standpoint of teaching a motor behavior. Most clinicians viewed speech sound errors as an individual's inability to produce the complex motor skills required for the articulation of speech sounds. Since the 1970s, clinicians have also viewed phonologic disorders from a more linguistic (phonological) perspective. The linguistic perspective is based on the recognition that some individuals produce phonologic errors because they have not learned to use certain phonologic rules, especially sound contrasts, in accord with the adult norm. In other words, many error productions reflect a client's lack of rules for appropriate sound usage rather than an inability to produce the adult sounds.

Although it is convenient to dichotomize **motor/articulation** and **linguistic/phonologic** aspects of phonology for organization purposes, normal sound usage involves both the production of sounds at a motor level and their use in accordance with the rules of the language. Thus, the two skills are intertwined and may be described as two sides of the same coin. At a clinical level, it is often difficult or impossible to determine whether a client's errors reflect a lack of motor skills to produce a sound, a lack of linguistic knowledge, or deficiencies in both. It may be that, in a given client, some errors relate to one factor, some to another, and some to both.

Even though a disorder may be perceived as relating primarily to either the motor or linguistic aspects of phonology, instructional programs typically involve elements of both. It should be recognized that although it is often difficult to determine whether a given instructional procedure is primarily a motor-based or a linguistic-based technique, some activities undoubtedly assist the client in both the development of linguistic knowledge and the development of appropriate motor skills. Both motor and linguistic aspects of phonology are a part of most therapy programs. One notable exception is the case of residual errors (e.g., /r/, /l/, /s/) where a motor approach is the treatment of choice since the "higher level" linguistic aspects of the sound can be assumed (e.g., the child uses distorted or lateralized [s] in situations where /s/ is the target). By careful observation of a client and the nature of his or her problem, the clinician may be able to determine when one type of intervention should be emphasized.

Although we sometimes categorize the treatment approaches presented in this chapter as primarily motor or linguistic, that does not mean that the approaches were necessarily developed from a particular theoretical perspective. Many phonologic treatment approaches have emerged from pragmatic origins and continue to be used simply because "they work." In the pages that follow, several approaches to remediation are described. Some of these can be related to theory, some are atheoretical, and others lie somewhere in between. In the summary of each approach, we have presented a "Background Statement" that reflects our perception of the theoretical perspective from which the approach has emerged. A challenge for the future is to develop, refine, and revise theories that provide rationale, support, explanations, and direction for intervention procedures.

Treatment Continuum

The treatment process can be viewed as a continuum comprising three stages-**establishment**, facilitation of **generalization**, and **maintenance**. This continuum, which comes from the motor learning literature, is applicable to most types of speech and language disorders and constitutes a framework for a wide variety of specific teaching techniques and procedures. The goal of the first phase of instruction, called *establishment*, is to elicit target behaviors from a client and then stabilize such behaviors at a voluntary level, and/or establish phonologic contrasts. Establishment procedures are often based on production tasks, as in the example of a clinician teaching a child who does not produce /l/ where to place his tongue to say /l/. In addition, for a child who can say /l/ but deletes it in the final position (e.g., *bow* for *bowl*), the contrast between word-pairs, such as *bow* and *bowl*, may need to be taught during the establishment phase. Once the client is able to readily produce the correct form of an error sound and is aware of how it is used contrastively, he or she is ready to move into the generalization phase of instruction.

The second phase of instruction is called *generalization*. As discussed in Chapter 6, it is designed to facilitate transfer or carryover of behavior at several levels—positional generalization, contextual generalization, linguistic unit generalization, sound and feature generalization, and situational generalization. The treatment process includes instructional activities or strategies designed to facilitate generalization of correct sound productions to sound contrasts, words, and speaking situations that have not been specifically trained. An example of a context generalization activity would be practicing /s/ in a few key words with high vowels (e.g., *see, sit, seek*) and then determining whether /s/ is produced correctly in words where /s/ is followed by low vowels (e.g., *soft, sock, sat*). An example of a situational generalization activity would be practicing /l/ in sentences in the treatment setting and then observing whether the child uses /l/ in sentences produced in his or her classroom or home.

The third and final phase of remediation, *maintenance*, is designed to stabilize and facilitate retention of those behaviors acquired during the establishment and generalization phases. Instructional activities related to the generalization and maintenance phases of treatment generally overlap. Frequency and duration of instruction are often reduced during maintenance, and the client assumes increased responsibility for "maintaining" correct speech patterns. The client may also engage in specific activities designed to habituate or automatize particular speech patterns. A maintenance activity may consist of a client's keeping track of his or her /s/ productions at mealtime or use of r-clusters during five-minute phone conversations every evening for a week.

A commonly used or traditional approach to remediation has been to focus on correcting one or two sounds, moving them through the treatment continuum to the maintenance phase, and then initiating the correction of other sound(s). As indicated earlier, many clinicians prefer to focus on several error sounds or phonologic patterns simultaneously, proceeding along the treatment continuum with several segments or patterns.

Clients may enter the treatment continuum at different points, the exact point being determined by the individual's articulatory/phonological skills. Consider these two examples: Mark is able to produce a sound correctly in words and is able to perceive the target contrastively. Mark therefore begins instruction at the generalization stage, and would likely focus on incorporating target words into phrases. Kristy is able to produce a sound imitatively in syllables, perceives the sound contrast in word-pairs, but fails to incorporate the target production of the sound into words. She also enters the treatment continuum at the generalization stage, but at an earlier point than Mark. In her case, the clinician will seek to establish the target sound in a set of target words, selected on the basis perhaps of facilitating context, or even vocabulary items used in her classroom. For Mark, the clinician will facilitate generalization to phrases, including his usage in phrases not worked on in therapy. For Kristy, the clinician will facilitate generalization from syllables to words, including words not specifically focused on in a therapy session. The clinician must identify not only the appropriate phase of the treatment continuum but also the appropriate level within a phase at which to begin instruction.

Motor Learning Principles

The remediation approaches described in the next two major sections of this chapter were designed to focus primarily on the motor skills involved in producing target sounds and frequently include perceptual tasks as part of the treatment procedures. Most of them represent variations of what is often referred to as a traditional approach or motor-based approach to remediation. Remediation based on an articulation/phonetic or motor perspective views phonologic errors as motor based, with treatment focused on the placement and movement of the articulators in combination with audiology stimulation, (e.g., ear training and auditory bombardment). This remediation approach involves the selection of a target speech sound or sounds, with instruction proceeding through a sequence of increasingly complex linguistic units (e.g., isolation, syllables, words, phrases) until target sounds are used appropriately in spontaneous conversation. Thus, speech production is viewed as a learned motor skill, with remediation requiring repetitive practice at increasingly complex motor and linguistic levels until the targeted articulatory gesture becomes automatic.

Ruscello (1984) has indicated that phonological errors may be modified in two ways when viewed from a motor perspective: (1) movements may be taught to replace incorrect movements, or (2) movements may be taught where they were formerly absent. On the basis of the literature related to motor skill learning, Ruscello has outlined the following critical features in motor skill development:

1. *Cognitive analysis.* A mental or cognitive analysis is important in the early phase of movement formation. In this process, the learner evaluates his or her anticipated performance mentally and then incorporates those adjustments necessary for appropriate execution of the movement. Once stabilization of the movement occurs, cognitive planning is minimized. This internalization of a skilled movement is thought to contribute to the generalization of skilled movement across a variety of contexts. Based on experimental data, Ruscello and Shelton (1979) reported that such mental planning was helpful in the acquisition of articulatory skills in a treatment paradigm.

2. *Practice.* Practice is the key variable thought necessary for mastery of any skilled motor behavior. As the learner practices a particular motor skill, modifications based on internal and/or external feedback are made so that accuracy of performance is increased. A motor skill is best practiced in limited contexts until correct execution of the movement is achieved. Early treatment sessions involve discrete productions, such as isolated sound or word practice, while later sessions introduce more advanced tasks in the context of continuous discourse.

3. *Stages of motor skill development.* Initially there is a sluggishness in the execution of motor skills because the learner is acquiring the movement. With practice, the motor skill is perfected and stabilized. Ultimately, the skill becomes a part of the learner's repertoire of skilled movements and becomes automatic for the speaker.

4. *Feedback.* Sensory feedback processes (internal and external) are described in the motor learning literature as being of great importance in the early development of a skill. When the individual perfects a skill pattern through practice, the error response is diminished and feedback becomes less important.

Teaching Sounds: Establishment of Target Behaviors

As stated earlier, the first phase of remediation for clients who do not produce target behaviors upon demand, or who have perceptual and/or production difficulty with particular adult phonologic contrasts, is called *establishment*. While the teaching of sounds may be viewed as motor oriented therapy, perceptual training (i.e., discrimination training, minimal pairs contrasts, and auditory bombardment) may be incorporated in both motor and linguistic oriented treatments. During the establishment phase of instruction, the clinician seeks to teach target behaviors and establish the awareness of phonological contrasts. Thus, the focus in this treatment phase is usually the production of a sound in isolation, syllables, words, and/or discrimination of a sound and the perception of sound contrasts in words. Clients who enter the treatment continuum at the establishment phase often include those who (1) do not have a specific sound in their repertoire and are not stimulable, (2) produce a sound in their repertoire, but only in a limited number of phonetic contexts, and are unable to readily produce the segment on demand, (3) do not perceive the sound in minimal pairs, and (4) produce a sound on demand but do not easily incorporate the sound into syllabic units, particularly combining the consonant with a following or preceding vowel.

Two basic teaching strategies are used to establish sound productions. The first involves discrimination/perceptual training prior to direct production training. The second involves initiating treatment with a production focus and makes the assumption that the client learns to discriminate and perceive the sound as an indirect benefit of production training. Perceptual training may be described as including minimal contrast training (e.g., sorting word-pairs such as *two* and *tooth* into two categories that reflect the presence of the final consonant and the deletion of the final consonant) as well as traditional discrimination tasks (e.g., discrimination of [s] from [θ]).

Discrimination/Ear Training and Perceptual Training of Sound Contrasts

The type of perceptual training that historically was used most commonly is called *ear training* or *speech sound discrimination training*. Instructional tasks designed to teach discrimination stem from the traditional motor approach to articulation treatment and typically involve making same-different judgments about what is heard (e.g., "Tell me if these are the same or different—*rake-wake*").

Van Riper and Emerick (1984), Winitz (1975, 1984), Powers (1971), and Weber (1970) recommended that discrimination training occur prior to production training during the establishment phase of the treatment continuum. Only sounds produced in error should be included in speech sound discrimination training since, as discussed in Chapter 4, little, if any, relationship has been reported between an individual's misarticulation of speech sounds and performance on general speech sound discrimination tasks (Locke, 1980).

Traditionally, speech sound discrimination training has focused on judgments of external (clinician produced) speech sound stimuli. Speech sound discrimination training procedures are often sequenced so that the client goes from judgments of another speaker's productions to judgments of one's own sound productions.

Winitz (1984) suggested that auditory discrimination training precede articulation production training and also be concurrent with production training at each stage of production (e.g., isolation, syllable, word, sentence, conversation) until the client can make the appropriate speech sound discrimination easily at that level. The idea that discrimination training should precede production training is based on the assumption that certain perceptual distinctions are prerequisites for establishing the production of a speech sound in the child's phonologic system although this assumption is not universally accepted.

The extent to which perceptual instruction is an inherent aspect of production training is not clear. For example, when a client is asked to say *house* and he or she says "*hout*," the clinician may say "no, not *hout* but *house*." In this instance, although instruction is production oriented, perceptual training is an inherent part of the task.

A critical question that remains to be answered is whether or not speech sound discrimination/perceptual training has a positive impact on the establishment or production of a target sound. Williams and McReynolds (1975) reported that when children were taught to produce a sound, they also learned to discriminate the sound. They also found that sound discrimination training alone did not result in improvement in production. Rvachew (1994) reported that an interpersonal (external monitoring) speech perception training program involving a computer based word-pair training program facilitated sound production learning. This study varied from earlier studies, however, in that subjects received both production and perceptual training simultaneously, rather than one preceding or following the other. Rvachew also reported that perceptual training was most effective for subjects who learned to produce the correct form of their error sound (e.g., became stimulable) during the course of instruction. Although there is a lack of evidence about the precise nature of the relationship between sound discrimination and the establishment of correct productions, it has frequently been assumed that perceptual training is an inherent part of production treatment.

Methodology for Traditional Discrimination/Ear Training (Van Riper and Erickson, 1996)

1. *Identification*. Call the client's attention to the target sound—what it sounds like, what it looks like as you observe the lips and mouth, and as best you can help them be aware of kinesthetic sensations—what it feels like inside the mouth. For some children, it may help to label the sound and have an appropriate picture or object to go with the sound (e.g., /f/ is the angry cat sound; /t/ is the ticking sound; /k/ is the throaty sound).

   After auditorily stimulating the child with repeated productions of the target sound, then ask the child to raise their hand, ring a bell, or otherwise indicate when they hear the target sound in isolation. Intermingle the target with other sounds. Initially the other sounds should have several feature differences from the target in terms of voicing, manner, and place of production (e.g., /s/ and /m/). However, as instruction progresses, the number of feature contrasts between the target and the other sounds should be fewer (e.g., /s/ and /θ/).

2. *Isolation*. In this activity, have the client again listen for the target sound, by identifying it in increasingly complex environments. Begin by having them raise their hand, show a happy face or otherwise indicate they hear the sound in a word (begin with the initial position). Progress to hearing it in phrases and sentences. This step might also include practice identifying the presence of a sound at the middle or end of the word. Note that this step is very difficult for young children before they have learned to read, and is not usually included unless the child has a good grasp of the concept's beginning and end.

3. *Stimulation*. In this activity, the client is provided an appropriate auditory model of the target sound in both isolation and words. This activity might include limited amplification and varying stress and duration of the target sound. This type of activity is advocated by Hodson and Paden (1991) as part of the cycles approach to remediation and in the treatment program is referred to as "auditory bombardment."

4. *Discrimination*. Ask the client to make judgments of correct and incorrect productions you produce, in increasingly complex contexts (i.e., words, phrases, sentences). In this activity, the client is comparing someone else's production with his or her own internal image of the correct form of a sound. For example, if a child substitutes /θ/ for /s/, the clinician might say: "Here is a picture of a thun. Did I say that word right? Did you see my tongue peeking out at the beginning of the word? Did you hear /θ/ instead of /s/? See if I name this picture rightly (picture of school): thcool, thcool. Did I say that correctly?"

Making judgments of another speaker is an easier task than making judgments about one's own productions. Winitz (1975) suggested that for clients who are not stimulable for a particular sound, speech sound discrimination such as that presented above is an important prerequisite to motor production. As indicated earlier, however, this concept has not been demonstrated by empirical research.

Methodology for Perceptual Training of Sound Contrasts

One aspect of the influence of linguistics on clinical phonology has been its impact on the nature of perceptual training that should either precede or be a part of phonological treatment. Rather than focus on discrimination between sounds, the phonological perspective suggests that perceptual training should focus on minimal pair contrast training. This training was proposed by LaRiviere, Winitz, Reeds, and Herriman (1974), and focuses on the client's differentiation of minimally contrasting word pairs. They recommended that when consonant clusters are reduced, the child be taught to sort contrasting word pairs (e.g., *led-sled*) into categories that reflect simplification of a consonant cluster and those that reflect appropriate production of the target consonant cluster (e.g., sick versus stick). Another example of such training is a task for final consonant deletion in which the client picks up pictures of "tea" and "teeth" as they are randomly named by the clinician. The intent of this training is to develop a perceptual awareness of differences between minimal pairs (in this case, the presence or absence of a final consonant in the word) and serve to establish the appropriate phonologic contrasts. Perceptual training is widely employed, and a method for using it is presented below. The topic is further described later in this chapter when minimal pair intervention strategies are discussed.

1. *Introduction of a minimal pair*. Present to the client a word that contains a target sound. For example, if the child is substituting /t/ for the fricative /ʃ/, the word *shoe* might be used in a perceptual training activity. The child listens as the clinician points to five identical pictures of a shoe, and names each one.

   Next, present to the client a second word, along with associated pictures of the word, which contains a contrasting sound that is very different from the target sound (i.e., has several different features from the target sound.) For example, *shoe* might be contrasted with *boo* (ghost picture). The phonemes /ʃ/ and /b/ differ in voicing, manner, and place of articulation. For this step, the clinician will identify the original five pictures of a shoe plus the five pictures of "boo."

2. *Contrast training*. Practice differentiating the two contrasting words at a perceptual level. Line up the ten pictures, five of which are of shoe, and five of boo. Ask the

client to hand you the picture you name. Make random requests for either *boo* or *shoe*. If the child can readily do this, he or she has established at a perceptual level the contrast between /ʃ/ and /b/. If the child has difficulty with this task, this activity should be repeated, possibly with different words. Once the child can do this task, contrast training should be repeated with a minimal pair involving the target and error sound (e.g., *shoe-toe*; *shop-top*).

When the clinician is satisfied that the client can discriminate the target sound from other sounds and that he or she can perceive the target in minimal pairs involving the target sound and error sound, the client is ready for production training. It should be pointed out that in our experience, many children readily discriminate accurately through external monitoring tasks, that is, discriminate the clinician's productions although they may not produce the contrast.

In summary, many speech clinicians teach their clients to perceive the distinction between the target and error sounds or to identify phonemic contrasts as part of the establishment process. Such activities may precede and/or accompany production training. As stated earlier, routine discrimination/perceptual training in treatment has been questioned because many individuals with phonologic disorders do not reflect discrimination problems. In addition, production training, unaccompanied by direct perceptual training, has been shown to modify phonologic errors. The type of perceptual training that appears most useful during the establishment phase is that of phonemic contrast training, as described above.

Production Training

For many clients, clinicians begin phonologic intervention at the establishment phase and focus on helping a client learn to produce a target sound. Whether or not perceptual training precedes or is interwoven with production training, the goal during this phase of training is to elicit a target sound from a client and stabilize it at a voluntary level.

When a sound is not in a person's repertoire, it is sometimes taught in isolation or syllables rather than words. It should be remembered that some speech sounds, such as stops, are difficult to teach in isolation since stops by their physical nature are produced in combination with vowels or vowel approximations. Glides, likewise, involve production of more than the glide when they are produced. Fricatives can be taught in isolation since they are sounds that can be sustained (e.g., s-s-s-s-s-s). Stops and glides are usually taught in CV contexts (e.g., stop + schwa = /gə/).

Whether sounds should be taught initially in isolation, syllables, or words is a matter of some controversy. McDonald (1964) urged that syllables be used in production training since the syllable is the basic unit of motor speech production. Some clinicians (e.g., Van Riper and Emerick, 1984) argued that since isolated sounds are the least complex units of production and afford the least interference between the client's habitual speech sound error and the learning of a correct (adult) production, they should be taught first. Words sometimes elicit interference from old error patterns and in such cases may not be a good place to initiate instruction. Others advocate words (lexical items) as the best place to begin instruction because the client can benefit from contextual influences in meaningful productions, and because of the communicative benefits that accrue from the use of "real words." The clinician can determine the level of production that is most facilitative for correct production and then determine whether interference from previous learning is a problem.

Four methods are commonly employed by speech-language clinicians to establish the motoric production of a target sound: imitation, phonetic placement, successive approximation, and contextual utilization. Each of these approaches is discussed below:

1. *Imitation.*   We recommend that the clinician attempt to elicit responses through imitation as an initial instructional method for production training. Usually the clinician presents several auditory models of the desired behavior (typically a sound in isolation, syllables, or words), instructs the client to watch his or her mouth and listen to the sound that is being said, and then asks the client to repeat the target behavior. Sometimes, the clinician may wish to amplify the model through an auditory trainer.

Procedures for Eliciting a Sound Through Imitation

CLINICIAN: Watch my mouth and listen while I say this sound—/θ/ (repeat it several times). Now you say it.
CLINICIAN: That's right, I heard the /θ/ sound. Now say this—/θa/ (repeat it several times).
CLINICIAN: Good, now say /θi/. (Proceed to have the client combine /θ/ and a couple of other vowels.)
CLINICIAN: Now say *thumb* (repeat it several times).

Productions are sometimes tape recorded by the clinician so that the client's productions may be played back and he or she can evaluate his or her productions. Clients may also be asked to focus on how a sound feels during correct production and to modify their productions to maintain this kinesthetic awareness.

When an individual can imitate a target sound, the goal during establishment is to simply stabilize target productions. Subsequent instruction will begin at the most complex linguistic level at which the client is able to imitate, whether it be isolation, syllables, or words. The level at which a client can imitate may already have been determined during stimulability testing, but it should be rechecked at the initiation of instruction. Even if the client was not stimulable on a sound during assessment, it is recommended that the clinician begin remediation by asking the client to imitate target productions using auditory, visual, and tactile cues.

2. *Phonetic placement.*   When the client is unable to imitate a target sound, the clinician typically begins to cue or instruct the client regarding where to place his or her articulators to produce a particular sound. This type of instruction is called phonetic placement.

Procedures for Using the Phonetic Placement Technique to Teach Sounds

    a. Instruct the client where to place the articulators to produce a specific speech sound (e.g., for /f/, tell the client to place his or her upper teeth on his or her lower lip and blow air over the lip; for /sh/, tell the client to pull the tongue back from the upper teeth past the rough part of the palate, make a groove in the tongue, round the lips, and blow air).

b. Provide visual and tactile cues to supplement verbal description (e.g., model the correct sound, and provide verbal cueing as the client attempts the sounds: "Remember to lightly touch the lower lip as you blow air for /f/; remember the groove as you blow air for the /ʃ/.").

c. It may be helpful, depending on the maturity level of the client, to analyze and describe differences between the error production and the target production. Sometimes clinicians like to use pictures or drawings reflecting placement of the articulators as part of the instruction.

The phonetic placement method has probably been used as long as anyone has attempted to modify speech patterns. Over three-fourths of a century ago, Scripture and Jackson (1927) published *A Manual of Exercises for the Correction of Speech Disorders,* which included phonetic placement techniques for speech instruction. These authors suggested:

a. Mirror work

b. Drawings designed to show the position of the articulators for the production of specific sounds

c. "Mouth gymnastics"; that is, movements of the articulators (lips and tongue) in response to models and verbal cues and instructions

d. The use of tongue blades to teach placement of sounds, and straws to help direct the airstream

The phonetic placement approach involves explanations and descriptions of idealized phoneme productions. The verbal explanations provided to the client include descriptions of motor gestures or movements and the appropriate points of articulatory contact (tongue, jaw, lip, and velum) involved in producing the target segments. This approach to teaching sounds frequently is used alone or in combination with imitation, plus successive approximation and context utilization (described below). The Appendix describes techniques for teaching various consonants, some of which utilize phonetic placement cues.

Application of the Phonetic Placement Procedure for Teaching /s/

a. Raise the tongue so that its sides are firmly in contact with the inner surface of the upper back teeth.

b. Slightly groove the tongue along the midline. Insert a straw along the midline of the tongue to provide the client a tactile cue as to the place to form the groove.

c. Place the tip of the tongue immediately behind the upper or lower teeth. Show the client in a mirror where to place the tongue tip.

d. Bring the front teeth (central incisors) into alignment (as much as possible) so that a narrow small space between the rows of teeth is formed.

e. Direct the airstream along the groove of the tongue toward the cutting edges of the teeth.

3. *Successive approximation.*   Another procedure for teaching sounds that is in some respects an extension of using phonetic placement cues involves shaping a new sound from one that is already in a client's repertoire, or even a behavior the client can perform, such as elevating the tongue. Complex behavioral responses such as speech sound productions often need to be broken down into a series of successive steps or approximations that lead to the production of the target behavior(s). A teaching method that utilizes successive approximation is termed **shaping**. The first step in shaping is to identify an initial response that the client can produce and one that is related to the terminal goal. One common way that this method can be initiated is by the modification of other speech sounds already in the repertoire. Instructional steps move successfully through a series of graded steps or approximations, each progressively closer to the target behavior. Shaping has been found to be an efficient method for teaching complex behavioral tasks but requires careful planning in the sequencing of events to be used for treatment.

Shaping Procedure for Teaching /s/

a. Make [t] (the alveolar place of constriction is similar for both /t/ and /s/).
b. Make [t] with a strong aspiration on the release, prior to the onset of the vowel.
c. Prolong the strongly aspirated release.
d. Remove the tip of the tongue slowly during the release from the alveolar ridge to make a [ts] cluster.
e. Prolong the [s] portion of the [ts] cluster in a word like oats.
f. Practice prolonging the last portion of the [ts] production.
g. Practice "sneaking up quietly" on the /s/ (delete /t/).
h. Produce /s/.

Shaping Procedure for Teaching /ɝ/ (Shriberg, 1975)

a. Stick your tongue out (model provided).
b. Stick your tongue out and touch the tip of your finger (model provided).
c. Put your finger on the bumpy place right behind your top teeth (model provided).
d. Now put the tip of your tongue "lightly" on that bumpy place (model provided).
e. Now put your tongue tip there again, and say [l] (model provided).
f. Say [l] each time I hold up my finger (clinician holds up finger).
g. Now say [l] for as long as I hold my finger up, like this: (model provided for five seconds). Ready. Go.
h. Say a long [l] but this time as you are saying it, drag the tip of your tongue slowly back along the roof of your mouth—so far back that you have to drop it. (Accompany instructions with hand gestures of moving fingertips back slowly, palm up.) (104)

These examples for /s/ and /ɝ/ reflect ways that clinicians capitalize on successive approximations: by shaping behavior from a sound in the client's repertoire (e.g., /t/), and by shaping from a nonphonetic behavior in the client's repertoire (e.g., protruded tongue). Once the client produces a sound that is close to the target, the clinician can use other techniques, such as auditory stimulation, imitation, and phonetic placement cues, to reach the target production. Descriptions of other ways to elicit various sounds are provided in the Appendix and are frequently discussed on the internet phonology listserv (www .phonologicaltherapy@yahoogroups.com).

4. *Contextual utilization.* Another procedure used to establish a sound involves isolating a target sound from a particular phonetic context in which a client may happen to produce a sound correctly, even though he or she typically produces the sound in error. As indicated in Chapter 5, the assessment chapter, correct sound productions can sometimes be elicited through contextual testing since sounds are affected by phonetic and positional context, and some contexts may facilitate the correct production of a particular sound. In Chapter 5, contextual testing was recommended for some clients selected for remediation. The intent of such testing is to identify environments where correct production of target behaviors occurs.

Correct consonant productions may occasionally be observed in clusters even when absent in singletons. Therefore, clusters should be included in contextual testing. Curtis and Hardy (1959) reported that more correct responses of /r/ were elicited in consonant clusters than in consonant singletons. It is of interest that Williams (1991) reported when teaching /s/ in clusters, the sound generalized to /s/ in singletons. If a particular context can be found in which the target behavior is produced correctly, it can be used to facilitate correct production in other contexts.

Procedures for Teaching Sounds through Context Utilization

If /s/ is produced correctly in the context of the word pair "bright sun," the /t/ preceding the /s/ may be viewed as a facilitating context.

   a. Ask the client to say *bright sun* slowly and prolong the /s/. Demonstrate what you
       mean by saying the two words and extending the duration of /s/ (e.g., *bright—ssssss-
       sun*).
   b. Next ask the client to repeat *bright—ssssssink*, then *hot—ssssssea*. Other facilitating
       pairs may be used to extend and stabilize the /s/ production.
   c. Ask the client to just say /s/ without the "lead-in."

Using phonetic/linguistic context as a method to establish a sound allows the clinician to capitalize on a behavior that may already be in the client's repertoire. This procedure also represents a form of shaping, because one is using context to help the client isolate and stabilize production of an individual phoneme.

Establishment Guidelines

Individual variations among clients preclude a detailed set of specific instructions applicable to all clients; however, the following are general guidelines for establishment:

   1. Perceptual training, particularly contrast training employing minimal pairs, is sug-
       gested as part of establishment when there is evidence that the client is unable to per-
       ceive appropriate phonologic contrasts or that the error pattern is based on a
       phonologic rule.
   2. When teaching production of a target sound, look for the target sound in the client's
       response repertoire through stimulability (imitation) testing, contextual testing
       (including consonant clusters, other word-positions, and phonetic contexts), and

observation of a connected speech sample. The recommended sequence for eliciting sounds that cannot be produced on demand, is (a) imitation (verbal stimulation), (b) phonetic placement, (c) successive approximation (shaping), and (d) contextual utilization. Stabilize correct productions and use them as a starting point for more complex linguistic units and contexts.

Beyond Teaching Sounds: Treatment Approaches with a Motor Emphasis

Traditional Approach

While teaching a sound may be the first step in intervention, correction of phonologic errors involves stages of the treatment continuum that go beyond establishment. Several treatment approaches are designed to move a client through a multistep process toward correct production of target sounds. The **traditional approach** to articulation therapy was formulated during the early decades of the 1900s by pioneering clinicians of the field. By the late 1930s, Charles Van Riper had assimilated these treatment techniques into an overall plan for treating articulation disorders and published them in his text entitled *Speech Correction: Principles and Methods* (originally published in 1939 and modified in subsequent editions). As an outgrowth of his writings, the traditional approach is sometimes referred to as the "Van Riper method."

The traditional approach is motor oriented and was developed at a time when those receiving treatment were typically school-age clients, often with residual errors. At that time, clinicians were seeing few children with language disorders and caseloads included more children with mild disorders than at present. However, the traditional approach was successfully used with clients representing ranges of severity level. The traditional approach to articulation therapy is still widely used and is appropriate for individuals with residual errors that typically are articulatory in nature.

The traditional approach progresses from the speaker's identification of error productions to the establishment of correct productions, and then moves on to generalization and finally to maintenance. As Van Riper and Emerick (1984) stated:

> The hallmark of traditional articulation therapy lies in its sequencing of activities for (1) sensory-perceptual training, which concentrates on identifying the standard sound and discriminating it from its error through scanning and comparing; (2) varying and correcting the various productions of the sound until it is produced correctly; (3) strengthening and stabilizing the correct production; and finally (4) transferring the new speech skill to everyday communication situations. This process is usually carried out first for the standard sound in isolation, then in the syllable, then in a word, and finally in sentences (206).

A characteristic of the traditional approach is its emphasis on perceptual training. During this part of therapy, the client is not required to produce the sound, but rather, instruction is designed to provide a perceptual standard by which the client can contrast his or her own productions. Thus, perceptual training becomes a precursor to production training. Procedures for doing perceptual training were presented earlier in this chapter in our discussion of methods for teaching sounds and will not be repeated here.

The primary ingredient of traditional instruction is production training, with the focus on helping a client learn to produce a sound on demand. Production training usually includes four sequential instructional phases wherein a target sound is (1) produced in isolation (the target sound is elicited in isolation or, in the case of stops and certain glides, in a CV context such as /pa/; (2) produced in syllables (the sound is produced in CV, VC, and VCV syllables); (3) produced in words (the target sound is produced in a word or lexical context in initial, final, and medial positions); and (4) produced in increasingly complex syntactic utterances (i.e., phrases, sentences, conversational speech).

Instructional Steps for Traditional Production Training (Secord, 1989; Van Riper and Erickson, 1996)

1. *Isolation.* The first step in the traditional method is to teach a client to produce a sound in isolation. An explanation for beginning with production of the target sound in isolation is the assumption that the articulatory gestures of a sound are most easily learned when the sound is highly identifiable and in the least complex context. The goal at this level is to develop a consistently correct response. Specific techniques for teaching sounds were discussed above and are included in the Appendix. It should be pointed out that training should begin at whatever level of sound complexity a child can produce—isolation, syllables, or words.

2. *Nonsense syllables.* The second step involves teaching the client to produce a sound in a syllable. The goal at this step is consistently correct productions in a variety of nonsense syllable contexts. A suggested sequence for syllable practice is CV, VC, VCV, and CVC. It is also suggested that the transition from the consonant to the vowel should be accomplished with sounds that are similar in place of articulation. For example, an alveolar consonant such as /s/ should be facilitated in a high front vowel context, as in [si]. The clinician might also wish to use the target sound in nonsense clusters.

3. *Words.* The third step involves having a client produce a sound in meaningful units, that is, words. This step begins once the client can consistently produce the target sound in nonsense syllables. Instructions at this level should begin with monosyllabic words, with the target consonant (assuming instruction is focusing on consonants as opposed to vowels) in the prevocalic position (CV). Instruction then moves to VC, CVC, CVCV, monosyllabic words with clusters, followed by more complex word forms. Table 7.1 reflects a hierarchy of phoneme production complexity at the word level as presented by Secord (1989).

Once a core group of words is established in which the client is readily able to produce the target sound, the clinician seeks to expand the small set of core words to a somewhat larger set of training words. Usually target words are selected on the basis of meaningfulness to the client (e.g., family names, places, social expressions, words from the academic curriculum), but other factors such as phonetic context and syllable complexity should also be taken into consideration, just as they were for the initial set of core words.

TABLE 7.1   Substages of Word Level Stabilization Training (Secord, 1989)

Substage	Syllables	Examples for /s/
1. Initial prevocalic words	1	*sun, sign, say*
2. Final postvocalic words	1	*glass, miss, pass*
3. Medial intervocalic words	2	*kissing, lassie, racer*
4. Initial blends/clusters	1	*star, spoon, skate*
5. Final blends/clusters	1	*lost, lips, rocks*
6. Medial blends/clusters	2	*whisper, outside, ice-skate*
7. All word positions	1–2	*(any of the above)*
8. All word positions	any	*signaling, eraser, therapist*
9. All word positions; multiple targets	any	*necessary, successful*

4. *Phrases*. Once the client can easily produce a target sound in words, instruction shifts from single-word productions to practicing a target sound in two- to four-word phrases. This level of production represents a complexity level between single words and sentence level productions. This is especially true if carrier phrases are employed. *Carrier phrases* are phrases where only a single word is added with each repetition (e.g., I see the *car*; I see the *cup*; I see the *cane*.). In phrase level productions, one should begin with phrases where only one word contains the target sound. As the client produces a target sound in a single word, the clinician may wish to add a second word in the phrase that contains the target sound.

5. *Sentences*. An extension of phrase level productions is sentence level practice. Just as practice at other levels has involved careful sequencing of task complexity, this principle also holds at this level. Consideration should be given to factors such as phonetic context, syllable structure of words, and number of words in the sentence. The following sequence of sentence levels is suggested:

   a. Simple short sentence with one instance of the target sound.
   b. Sentences of various lengths with one instance of the target sound.
   c. Simple short sentences with two or more instances of the target sound.
   d. Sentences of various lengths with two or more instances of the target sound.

6. *Conversation*. The final step in production training involves using a target sound in everyday speech. At this point, the clinician is seeking to facilitate generalization of productions that have already proceeded through more structured production tasks. Initially, generalization situations are structured so that the client produces his or her sound correctly in situations where the speech is monitored. Activities such as role playing, talking about future plans, attempting to get information, interviewing, and oral reading can be used at this level. Following structured conversations, subsequent activities are more spontaneous and free and sometimes characterized as "off-guard" type conversations. The intent is to provide activities to facilitate transfer that approximates real-life situations. Activities should include speaking situations where the client focuses not on self-monitoring but on what he or she says. Telling personal experiences, talking about topics that evoke strong feelings, and taking part in group

discussions are used at this stage of instruction. Some clinicians include "negative practice" to help to stabilize a new response. In negative practice, a client deliberately produces a target sound incorrectly and then contrasts it to a correct production; Van Riper and Erickson (1996) stated that such deliberate productions of error sounds increased the rate of learning.

At this point, the clinician also seeks to facilitate the carryover of conversation to situations beyond the therapy environment. It is suggested that such situational generalization be encouraged once the client can produce a target sound at the word level. By encouraging transfer in earlier stages of instruction, it is assumed that generalization beyond the word level will be significantly enhanced and will perhaps decrease the amount of time needed at the phrase, sentence, and conversational levels.

Summary of the Traditional Approach

Background Statement.   The underlying assumptions of the traditional approach to remediation include the following: (1) Faulty perception of speech sounds may be related to phonological errors, and (2) phonological errors may be viewed as inadequate motor production of speech sounds. Thus, the traditional approach relies heavily on motor production practice combined with activities related to discrimination/perceptual training.

Unique Features.   The traditional approach to articulation remediation, until the 1980s, constituted the basic methodology employed by most clinicians for articulation instruction and is still widely used today. The traditional method focuses on motor learning of individual speech sounds. The approach provides a complete instructional sequence for correcting articulatory errors. The approach can be modified to fit the needs of clients of all ages. Perceptual training is recommended as a precursor to or an accompaniment of direct work on sounds.

Strengths and Limitations.   This approach has been widely used over time and forms the basis of several current treatment approaches. Its widespread usage is likely related to the logical sequence of training tasks, the success that accrues through motor practice, and the adaptability and applicability of the approach. It may not, however, be the most efficacious approach for clients with multiple errors.

Research Support.   This approach has stood the test of time because it has "worked" for many clinicians, with many clients. Many investigators have reported phonological change in association with intervention that has been based on this approach; however, comparative studies between the "traditional approach" and others are limited. The emphasis on external discrimination training as part of the treatment process for all children has been questioned because of the difficulty involved in separating discrimination training and production training, as well as the lack of data to support its effectiveness. The traditional approach is appropriate for the treatment of clients who have a limited number of errors that are articulatory based. Elements of this approach (e.g., increasing the linguistic complexity of the training tasks by moving from words to phrases and sentences) are also utilized in many linguistic approaches to remediation.

Programmed Articulation Instruction: A Detailed Example of Sequencing Goals Based on the Traditional Method

During the 1970s many efforts were made to apply principles of behavior modification and programmed instruction to speech intervention. Using the traditional approach to treating articulation disorders as the point of reference, Baker and Ryan (1971) developed the following outline for treating consonant sounds (see Tables 7.2 and 7.3). It is presented here to provide you with a detailed description not only of programmed instruction, but also how goals can be sequenced in traditional articulation therapy.

TABLE 7.2   Establishment Phase: Programmed Conditioning for Articulation

Step		Stimulus	Response	Schedule of Reinforcement
Series A		Take Criterion Test Placement Start		
	1	Sound in isolation	Sound	
Series B	1	Sound in nonsense syllable, random presentation of short vowels (a, e, i, o, u) with X* in initial position (Xa)	Syllable	
	2	Sound in nonsense syllable, random presentation of short vowels (a, e, i, o, u) with X in final position (aX)	Syllable	
	3	Sound in nonsense syllable, random presentation of short vowels (a, e, i, o, u) with X in medial position (aXa)	Syllable	100% (continuous)
Series C	1	Word with X in initial position	Word	50%
	2	Word with X in final position	Word	50%
	3	Word with X in medial position	Word	50%
Series D	1	Word with X in initial position appearing randomly in 2- or 3-word phrase	Phrase	50%
	2	Word with X in final position appearing randomly in 2- or 3-word phrase	Phrase	50%
	3	Word with X in medial position appearing randomly in 2- or 3-word phrase	Phrase	50%
Series E	1	Word with X in initial position appearing randomly in 4- to 6-word sentence	Sentence	50%
	2	Word with X in final position appearing randomly in 4- to 6-word sentence	Sentence	50%
	3	Word with X in medial position appearing randomly in 4- to 6-word sentence	Sentence	50%
Series F	1	Contextual reading material (If nonreader, go to series G-2.)	Reads a sentence	100%

TABLE 7.2 *(Continued)*

Step		Stimulus	Response	Schedule of Reinforcement
Series G	1	Story: Instruct to read silently and then tell a story about it.	Reads story silently Tells what he/she reads in phrases and sentences	100%
	2	Pictures: (Instructor models first picture by telling short story about the picture.)	Tells story about picture in sentences	100%
Series H	1	Conversation	Conversation	100%
	2	Conversation End of Program Stop Take Criterion Test Go to Transfer Program Series B. Begin Program again with New Sound(s).	Conversation	10%

Source: Used with permission of Monterey Learning Systems, 900 Welch Road, Palo Alto, Calif.

*X = target sound

TABLE 7.3 **Transfer Phase: Programmed Conditioning for Articulation**

Step		Stimulus	Response	Schedule of Reinforcement
Series A		Child working with parent at home:		
	1	Says word containing X	Repeats word	100%
	2	Says phrase containing word with X	Repeats phrase	100%
	3	Says sentence containing word with X	Repeats sentence	100%
	4	Reading material or pictures	Reads or tells about pictures	100%
	5	Conversation	Conversation	100%
Series B		Take Transfer Criterion Test Different physical settings with the clinician:		
	1	Outside clinic (outside the door)	Conversation	100%
	2	Outside clinic (down the hall)	Conversation	100%
	3	Outside clinic (outside the building or in another room)	Conversation	100%
	4	Playground or cafeteria or off school or clinic grounds	Conversation	100%
	5	Outside classroom	Conversation	100%

(continues)

TABLE 7.3   *(Continued)*

Step		Stimulus	Response	Schedule of Reinforcement
Series		In the classroom:		
C	1	With clinician in classroom	Conversation	100%
	2	With clinician and teacher in classroom	Conversation	100%
	3	Small-group activity	Conversation	100%
	4	Large-group activity	Conversation	100%
	5	"Speech" or "Show and Tell" in front of class	Conversation or monologue	100%
		Take Transfer Criterion Test		
		End of Program		
		Stop		
		Go to Maintenance		

Source: Used with permission of Monterey Learning Systems.

Summary of the Programmed Conditioning for Articulation

Background Statement.   This behavioral program views remediation from the perspective that speech sounds are learned motor behaviors. Instruction involves a progression of motor skills and employs behavioral principles that are used in modifying behaviors. Instruction consists of several series of small, sequential steps associated with contingent reinforcement. Thus, this program represents a formal programmed approach to instruction that is based on behavioral conditioning.

Unique Features.   The detailed, step-by-step instructions for correcting misarticulations provide the clinician with what some might call a "recipe" for sequencing therapy. The scope of the program, which moves from establishment to transfer to maintenance, including a home program, is more comprehensive than most programs. As with all programmed instruction, the course of treatment is based on data that accrue from tabulation of responses made by the client.

Strengths and Limitations.   The reason this program is included in this text is that it provides clinicians or instructional aides with a systematic, step-by-step instructional procedure that takes a client from establishment of a sound to consistent production of that sound. The emphasis on numerous responses per session ensures much repetition and motor practice. Program methodology relies heavily on imitation, which may become tedious for some clients and clinicians. The inclusion of branching steps allows some individualization of the program, but the basic assumption is that the program is particularly suitable for school-age children and adults with residual errors.

Research Support.   Data to support the program have been reported by Baker and Ryan (1971) and Gray (1974). These investigators reported that significant gains can be achieved by subjects when comparing pretest and posttest scores for all phases of the program. However, experiments that have included control groups or compared studies with other treatment programs have not been reported.

Context Utilization Approaches

Contextual or sensory-motor based approaches to intervention have been advocated by some clinical phonologists (McDonald, 1964; Hoffman, Schuckers, and Daniloff, 1989). Treatment suggestions related to these approaches are based on the recognition that speech sounds are not produced in isolation, but rather in syllable-based contexts, and that certain phonetic contexts may be facilitative of correct sound usage. McDonald suggested that instruction for articulatory errors be initiated in a context(s) where the error sound can be produced correctly. He provided an example of a child with a defective /s/ who produced [s] correctly in the context of *watchsun*. He suggested the following sequence of instructions after *watchsun* was identified as a context where /s/ was correctly produced: (1) Say *watchsun* with "slow-motion" speed; (2) say *watchsun* with equal stress on both syllables, then with primary stress on the first syllable, and then with primary stress on the second syllable; (3) say *watchs* and prolong [s] until a signal is given to complete the bisyllable with [ʌn]; (4) say short sentences with the same facilitating context such as "Watch, sun will burn you." The sequence is repeated with other sentences and stress patterns. The meaningfulness of the sentence is not important since the primary focus of the activity is the movement sequences.

Following the above steps, the client is instructed to alter the movement patterns associated with the correct /s/ by changing the vowel following the segment in a suggested a sequence such as:

watch-sun	*watch-sat*
watch-sea	*watch-soon*
watch-sit	*watch-sew*
watch-send	*watch-saw*

The next step is to practice words that include a second contextual modification. Using the previous example, segments preceding and following /tʃ/ would be altered. Words like *teach*, *reach*, *pitch*, *catch*, and *beach* would be used in combination with one-syllable words beginning with /s/ and followed by a variety of vowels (such as *sand*, *sun*, *said*, and *soon*). Practice is then conducted with various combinations of the words that terminate with /tʃ/ in combination with words that begin with /s/ (for example, *teachsun*). Various sound combinations are practiced with different rates and stress patterns and should eventually be practiced in sentence contexts.

The next phase of instruction is directed toward a phonetic context other than [tʃ] in which the /s/ is correct, and then vary the phonetic context, rate of speech, and syllable stress in alternative contexts. Situational transfer procedures and activities are similar to those used with other treatment systems.

Hoffman et al. (1989) described another variation of a contextual approach that involves a sequenced set of production-based training tasks designed to facilitate the automatization of articulator performance. The basic assumption behind their suggestions is that "revision of over learned, highly automatic behavior is possible through carefully planned and executed performance rehearsal" (248). They also indicated that once *inappropriate* articulatory patterns are automatized or habituated, the process of revising those behaviors may differ from development of the original behavior. Intervention is seen as involving instruction and practice of motor articulatory adjustments to replace previously learned (incorrect) productions. The paragraphs that follow present the sequence of tasks and instructional activities these authors suggest.

Prior to working directly on error targets, the clinician elicits, via imitation, sound segments that the client can produce correctly. Such "stimulability tasks" provide the client with an opportunity to experience success in a speech task as well as the opportunity to observe and imitate the clinician's productions. It is suggested that the clinician not only model the correct form of sounds in the child's repertoire but also distort such productions through excessive movements (e.g., lip rounding for /m, p, f/) for the purpose of giving the client the opportunity to practice manipulation of the articulators in response to the clinician's model. Such activity will hopefully facilitate the client's skill at identifying, comparing, and discriminating the clinician's and his/her own sound productions.

Following stimulability tasks, the clinician and client work together to employ the articulatory adjustments necessary for correct target sound production. It is suggested that the clinician be able to repeat sentences using error productions similar to those of the client in order to be aware of the motoric acts involved in the client's misarticulations. Instead of focusing instruction on correct target sound productions, the emphasis is on doing interesting things with the speech mechanism; at this stage, children are encouraged to view their productions in the mirror and listen to themselves on audio/video tapes.

Rehearsal involves four levels of complexity: nonsymbolic units, words and word pairs, sounds in sentences, and narratives. Once the narrative level is reached, rehearsal can include a mixture of the four levels.

Practice with nonsymbolic units (the authors use the term *nonsymbolic* rather than *nonsense syllables*) provides for manipulation of articulatory gestures that were begun during pretraining. Nonsymbolic instruction focuses on target productions in VC, CV, VCV, and VCCV syllables. It is asserted that production of nonsymbolic units imposes minimal constraints on the speaker by allowing him or her to focus on the speech task rather than morphology, syntax, and semantics. Table 7.4 reflects nonsymbolic sound unit rehearsal matrices. The authors suggest that motoric success at this rudimentary level facilitates success at more linguistically and socially complex levels.

Word and word-pair practice is the next step in the program. Initial targets should reflect a transition from nonsymbolic units to meaningful units that encompass the nonsymbolic syllables already practiced. Practice activities at this level are designed to encourage the client to assume responsibility for recognizing and judging the adequacy of his or her performance. Table 7.5 reflects a list of words and word-pairs by word-position that might be used at this level.

The next step in the program involves *sounds in context* in what are termed *rehearsal sentences*. At this stage the client repeats the clinician's model of sentences that includes words practiced at the word level. As in target word selection, it is important that sentences selected for imitation are appropriate for the client's age, abilities, and interests.

TABLE 7.4 **Nonsymbolic Sound Unit Rehearsal Matrices**

V	C		V	C	V		C	V		V	C	C	V
i	s		i	s	i		s	i		i	t	s	i
a	s		i	s	a		s	a		i	t	s	a
u	s		i	s	u		s	u		i	t	s	u
æ	s		i	s	æ		s	æ		i	t	s	æ
			a	s	i					a	t	s	i
			a	s	a					a	t	s	a
			a	s	u					a	t	s	u
			a	s	æ					a	t	s	æ
			u	s	i					u	t	s	i
			u	s	a					u	t	s	a
			u	s	u					u	t	s	u
			u	s	æ					u	t	s	æ
			æ	s	i					æ	t	s	i
			æ	s	a					æ	t	s	a
			æ	s	u					æ	t	s	u
			æ	s	a					æ	t	s	a

A second phase of this level consists of presenting a stimulus word containing the target segment to the client, then requiring the client to repeat the word, and then embedding it in a spontaneously generated sentence.

The final step in this program involves using a target sound in narratives. This activity employs stories that can be illustrated, acted out, or read. A series of clinician-generated narratives are employed; for example for a preschool client, "This is Poky the turtle. Today is his birthday. He is 6 years old. He says, 'It's my birthday.' What does he say?" This is followed by the client saying "It's my birthday." Through such narratives, practice of the target sound is embedded in communicative tasks. The clinician may have a client practice individual sentences from these narratives for additional practice at the sentence level.

TABLE 7.5 **Word and Word-Pair List for [s]**

Prevocalic		Intervocalic	Postvocalic	
Initial	**Cluster**	**Medial**	**Final**	**Word-Pair**
Sam	scat	passing	pass	Jack sat
seed	ski	receive	niece	jeep seat
soup	scooter	loosen	loose	room soon
saw	scar	bossy	toss	cop saw
sit	skit	kissing	miss	lip sip
sign	sky	nicer	mice	right side

While this program has been presented as a series of steps or levels, the authors point out that these steps should overlap. Throughout the program the client is the primary judge of productions, describing the movement patterns, articulatory contacts, and adequacy of production of each target sound.

Summary of Contextually Based Approaches

Background Statement.   The theoretical concept underlying contextual approaches is that articulatory errors can be corrected by extensive motor practice of articulatory behaviors, with syllabic units as a basic building block for later motor practice at more complex levels. To employ this approach, a sound must be in the client's repertoire.

Unique Features.   The emphasis on imitated, repetitive productions is a unique aspect of this approach. The systematic variation of phonetic contexts in productions of both sounds produced correctly and error sounds targeted for remediation sets this approach apart from others. A major value of context testing is to identify contexts that may be useful in therapy.

Strengths and Limitations.   A major strength of this approach is that it builds on behaviors (segmental productions in particular phonetic contexts) that are in a client's repertoire and capitalizes on syllables plus auditory, tactile, and kinesthetic awareness of motor movements. It may be particularly useful for clients who use a sound inconsistently and need methodology to facilitate consistent production in other contexts. The concept of syllable practice and systematic variation of phonetic contexts and stress may be useful to any training method that includes syllable productions.

Research Support.   Contextual testing, designed to locate facilitating contexts, can be used with clients who have difficulty with stimulability. Published clinical investigations that provide support for the efficacy of using a context facilitation approach to intervention are lacking.

Summary of Motor Approaches to Remediation

The treatment approaches described on the previous pages focus on the development and habituation of the motor skills necessary for target sound productions, with the traditional approach to remediation forming the basis of these approaches. An underlying assumption is that motor practice leads to generalization of correct productions to untrained contexts and to automatization of behaviors. Motor approaches to remediation are especially appropriate for phonetically based errors but are frequently employed in combination with procedures that will later be described under linguistic-based approaches.

Remediation Guidelines for Motor Approaches

1. A motor approach to remediation is recommended as a teaching procedure for clients who evidence motor production problems with individual segments such as /s/, /l/, /r/, and other residual errors. It can also be incorporated into treatment programs for

clients reflecting linguistic or pattern-based errors, especially if the patterns reflect motor constraints (e.g., prevocalic voicing or certain cluster simplifications). Instruction should be initiated at the linguistic unit level (isolation, syllable, word) at which a client can produce target sounds.

2. Perceptual training, especially contrast training, is recommended as part of a motor remediation program, especially for those clients who evidence perceptual problems related to their error sounds.

3. Addressing multiple errors in a given treatment session (i.e., horizontal and cyclical approaches) is recommended for clients with multiple errors.

4. For clinicians who wish to follow a detailed treatment protocol based on a traditional treatment approach, the Programmed Conditioning for Articulation provides such a model.

Linguistic-Based Approaches to Intervention

A second category of treatment approaches to disordered speech is linguistic or phonologically based instruction. While motor approaches may be described as phonetically based and focus on teaching sounds one at a time, linguistic approaches are focused on teaching sound contrasts and appropriate phonological patterns in children with multiple errors. As such, linguistic-based intervention focuses on strategies for reorganizing the child's phonological system. Although a linguistic-based approach is most suitable for children with multiple speech sound errors, elements of the approach can be used in combination with more traditional approaches.

The primary focus of linguistic approaches to remediation is the establishment of adult phonological rules in a client's repertoire (e.g., distinctive features, contrast rules, and phonotactic rules). Treatment programs designed to facilitate acquisition of linguistic rules are not associated with a single unified method; however, two primary characteristics are associated with linguistically oriented phonological approaches. The first characteristic relates to the behaviors targeted for treatment, the second to the instructional procedures themselves.

As discussed in Chapter 5, selection of target behaviors is based on phonological errors as they relate to patterns that may describe the errors. Following pattern or phonological process identification, individual sound(s), called **exemplars**, are chosen that are likely to facilitate generalization from the exemplar to other sounds related to a particular error pattern. Treatment is then designed to facilitate the acquisition of appropriate sound contrasts and/or sequences, with the expectation that generalization will occur to other sounds that are part of the same pattern (e.g., in targeting final consonant deletion, teaching a couple of final consonants is assumed to generalize to other final consonants that are also deleted).

Most treatment protocols that are based on a linguistic model employ minimal contrast word-pairs, which involve minimal or maximal feature contrasts (Weiner, 1981; Gierut, 1989; Fey, 1992). For example, minimal pairs such as bu*s*-buc*k* and bu*s*-bu*t* represent minimal pairs with greater and lesser contrasts, respectively, because of the differences in place and manner of articulation between /s/ and /k/ (greater differences because of place and minimal contrasts), and /s/ and /t/ (lesser contrast because both /s/ and /t/ differ only in manner).

The primary focus of linguistic approaches has been to (1) establish sound and feature contrasts, and (2) replace error patterns with appropriate phonological patterns. Linguistic approaches have targeted elimination of homonyms (one word used for two referents; e.g., *shoe* used for both *chew* and *shoe*), establishment of new syllable and word shapes, and establishment of new sound classes and feature contrasts.

Distinctive Feature Approaches

Distinctive features may be considered subphonemic elements of phonemes that determine the linguistic contrasts between sounds and sound classes. In other words, unique bundles of distinctive features underlie the distinctions among phonemes in a language. For a review of information concerning distinctive features, refer to Chapters 1 and 5.

The intent of instructional programs based on distinctive features is to establish a feature that is lacking in a client's repertoire. For example, lack of frication may describe several sound production errors; for example, the client may use stops for fricatives. Distinctive feature instructional programs usually focus on the establishment of a particular feature through teaching a sound containing that feature, since features are part subphonemic units of sounds and cannot be taught independently. It is then assumed that the newly established feature will generalize from the exemplar to other members of the sound class in which the feature may be absent (e.g., + continuant generalizes from target /f/ to /θ/, /s/, and /ʃ/).

McReynolds and Bennett (1972) reported data indicating that features established in one sound (exemplar) will generalize to other sound segments in which the target feature is absent. They inferred from this finding that remediation based on distinctive features should be an efficient treatment approach since by teaching a feature in one sound you may correct several error sounds. As in other types of generalization, the nature and extent of feature generalization that takes place is highly variable. Generalization seems to be significantly influenced by the similarity between the sound selected for training and other error sounds (e.g., generalization occurs most rapidly across similar sounds or within sound classes). In general, the more features two sound segments share, the more potential there is for generalization to occur from one sound to the second sound.

McReynolds and Bennett (1972) described instructional procedures designed to teach a feature contrast that was absent in a child's productive repertoire. In Phase 1, production focused on nonsense syllables which contained the target feature (e.g., + continuant) in the initial position (e.g., *fɑ*). In Phase 2, the child was taught to produce a sound containing the target feature in the final position of a nonsense syllable (e.g., *ɑf*). Within each phase there were several steps. In Step 1, the child was instructed to produce a consonant in which this feature was lacking. In Step 2, the child was taught to contrastively produce two consonant sounds in syllables, the segment learned in Step 1, and a second consonant selected to contrast with the first. For example, if [+ continuant] was the feature contained in the first sound taught, [– continuant] was the feature selected for the second or contrast sound ([fi] vs. [pi],

[fa] vs. [pa], [fʌ] vs. [pʌ], and [fo] vs. [po]). Phase 2 was identical except for the position of the target sound. In the example above, the child used stops instead of fricatives/continuants (e.g., *fun* was said *tun*; *show* was said *toe*, etc.). In Phase 1, the client was taught the continuant /f/ and then was taught to produce it in the initial position of a nonsense syllable (e.g., fi, fæ, fa, fo). Step 2 focused on having the child produce pairs of nonsense syllables that reflected the + continuant/– continuant contrast (e.g., *fa-pa*; *fi-pi*). In Phase 2, the two steps were repeated except /f/ was taught in the final position (e.g., *af*; *af-if*).

Blache (1989) published a distinctive feature approach to remediation of phonological delay. The approach is organized into four basic steps:

Step 1. *Discussion of words.* Determine whether or not the child knows the meaning of lexical items (words) to be used in therapy. Once a minimal pair contrast has been selected to teach a distinctive feature, it is important to determine if the child understands both lexical items in the word-pair. For example, if the word-pair selected is the letter *T* and the word *key*, the child might be asked: "Which one opens the door? Which one is a letter of the alphabet? Which one goes into a lock? Which one do you write?" (See Figure 7.1.)

Step 2. *Discrimination testing and training.* The child is tested to determine if he or she can perceive the feature contrast. The clinician presents one word of a minimal pair, for example, *fan-pan* or *bear-pear*. The child is instructed to point to the picture that the clinician has named. A criterion of seven consecutive correct responses is used to determine that the child perceived the contrasting word-pairs.

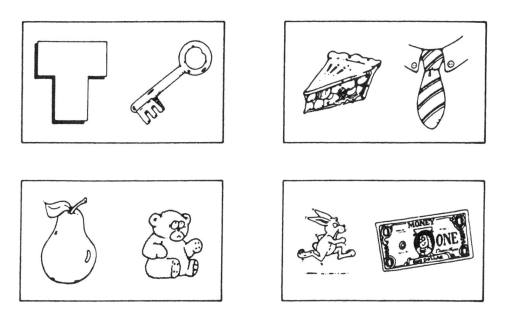

FIGURE 7.1 Exemplars Illustrating Six Different Distinctive Features Contrasts

Step 3. *Production training.* After the client has demonstrated that he or she perceives the minimal contrast, the next step is to establish the feature in a production task. In this step, the child is instructed to say the word and the clinician points to the picture of the word the client pronounced. The client should always be able to correctly pronounce one word of the pair but may not be able to pronounce the other member of the word-pair; thus, a correct production of an error sound may not be required at this stage. Production training continues until the client can use the target feature in a correct production of a target sound.

Step 4. *Carryover training.* Once the child is able to pronounce the target word, the word is placed in longer and more complex linguistic environments. The word is used with the indefinite article *a* in varied phonetic contexts, two-word expressions, three-word carrier phrases, and so on, until the word is used in meaningful social situations in the school and home.

A therapeutic model is recommended in which features that comprise the most salient contrasts are focused on first, followed by successive steps to finer distinctions. Blache (1989) identified the following feature comparisons occurring in the stop–nasal sound class, which proceed from larger to finer contrasts and are presented in Table 7.6. An example of a distinctive feature program designed to teach + frication was presented by Weiner and Bankson (1978) and is presented below:

1. Introduction of the concept of "dripping" sounds (stops) and "flowing" sounds (fricatives).
2. Identification of words that begin with dripping as compared to flowing sounds.
3. Imitation of words containing fricatives in the initial position, with such fricatives emphasized through duration of initial sound (e.g., *f-f-f-f*ish). Following his or her

TABLE 7.6   **Contrast Ordering for Stop–Nasal Sound Class**

No.	Pair	Feature	Sample Words
1.	[t-k]	front-back lingual	*tea-key, tape-cape, ten-Ken*
2.	[n-ŋ]	front-back lingual	*win-wing, fan-fang, ton-tongue*
3.	[p-b]	voiced-voiceless	*pea-bee, pig-big, pat-bat*
4.	[t-d]	voiced-voiceless	*toe-doe, time-dime, tot-dot*
5.	[k-g]	voiced-voiceless	*curl-girl, coat-goat, cap-gap*
6.	[b-m]	nasal-nonnasal	*beet-meat, bat-mat, bike-Mike*
7.	[d-n]	nasal-nonnasal	*D-knee, deck-neck, dot-knot*
8.	[g-ŋ]	nasal-nonnasal	*wig-wing, bag-bang, log-long*
9.	[b-d]	labial-lingual	*big-dig, bark-dark, bow-dough*
10.	[d-g]	front-back lingual	*deer-gear, date-gate, doe-go*

Source: "A Distinctive Feature Approach" by S.E. Blache, in *Assessment and Remediation of Articulatory and Phonological Disorders* (p. 377). N. Creaghead, P. Newman, and W. Secord, eds., Columbus, Ohio: Charles E. Merrill, 1989.

production, the client was required to judge whether the word began with a dripping or flowing sound. Feedback was provided for both production and identification.

4. Repetition of Step 3 without exaggeration of the word-initial fricative.
5. Presentation of a 20-item picture-naming task in which each item began with a fricative.

These investigators reported that as a result of this instructional program, a subject who used stops for fricatives learned to use fricatives in single-word responses.

Summary of Distinctive Feature Approaches

Background Statement.   Distinctive feature approaches to phonological remediation are based on the theory that speech sounds are comprised of bundles of features, each phoneme having a unique and individual set of features that characterize segmental productions. Further, if a client has several sounds in error, an efficient instructional strategy may be to identify or teach an exemplar that contains the absent feature(s), and monitor generalization from that exemplar to other sounds in the same class (i.e., containing the same feature) that are in error.

Unique Features.   This approach is designed to capitalize on patterns (features) of commonalities among error productions. Although features are taught in sounds, feature analysis and remediation represent an endeavor to correct several sounds simultaneously by teaching a feature in one target sound with the assumption that it will generalize to other sounds containing the target feature.

Strengths and Limitations.   An attraction of therapy based on distinctive features is the targeting of phonological patterns that may underlie several individual errors. A major limitation, as pointed out in earlier discussion, is that distinctive features were not designed for clinical intervention. Rather, features were derived as a classification system in order to describe the sound segments across language systems. As a result, some sounds produced by individuals with phonological disorders cannot be described within this framework. The feature classification systems that have been applied clinically tend to be useful for sound substitutions, but difficult to use with sound omissions and distortions. In spite of the fact that distinctive feature approaches are not frequently employed, they encompass the concepts of pattern analyses and treatment focused on linguistic contrasts.

Research Support.   Data to support a distinctive feature approach to therapy may be gleaned from studies that have included the treatment approaches described here. McReynolds and Bennett (1972) reported that all three of their subjects reflected distinctive feature generalization from the exemplar sounds to other sounds, although the amount of feature generalization varied across subjects. Similarly, Weiner and Bankson (1978) reported that their subject generalized [+ frication] to nontrained items. Costello and Onstein (1976) reported that their distinctive feature instructional approach was successful in teaching a subject to generalize the [+ continuant] feature. These data support the finding that feature generalization is seen with distinctive feature approaches to remediation.

The number of subjects involved in these studies was small, and additional data regarding the efficiency of this approach are needed.

Minimal Pair Contrast Therapy

A signature approach of linguistic-based remediation is **minimal pair contrast therapy**. Contrast therapy employs pairs of words that differ only by a single phoneme (e.g., *bat-pat*, *move-mood*, *sun-ton*). As stated earlier, the underlying concept of this type of therapy is that by focusing on word-pairs that typically differ by a single phonemic contrast, the client will be taught that different sounds signal different meanings in words. The phonemic contrasts are related either to feature differences between sounds (e.g., *pat-bat* differ by the voicing feature; *pat-fat* differ by the continuant feature), or syllable shape contrasts (e.g., *bow-boat* differ by the final sound; *key-ski* differ by the initial sound(s) in the syllable initiation—cluster vs. noncluster). Investigators have reported changes in children's phono- logical systems (Weiner, 1981; Elbert and Gierut, 1986; Gierut, 1989, 1990; Williams, 1991) following training with word-pair contrasts. Contrast therapy focuses on the establishment of sound contrasts necessary to differentiate one word from another. While this communication-oriented therapy emerged from a linguistic orientation, it is also used in traditional treatment approaches.

An example of a contrast approach to treatment can be observed through remediation strategies employed with a client who deletes final consonants. In this instance, stops may be produced correctly in word-initial position, but deleted in word-final position (lack of syllable closure). In such a circumstance, the clinician can assume that the final consonant deletions are probably not a production (phonetic) problem. Rather, final consonant deletion in this case likely reflects a conceptual rule related to syllable structure (use of the open syllable). Treatment for this rule would focus on getting the client to recognize that the presence of a consonant in word-final position is a necessary contrast to distinguish certain word-pairs in the language (e.g., *two-tooth*; *bee-beet*). In this instance, the motoric production of a target consonant is already within a child's productive repertoire, and thus motor production of the sound is not the primary focus of instruction. Rather, the focus of instruction is the development of cognitive awareness of final consonant contrasts/syllable closure.

The most commonly employed type of contrast training typically contrasts a substituted or deleted sound with a target sound. For example, if a client substitutes /t/ for /k/ in word-initial position, contrast training words might include *tea-key* and *top-cop*. Similarly, if a child deletes the final /t/, contrast pairs might include *bow-boat* and *see-seat*. Minimal contrast instruction is appropriate when two or more contrasting sounds in the adult language are collapsed into a single sound unit with the result that feature contrasts are not produced (e.g., /t/ replaced /k/), or segments are deleted, such as in final consonant deletions. Training is designed to establish sound contrasts that mark a difference in meaning. Such contrasts are typically selected for remediation because of their relationship to phonological patterns (processes) or error patterns seen in children's phonology (i.e., they become exemplars to facilitate generalization across sounds).

Minimal contrast instruction, as discussed earlier in this chapter, typically focuses first on perception of contrasts and then production of contrasts. A training task that focuses on perceptual training utilizing contrast pairs was first proposed by La Riviere et al. (1974).

In this procedure, subjects are taught to identify sound categories where the target sounds and errors are presented in word-pairs. For example, if a child deletes /s/ in /s/ clusters (cluster simplification), the clinician names several pictures representing minimal pair words like *spool-pool* or *spill-pill* to the client. The client is then required to pick up items named by the clinician, or perhaps sort each lexical item into one or two categories (/s/ singletons or /s/ clusters).

A production-based task would require the client to produce minimal pairs. For example, a client who deletes final consonants might ask the clinician to give him or her the picture of either a *bee* or a *beet*, then be reinforced by the clinician's response for the appropriate production. In this task, the client must be able to produce the distinction between *bee* and *beet*. As stated earlier, the reverse of this procedure (i.e., the clinician asks the client to give him or her certain pictures) can be used to establish perceptual contrasts (i.e., the distinction between *bee* and *beat*).

Weiner (1981) reported a study where minimal contrast training was used to reduce the frequency of selected phonological patterns. He used minimal pairs in activities where accurate word productions were required for the child to communicate successfully. For example, Weiner used a game to teach final [t] in a minimal contrast format. He placed into minimal pairs such words as *bow* and *boat*. Sample stimuli consisted of several pictures of *bow* and several pictures of *boat*. The instructions for the game were as follows:

> "We are going to play a game. The object of the game is to get me to pick up all the pictures of the *boat*. Every time you say boat, I will pick one up. When I have all five, you may paste a star on your paper." If the child said *bow*, the clinician picked up the *bow* picture. At times he would provide an instruction, e.g., "You keep saying *bow*. If you want me to pick up the *boat* picture, you must say the [t] sound at the end. Listen, *boat, boat, boat*. You try it. Okay. Let's begin again" (98).

He reported that such training established additional phonological contrasts in the child's repertoire and then generalization to nontrained words. A variety of word lists, e.g., Bleile (1995), and treatment materials, e.g., Bird and Higgins (1990); Palin (1992); Price and Scarry-Larkin (1999), are available commercially to assist clinicians in finding contrasting word pairs and pictures for treatment.

Protocol for Employing a Minimal Pair Training Procedure

1. Select a sound contrast to be trained based on the client's phonological errors. For example, if the child substitutes /t/ for /ʃ/ (stopping), one might select *tea-she, toe-show,* and *tape-shape* as target contrast words reflecting the stopping pattern. Select five pictures for each of the target words. (In this example, that would include a total of 30 pictures.)
2. Engage the client in minimal contrast training at a *perceptual* level (e.g., "I want you to pick up the pictures that I name. Pick up _____.").
3. Pretest the client's motor production of each of the target words containing the error sound, and if necessary instruct him or her in production of the target phoneme.
4. Have the client imitatively produce each target word.
5. Engage the client in minimal contrast training at a *production* level (e.g., "I want you to tell me which picture to pick up. Every time you say *toe*, I will pick up this picture.").

   6. Engage the client in a task that requires him or her to incorporate each of the contrast words in a carrier phrase (e.g., "I want you to point to a picture and name it by saying 'I found a _____'.").

   7. Continue the carrier phrase task, incorporating each of the contrasting words into the phrase (e.g., "I found a *tea* and a *she*.").

Clinicians can use their creativity and clinical knowledge to modify a protocol such as that just presented. As stated earlier, there are descriptions in the literature of minimal pair treatment approaches as well as several commercially available sets of materials designed to facilitate this treatment approach. It should be mentioned that for those instances where meaningful minimal pairs cannot be found to reflect a particular contrast, "near minimal pairs" are sometimes used (e.g., *van-shan*), wherein one word may not have meaning. In this instance, the clinician may point to an abstract drawing and, as in the example above, say, "This is a *shan*." Thus, the child is taught a nonsense but contrasting word to use in the minimal pair activity.

Thus far we have focused on using minimal pairs that involve error and target sound contrasts. Sometimes minimal pairs involve the target sound and another sound, not necessarily the error production. Often it may be helpful to work on contrasts between the target sound and one or more other sounds which contain several feature differences from the target. When choosing such word pairs, the sound contrasts may represent a minimal or maximal sound opposition. When sound contrasts in minimal pairs contrast by a single feature, this is referred to as *minimal opposition contrasts*. On the other hand, a *maximal opposition contrast* reflects several feature contrasts between a target sound and the second sound. For example, if a child replaces /ʃ/ with /t/, the target words might be *shoe* and *moo* rather than *shoe* and *two*. In this case, /ʃ/ and /m/ are more dissimilar than are /ʃ/ and /t/, and thus the phoneme contrasts reflect a greater number of feature differences (maximal opposition) rather than fewer feature differences (minimal opposition). An underlying assumption of the maximal contrast approach is that phonological oppositions of greater disparity will facilitate more change in the client's acquisition of feature contrasts and the contrast between the word pairs will be more salient and thus easier for the client to perceive. Examples of minimal and maximal oppositions are as follows:

Minimal Oppositions	*Feature Differences*
*s*un—*t*on	manner of production
*th*umb—*s*um	place of production
*ch*ew—*sh*oe	manner of production

Maximal Oppositions	*Feature Differences*
*ch*ain—*m*ain	manner of production, nasality, place of production
*c*an—*m*an	manner of production, place of production, nasality
*g*ear—*f*ear	manner of production, voicing, place of production

The treatment methodologies outlined earlier for minimal contrast therapy are applicable to maximal contrast training.

The use of maximal oppositions is supported by data from Gierut (1989, 1990). Her research indicated that for children with multiple errors, maximal contrast training facilitated a greater overall change in the phonological system than did minimal contrast training. In her research, the sound contrasted to the target sound was a phoneme that was already in the subject's phonological repertoire, not one that had to be taught before being used in the minimal pair. Nonetheless, by focusing on maximal oppositions, greater generalization to other sounds occurred than with minimal opposition minimal pairs.

Multiple Oppositions Therapy

A treatment methodology that represents a variation of the minimal contrast approach presented above is the multiple oppositions approach (Williams, 1993, 2000a, 2000b, 2003). *Multiple oppositions* is a treatment approach that simultaneously contrasts several target sounds with a comparison sound. This approach is in contrast to the singular contrastive approach (i.e., including either minimal or maximal oppositions), which addresses sound errors or collapses one at a time. The multiple oppositions approach is designed for children with multiple sound collapses characterized by severe to profound phonological impairments.

The underlying premise behind this approach is that multiple errors produced by children evidencing numerous phoneme collapses (i.e., one sound is used in place of two or more other sounds), are best treated with a "systematic" view as opposed to individual sound focus. The goal is to help a child reorganize his or her sound system by focusing on numerous minimal contrast pairs designed to help the child recognize the nature of his or her phoneme collapses. For example, if a child substitutes /t/ in the final word position for each of the following sounds—/k/, /tʃ/, /s/—treatment might focus on contrasting the word *bat* with *back*, *batch* with *bass*, or contrasting *ate* with *ache*, *H*, and *ace*. In these examples, instead of focusing on a single contrast (e.g., *bat-back*), the procedure would use three minimal pair contrasts in the same activity (i.e., *bat-back; bat-batch; bat-bass*). A treatment session might also include instructional activities related to additional phoneme collapses. Lessons are centered on words evidencing "multiple oppositions" related to error targets. Eventually instruction moves from focusing only on contrastive word pairs to using sounds in increasingly complex linguistic structures.

A list of a child's phoneme collapses followed by sets of contrasting training items focusing on multiple oppositions (Williams, 2000a, 2000b) can be found in Figure 7.2.

Data reported by Williams (1993, 2000a, 2000b) indicated that by using the enlarged treatment sets included in the multiple oppositions approach with severely impaired children, clinicians were able to expand the number of phonemic contrasts. She hypothesized that through such an approach, the greatest amount of change will occur in the smallest amount of time with the least effort.

Metaphon Therapy

Howell and Dean (1991) indicated that children with phonological disorders who fail to respond well to minimal pair therapy need to be taught the characteristics of sounds as a way to facilitate development of sound contrasts in their phonological repertoire. Instruction is

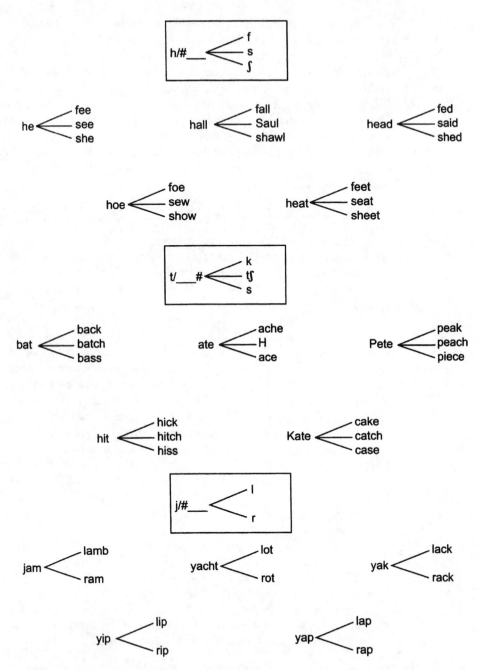

FIGURE 7.2   Phoneme Collapses with Related Minimal Pair Treatment Sets Focusing on Multiple Oppositions

designed to teach the awareness and skills necessary to succeed with minimal pair therapy. It structures treatment to facilitate children's development of metaphonological skills, that is, the ability to pay attention to the phonological structure of language. Investigators have reported that children with phonological disorders do not perform as well as their normal developing peers on metaphonological tasks (Kamhi, Friemoth-Lee, and Nelson, 1985). Metaphon therapy focuses on feature differences between sounds in order to develop an awareness that sounds can be classified by characteristics such as duration (*long-short*), manner (*noisy-whisper, stopping-flowing*), and place (*front-back*).

Therapy begins by teaching these basic concepts, followed by teaching how these concepts apply to sounds in general. Treatment then moves to identifying features across speech sounds and finally focuses on word pairs, which incorporate targeted sound contrasts. The second phase of therapy is designed to transfer the metaphonological knowledge gained in the first phase to communication situations wherein the client must convey his or her intended message through appropriate use of sound contrasts.

Summary of Minimal Pair Contrast Training

Background Statement.   The establishment of sound contrasts (contrast training) is a linguistic approach to phonological remediation. Instruction typically involves perceptual and production tasks of word-pairs that reflect phonemic contrasts described as minimal, maximal, or multiple oppositions. Contrast training procedures facilitate the reorganization of the phonological system to reduce the use of phonemic collapses and to establish additional phonemic contrasts and syllable shapes.

Unique Features.   Contrast training is communication oriented and requires the listener-speaker to select the appropriate word of the word-pair in order for communication intent to occur. That is, the listener-speaker must perceive and produce a particular phonemic contrast in order to communicate (act or get someone else to act appropriately) with the listener. It is focused on the ways sounds are used in the language (i.e., to signal contrasts in meaning).

Strengths and Limitations.   The approach is designed for clients who collapse sounds and do not contrast sounds consistent with the rules of the language. It is particularly useful with children who evidence numerous misarticulations or phonological rules that are not consistent with the adult standard. It is recommended for use with any client who needs to establish phonemic contrasts, regardless of whether errors have a motor component or not. By focusing on communication-oriented teaching activities, the training steps are generally less tedious than more drill-oriented activities including productions in increasingly complex linguistic utterances. Clinicians need to have a plan for fitting contrast training in with other treatment activities, including practice with increasingly complex linguistic utterances. Contrasting word-pairs can be focused on a single sound contrast pair or simultaneously on multiple contrasts.

Research Support.   Data to support the efficacy of contrast training are available (Ferrier and Davis, 1973; Weiner, 1981; Elbert and Gierut, 1986; Gierut, 1989, 1990; Williams,

1993, 2000a, 2000b). It is anticipated that research in this area will be ongoing and will assist in developing a stronger theoretical base for understanding and treating phonological disorders.

Cycles Approach

The cycles approach (Hodson and Paden, 1991) represents a linguistic approach designed for children with multiple sound errors. This approach targets deficient phonological patterns for instruction, uses sounds to teach appropriate phonological patterns, and moves through these targets in a sequential manner that is not based on a criterion level of performance before moving onto another sound and/or pattern. The cycles approach helps children to acquire appropriate phonological patterns, rather than focusing on helping children eliminate inappropriate patterns or deviations. The procedures followed in a cycles approach treatment session typically include (1) auditory stimulation of a target sound with amplification (the client focuses attention on auditory characteristics on the target sound); (2) production practice (to help the child develop new kinesthetic images); and (3) participation in experiential play activities involving picture and object naming tasks that incorporate the target pattern into word productions. A cycle is completed after a set of targeted phonological patterns (usually 60 minutes of instructional time) focusing on targets sounds related to the pattern that has been presented. Subsequent cycles incorporate patterns that continue to be averse to the adult standard.

The remediation plan is organized around treatment cycles that range from 5 to 16 weeks, depending on the client's number of deficient patterns and the number of stimulable phonemes within each pattern. Hodson's (1989) suggestions for treating behaviors through a cycles approach include the following:

> Each phoneme within a pattern should be targeted for approximately 60 minutes per cycle (i.e., one 60-minute, two 30-minute, or three 20-minute sessions) before progressing to the next phoneme in that pattern and then on to other phonological patterns. Each pattern is targeted for 2 to 6 hours, depending on the number of sounds targeted within that pattern. Furthermore, it is desirable to provide stimulation for two or more target *phonemes* (in successive weeks) within a pattern before changing to the next target *pattern* (i.e., each deficient phonological pattern is stimulated for two hours or more within each cycle). Only *one* phonological pattern should be targeted during any one session so that the client has an opportunity to focus, and patterns should not be intermingled (324).

A cycle is complete when all phonological patterns selected for remediation at a given point in time have been treated. Following completion of one cycle, a second cycle begins that will again cover those patterns not yet emerging and in need of further instruction. Phonological patterns are recycled until the targeted patterns emerge in spontaneous utterances. Hodson (1989) indicated that three to six cycles of phonological remediation, involving 30 to 40 hours of instruction (40 to 60 minutes per week) are usually required for a client with a disordered phonological system to become intelligible. Within each cycle, a pattern is the focus of instruction for 2 to 4 weeks, with a different phoneme targeted each week.

Hodson recommended that deviations (processes) targeted for remediation should occur in at least 40 percent of the instances in which the opportunity for their occurrence is present in the *Hodson Assessment of Phonological Patterns* (Hodson, 2003). Phonological patterns are targeted for remediation based on the child's "phonological deficiencies" and the patterns on which he or she is stimulable. Hodson and Paden (1991) identified the following as potential primary target patterns: early developing phonological patterns, posterior-anterior contrasts, /s/ clusters, and liquids. They identified secondary target patterns as voicing contrasts, vowel contrasts, singleton stridents, other consonant clusters, and residual context-related processes such as assimilation, metathesis, reduplication, and idiosyncratic rules.

An example of target selection and implementation of the cycles approach is the following. If fronting of velars occurs at least 40 percent of the time and if velars are stimulable, the appropriate use of velars could be selected as a target pattern for remediation. Initially, a target velar (e.g., final /k/) would be selected as an instructional target and, following the instructional sequence delineated below, activities related to this sound would be focused on for approximately one hour. Following work on this sound, a second velar (e.g., initial /g/) could be targeted. Following work on this pattern, a second pattern would be selected as part of this cycle (e.g., /s/ clusters).

The instructional sequence for each session is as follows:

1. *Review.* At the beginning of each session, the prior week's production practice word cards are reviewed.
2. *Listening activity.* This step requires listening for about 2 minutes while the clinician reads approximately 12 words containing the target sound. This auditory stimulation (called auditory bombardment) is done at the beginning and end of each session and includes the use of amplification (mild gain assistive listening device). The clinician may also demonstrate the error and contrast it with the target.
3. *Target word cards.* The client draws, colors, or pastes pictures of three to five target words for the lesson on large index cards. The name of the picture is written on each card.
4. *Production practice.* The client participates in experiential play production practice activities. The client is expected to have a very high success rate in terms of correct productions. Shifting activities every 5 to 7 minutes helps to maintain a child's interest in production practice. The client is also given the opportunity to use target words in conversation. Production practice incorporates auditory, tactual, and visual stimulation as needed for correct production at the word level. Usually five words per target sound are used in a single session. The client must produce the target pattern in words in order to get his or her turn.
5. *Stimulability probing.* The target phoneme in the next session for a given pattern is selected based on stimulability probing (checking to see what words a child can imitate), which occurs at this point in the treatment session.
6. *Listening activity.* Auditory bombardment with amplification is repeated, using the word list from the beginning of the session.
7. *Home program.* Parents are instructed to read the 12-item word list used in the auditory bombardment task to the child at least once a day. The five cards used during the session for production practice are also sent home for the child to practice daily.

The client is not required to meet a criterion level prior to moving on to treatment of other patterns within a cycle. When patterns persist, they are recycled for treatment at a later time.

Hodson (1994) reported that she also incorporates metaphonological or phonological awareness activities such as rhyming, syllable and phoneme segmentation, blending, and manipulation into treatment, because children who are unintelligible tend to have relatively poor rhyming and segmentation skills, which are important in the acquisition of literacy (see Chapter 9).

Summary of Cycles Approach

Background Statement.   The cycles approach is based on the phenomenon of gradualness (moving ahead, recycling, moving ahead) as observed in normal phonological acquisition. The emphasis on acquisition of phonological patterns stems from a linguistic perspective of phonological behavior. Production practice of target sounds along with auditory bombardment (listening tasks) reflects aspects of a more traditional approach to intervention.

Unique Features.   The most distinctive feature of this approach is its focus on shifting and cycling of remediation targets and the fact that a phoneme related to a particular pattern is focused on for a given length of time rather than a set criterion level of performance, with a new target being worked on after an hour of instructional time. Focusing on pattern *acquisition* rather than on elimination of inappropriate patterns is a developmentally sound way to conceptualize intervention.

Strengths and Limitations.   The attributes identified above are all strengths of this approach. Although it was designed for unintelligible children, aspects of this approach can be used with less severely impaired clients. The cycles approach has been adapted for use with children with cleft palate (Hodson, Chin, Redmond, and Simpson, 1983), developmental dyspraxia (Hodson and Paden, 1991), and recurrent otitis media and hearing impairments (Gordon-Brannan, Hodson, and Wynne, 1992), as well as developmental delay.

Research Support.   The authors have a wealth of clinical experience to support this approach to intervention and report good success with unintelligible children. This approach, like many others, represents a composite or "package" of various instructional components. However, it has seen widespread adoption among clinicians for unintelligible and phonologically delayed children.

Teaching Phonology Through Broader-Based Language Approaches

Children with severe phonologic disorders frequently have difficulty with other aspects of language (Camarata and Schwartz, 1985; Panagos and Prelock, 1982; Hoffman et al., 1989; Paul and Shriberg, 1982; Fey, Cleave, Ravida, Long, Dejmal, and Easton, 1994; Tyler, Lewis, Haskill, and Tolbert, 2002; Tyler and Watterson, 1991). The relationship between phonology and morphosyntax has been shown to be strong, and this relationship impacts clinical practice. Impairments of phonology that coexist with other language impairments suggest that many children have a generalized difficulty in the language learning process. Although the precise nature of the relationship between phonology and other aspects of language is unknown, it has been suggested that phonologic delay, especially when it coincides with other language impairments, can be at least partially remediated by employing a language-based intervention approach (Gray and Ryan, 1973; Matheny and Panagos, 1978; Hoffman, Norris, and Monjure, 1990; Tyler et al., 2002). Hoffman and colleagues (1990) stated that "descriptive research continues to show the importance of language organization levels that are higher than the word level upon sound production, suggesting that remediation of speech disorders outside of a more generalized context of language development may not be the most efficacious tack" (102). Others have indicated that the efficacy of a language-based approach to treating phonological disorders may be related to the degree of severity of the phonological impairment (Fey et al., 1994; Tyler and Watterson, 1991), although results reported by Tyler and colleagues (2002) did not support this view. However, many clinicians use a language-based approach to remediation for children with mild phonological problems and language delay/disorders, while for those with more severe phonological disorders, instruction may need to be focused specifically on phonology as well as the language problem. It may be that as children with severe phonological disorders progress in treatment, instruction may be more language based. The following paragraphs delineate possible ways to use language-based therapy to ameliorate a phonological disorder.

Norris and Hoffman (1990) described a storytelling language-based approach to phonologic intervention based on client generation of narratives. Preschool children constructed verbal stories in response to pictures from action-oriented children's stories and shared these with a listener(s). The clinician's primary role was to engage the child in constructing and talking about the pictures. The goal for each child was to produce meaningful linguistic units, syllable shapes, phonemes, and gestures that are shared with a listener. The clinician seeks to expand each child's language-processing ability by asking children to produce utterances that exceed their current level of functioning.

Norris and Hoffman (1990) also suggested that language-oriented intervention should be naturalistic and interactive as the clinician seeks to simultaneously improve semantic, syntactic, and phonologic knowledge. In terms of treatment priorities, phonology is the last component emphasized since intelligibility is a concern only after children have expressive language. Such child-clinician interactions should be based on spontaneous events or utterances and communicative situations that arise in the context of daily play routines and instructional activities. They outline three steps for intervention:

1. Provide appropriate organization of the environment/stimulus materials for the child to attend to, which enables the clinician to alter language complexity systematically throughout the course of therapy.
2. Provide a communicative opportunity, including scaffolding strategies that consist of various types of prompts, questions, information, and restatements that provide support to the child who is actively engaging in the process of communicating a message.

3. Provide consequences or feedback directly related to the effectiveness of the child's communication.

Norris and Hoffman (1990) described an "interactive storytelling" technique in which the clinician points to a picture and models language for the client, then gives the child an opportunity to talk about the event. If the child miscommunicates the idea, the adult provides feedback designed to assist the child in reformulating the message. The clinician can use three primary responses with the child:

1. *Clarification.* When the child's explanation is unclear, inaccurate, or poorly stated, the clinician asks for a clarification. The clinician then supplies relevant information to be incorporated in the child's response, restates the event using a variety of language forms, and asks the child to recommunicate the event. Hoffman and colleagues (1990) presented the following example of this type of response: If a child described a picture of a man cooking at a grill by saying, "Him eating," the clinician might say:

   No, that's not what I see happening. The man isn't eating yet, he's cooking the food. See his fork, he is using it to turn the food. I see him—he is cooking the food. He will eat when he's done cooking, but right now the food is cooking on the grill. He is cooking the food so that they can eat (105).

   Then the clinician provides an opportunity for the child to restate the information (e.g., " . . .so tell that part of the story again"). Thus, feedback is based on meaning rather than structure.

2. *Adding events.* If the child adequately reports an event, the clinician points out another event to incorporate in the story using a variety of language models. The child is then given the opportunity to retell the story. In an example from Hoffman and colleagues (1990), the clinician points to specific features in the picture and says something like:

   That's right, the man is cooking. He is the dad and he is cooking the hamburgers for lunch. Mom is putting plates on the table. Dad will put the hamburgers on the plates. So you explain the story to the puppet (105).

3. *Increasing complexity.* If the child adequately describes a series of events, the clinician seeks to increase the complexity of the child's story by pointing out relationships among events such as motives of the characters, cause-effect relationships among the individual events, time and space relationships, and predictions. The child is given the opportunity again to reformulate his or her own version of the story. Another example from these authors is: If the child said, "The daddy is cooking hamburgers and the mommy is setting the table," the clinician might prompt the child to link these two events in time and space by saying:

   That's right, mommy and daddy are making lunch for the family. When daddy finishes cooking the hamburgers he will put them on the plates, so tell that part of the story to the puppet (105).

As discussed in Chapter 5, investigators who have studied the effect that language-based intervention has on disordered phonology have reported conflicting results. In a study conducted by Fey and colleagues (1994), 30 preschool children displaying mild to severe speech and language impairments received either clinician or parental language intervention. Treatment in both settings focused on language-based stimulation in highly naturalistic tasks that were designed to facilitate grammar (i.e., making sandwiches, planting beans, play, etc.).

Baseline and treatment measures of phonology and expressive grammar were obtained at regular intervals. The results indicated that although gains in the children's grammatical output were observed, phonologic gains remained insignificant. Fey and colleagues (1994) stated: "We found no support for our prediction that effective facilitation of grammar would lead to spontaneous improvements in phonological output in children with speech and language impairments" (605).

Fey and colleagues (1994) indicated that the lack of an indirect effect of language-based intervention on phonology could have resulted from the intervention style employed and the severity level of the speech and language impairments. Their subjects appeared to be more severely involved than those of Hoffman et al. (1990). Fey and colleagues (1994) concurred with the findings of Tyler and Sandoval (1994), who also reported that language-based instruction had little effect on children with moderate to severe problems in both domains. Both of these studies concluded that clinical attention needed to be focused on both speech and language when impairments in these areas coexisted. This could be accomplished by simultaneously treating phonology and grammar (integration) or by shifting intervention focus from one area to another (alternating language and phonology instruction).

An investigation by Tyler et al. (2002) suggests that the matter of cross-domain generalization between language and phonology is not yet resolved. These investigators, using children with moderate to severe language and phonological disorders, studied the extent to which intervention focused on morphosyntax facilitates gains in phonology, and conversely, the extent to which intervention focused on phonology facilitates gains in morphosyntax. In contrast to previous studies, their data indicated that intervention focusing on morphosyntax resulted in phonological improvement; however, the reverse did not occur. These investigators employed a 12-week block of morphosyntactic instruction and a 12-week block of phonological instruction with two groups, counterbalancing the order in which the blocks were presented. These authors suggested that clinicians should consider targeting morphosyntax first when using a block intervention sequence for children with concomitant morphosyntactic and phonological impairments. Issues of sample size, degree of severity, and type of instruction appear to have influenced the nature of research findings in the area of cross-domain generalization and may account for the conflicting findings.

Summary of Teaching Phonology Through Broader-Based Language Approaches

Background Statement.   Language-based approaches are generally founded on two basic premises: (1) phonology is a part of the overall language system and should be treated in a language/communication context; and (2) improvement in phonologic behaviors occurs when instruction is focused on higher levels of language (morphosyntax, semantics).

Unique Features.   This approach emphasizes a communication-oriented therapy that focuses on narratives, semantics, and syntax on the assumption that such emphasis will facilitate phonological development/remediation.

Strengths and Limitations.   From a theoretical perspective, the rationale behind this approach is attractive (i.e., teaching higher-level language communication context will result in phonological improvement). Research results are conflicting concerning the validity of this approach with clients evidencing moderate to severe phonological impairment. Nonetheless, for some phonology clients, this concept is useful. In addition, when any client is at the point in treatment where carryover of connected speech is the goal, these approaches can be used.

Research Support.   Preliminary data from Hoffman and colleagues (1990) suggested that a whole language approach was a more efficacious approach to language-phonology intervention than was phonologic intervention alone, but their subjects appeared to have mild phonologic delay and were small in number (one set of twins). Research of Fey and colleagues (1994) and Tyler and Sandoval (1994) indicated that for children with more severe phonological impairments, direct instruction in phonology may be necessary to see improvement in phonologic behavior. However, Tyler and colleagues (2002) reported that a morphosyntactic intervention approach, delivered in a 12-week block, resulted in cross-domain (i.e., morphosyntax to phonology) improvement.

Remediation Guidelines for Linguistic Approaches

1. A linguistic approach, particularly the use of minimal pairs, is recommended when there are multiple sound errors that reflect phonologic error patterns. This approach is particularly useful with young children who are unintelligible.
2. Once error patterns have been identified, a review of the child's phonetic inventory will assist in the identification of target sounds (exemplars) to facilitate correct pattern usage. This review usually includes stimulability and may also include facilitative contexts, frequency of occurrence, and developmental appropriateness.
3. Selection of training words should reflect the syllabic word shapes the child uses. For example, if the child uses only CV and CVCV syllable shapes, multisyllabic target words would not be targeted. This guideline is inappropriate if the focus on remediation is on syllable structure simplifications and/or word structure complexity.
4. Treatment efficiency may be increased by selecting target words that facilitate the reduction of two or more patterns simultaneously. For example, if a child uses stopping and deletes final fricatives, the selection of a final fricative for training may aid in the simultaneous reduction of the processes of stopping and final consonant deletions.
5. When phonologic errors reflect errors in several sound classes (e.g., final consonant deletion may affect stops, fricatives, and nasals), select exemplars that reflect different sound classes.
6. Instruction related to phonologic patterns may focus on appropriate use of a phonologic rule and less on the phonetic accuracy of sounds used in treatment. For exam-

ple, if a child deletes final consonants but learns to say [dɔd] for [dɔg], the /d/ for /g/ replacement might be overlooked during the *initial* stage of instruction because the child has begun to change his or her phonologic system to incorporate final consonant productions.

7. Minimal contrast therapy usually focuses on both perception and production. When using contrast therapy, minimal pairs with maximal feature differences between contrasting sounds (maximal oppositions) may be a more efficient way to establish contrasts and impact the child's entire sound system than are word-pairs that reflect few feature differences (minimal oppositions).

8. For children with many sound collapses, a multiple oppositions approach may be an efficient way to impact the child's overall sound system.

9. Teaching behaviors from a linguistic perspective often incorporates selected methods used in more traditional approaches.

10. Treatment focused on morphosyntax and other aspects of language may result in positive changes in phonology. For example, working on plural and morphological endings may reduce the deletion of final consonants, thereby indicating that in such cases the perceived phonological error is in reality a morphological rule.

11. Correction of phonologic errors based on treatment of language behavior may or may not be an effective strategy for facilitating changes in the phonology of a child with moderate or severe phonologic impairment. More encouraging results have been reported in children with mild phonological delay.

12. The cycles approach has been shown to be an effective way to treat children with multiple errors.

Oral-Motor Activities as Part of Articulation Instruction

Background

Some clinicians advocate the use of oral-motor training as a precursor to teaching sounds or to supplement articulation instruction. The rationale behind this concept has been that immature or deficient oral-motor control and/or strength may underlie poor articulation, and that differential control of the articulators is necessary before the rapid, precise, and sequential movements involved in correct articulatory productions can be performed. Thus, remediation for articulation disorders should consider including oral-motor instruction as part of a therapy program. Although many clinical phonologists would concur with this basic concept, the question has been raised as to whether or not children identified as having a functional articulatory disorder (disorder of unknown etiology) lack the basic oral-motor skills necessary for articulation. Based on the fact that most clients learn correct speech sound productions without oral-motor training, such exercises have been called into question. In addition, definitive data are lacking to support the use of oral-motor activities as a part of articulation therapy. See Forrest (2002) for a critical critique of such techniques.

During the 1990s, some speech-language pathologists evidenced a renewed interest in oral-motor instruction and advocated that clinical practice with some children evidencing articulation disorders should employ oral-motor training activities as a part of therapy. It should be pointed out that oral-motor instruction is advocated not only for articulation disorders but also for disorders of developmental apraxia, feeding, swallowing, and other oral-myofunctional disorders (Marshalla, 1996). There are those who see oral-motor exercises as a useful precursor to phonological instruction for children with severe phonological impairments. In the following paragraphs, we present the rationale behind this approach and highlight aspects of this type of training and the types of clients for whom such an approach may be of value.

Rationale

Motor pattern development in children progresses from gross generalized reflexive patterns toward movements requiring finer motor control. In terms of speech sound productions, jaw movements become differentiated from head movements, lip and tongue movements become differentiated from the jaw, the tongue tip from the tongue body, the tongue back from the tongue body, and the tongue's lateral margins from the tongue body. Differentiated use of each articulator is necessary for normal speech. Correct positioning of the tongue and lips is based on stability of the jaw and the tongue's ability to remain in a neutral position in relation to the jaw. Green, Moore, Higashikawa, and Steeve (2000) studied lip and jaw coordination in the development of speech motor control and reported the following during the first years of life: (1) prevalence of jaw movement during speech, (2) poor lip and jaw coupling, (3) poor lip control, and (4) poor upper and lower lip movement independence. As the child gets older, he or she develops independent movement of the tongue tip/blade and tongue body, which is necessary for the co-articulation of speech sound productions. It is hypothesized that differentiated movements of the oral structures are necessary for normal articulatory functioning, and when they are lacking, oral-motor instruction may be appropriate.

Assessment

Before a client with a phonological disorder is a candidate to receive oral-motor instruction as a component of articulation therapy, the clinician must determine that there is a deficiency in terms of oral-motor awareness and skills. In Chapters 4 and 5, procedures for examining the speech mechanism were identified. These activities constitute a basic framework for oral-motor assessment. In assessing the need for oral-motor instruction, the clinician will want to ascertain whether the child is sensitive to and/or aware of the parts of the tongue, including the tip, blade, back, and sides; whether or not the client can elevate the tongue to the palate with the jaw open but remaining stable; whether the child can protrude the tongue independently of movement of the lips and jaw; and whether the tip of the tongue can be held on the palate with independent movement of the lips and/or jaw. These activities are used to determine whether or not the client has the awareness and differentiated movement of the jaw, lips, and tongue necessary for speech. As ways to observe functioning of the articulators, Meyer (2000) suggested that one can ask clients to alternately pucker their lips and smile, open their mouth and stick out the tongue, elevate the tongue to touch the nose, try to touch the chin with the tongue, and/or move the tongue from side to side. Speech-related tasks include the diadokokinetic assessment discussed in Chapter 5 (e.g., tasks involving the lips (pʌpʌpʌ); lips and tongue (pʌtʌkʌ); having the client repeat words and phrases involving the tongue tip—I like licorice). Procedures such as these are examples of how the clinician can employ speech mechanism activities to observe awareness, strength, independence, and coordination of the articulators.

Treatment

For clients who evidence oral-motor deficiencies related to their speech problems, guidelines for oral-motor instructional activities from Marshalla (1996) and Meyer (2000) may be helpful. Their suggestions are part of programs designed to address not only articulation but also oral-myofunctional disorders related to swallowing, drinking, and feeding. These authors suggested brushing the tip and sides of the tongue to increase tactile awareness of the oral areas; activities to help stabilize the jaw, such as having the child hold a tongue depressor between his or her teeth while speaking, having the client open his or her mouth and move the tongue up and down without moving the jaw, and having the child say "guh" like a frog without allowing the jaw/chin to move. Having a child say "giddy-up" can increase awareness of lateral tongue muscles. These suggestions represent a sampling of what can be included in oral-motor instruction.

Summary

A central concern for speech-language pathologists is twofold: (1) Are there data to support the need to engage in oral-motor activities as part of articulation/phonological instruction (2) If so, what procedures are recommended? With regard to the first concern, it is our impression that there are limited data to support oral-motor instruction as a part of articulation therapy. Clinicians who deal with oral-motor deficiencies and related articulation impairments report success with oral-motor therapy. It is likely that such clients have a history of delayed or unusual oral-motor development and may benefit from the type of awareness, stabilization, and oral-motor instruction described above. These children are identified through their medical history, case history, speech mechanism examination, and articulation/phonological assessment. We caution against jumping on the "bandwagon" of those who see oral-motor activities as a panacea for children with severe phonological disorders. Careful evaluation including, among other things, determining whether a severe problem relates to phonological rules, faulty phonological perception, developmental verbal dyspraxia, and/or deficiencies of oral-motor behavior, should be taken into consideration before embarking on such a treatment program.

Intervention for Children with Developmental Verbal Dyspraxia (DVD)

The topic of developmental verbal dyspraxia (DVD) was introduced in Chapter 4 in our discussion of factors related to the presence of phonologic disorders. In this section, we add to the historical and descriptive background presented in that chapter by addressing issues relevant to clinical intervention with this subpopulation of individuals with phonological impairment.

DVD appears to involve both motor and linguistic components, with wide variation in symptoms across children. Aram (1984) suggested that DVD be viewed as a syndrome that includes a severe and persistent phonologic disorder coupled with an expressive syntactic disorder, with variable neurological and articulatory findings. Ball (1999) identified social and behavioral components along with co-occurring articulation, language, and intelligibility impairments. Velleman and Strand (1994) proposed a hierarchical hypothesis of DVD, suggesting that children may be capable of producing the individual aspects of speech production (i.e., articulatory postures, phonemes, words), but have great difficulty "bridging among the various elements that constitute language performance" (120). Shriberg, Aram, and Kwiatkowski (1997), as reported earlier, added that phrasal stress is a linguistic variable that also characterizes this population. Although data suggest that the "syndrome" includes not only difficulty with phonology, but also with other aspects of language, the most commonly employed methodology for treating this population has focused on motor planning for producing syllables in the stream of speech.

Assessment

Assessment of this population is not unlike that used with any child with a phonologic disability and, in addition to a standard articulation/phonological battery, typically includes a case history, a hearing screening, and a screening for other areas of communication (language, voice, fluency). There are, however, specific aspects of evaluation of the DVD population that warrant elaboration.

The oral mechanism examination should be thorough and include an assessment of strength, tone, and stability of the oral structures (e.g., can the child move the tongue independently of the mandible? Does the child do anything special to stabilize the mandible, such as thrust it forward?). A review of the child's feeding history may be of interest in this regard. Young children, in particular, may exhibit uncoordinated feeding patterns without dysphagia. Overall motor skills, both automatic and volitional, including the ability to perform imitative and rapidly alternating tongue movements, plus diadochokinetic rates should be a part of the assessment. Velleman and Strand (1994), in a review of the literature, suggested that DVD children have difficulty with transitions between sounds. While static articulatory positions (sounds in isolation) may be produced correctly, rapid combinations of movements frequently are difficult for this population. The rapid successive movements (e.g., syllable to syllable) of connected speech entail constant approximations of specific articulatory targets because there are no absolute or static positions associated with speech sounds. For children with DVD, the inherent dynamic overlapping movement involved in producing sequential motor speech elements is a problem. Velleman and Strand (1994) indicated that sequencing difficulties may not manifest themselves in phonemic sequencing errors per se, but rather are more evident at the articulatory level, affecting the relative timing of glottal and articulatory gestures. These latter factors result in perceived errors of voicing and vowels, especially diphthongs.

Strand and McCauley (1999) proposed using an utterance hierarchy for assessment. In their example, evaluation proceeds among levels of utterance types, for example, connected speech from conversation, picture description, and narrative; diadochokinetic tasks; imitative utterances including vowels (V), consonant-vowel (CV), and vowel-consonant (VC) combinations; CVC when the first and last phoneme are the same and when they are different; repetition of words of increasing length, multisyllabic words, phrases, and sentences of increasing length.

In analyzing speech performance, the clinician must keep in mind the nature of DVD as a disorder involving the hierarchical levels of speech and language, including motor planning for syllable sequencing. Movements, transitions, and timing should be observed as speech is produced at a variety of linguistic levels from simple to complex. For children with a limited verbal repertoire, an independent phonological analysis of a speech/language sample is recommended. For those with more normal verbal skills, a traditional phonologic assessment battery (relational analysis) is recommended, with particular attention to the analysis of speech sounds within syllabic units. In this instance, a connected speech sample is critical because it will allow the examiner to review syllable and word shapes produced by the child. Phonologic assessment should also include imitation of words that increase in number of syllables (e.g., *please, pleasing, pleasingly*).

Because children with DVD evidence problems with the dynamic organization of communication efforts, it is not unusual for problems to be present with the suprasegmental (e.g., phrasal stress) aspects of speech. Coordinating the laryngeal and respiratory systems with the oral mechanism is often very difficult. This problem may result in difficulty with varying intonation contours, modulation of loudness, and maintaining proper resonance. Vowels may be prolonged because the child needs time to organize coordination for the next series of speech sound movements.

In an assessment of children with suspected DVD, the clinician should be sensitive not only to apraxia but also to a possible dysarthria. It may be prudent to refer more seriously impaired children with suspected dysarthria and/or DVD to a pediatric neurologist to determine the status of current neurological functioning. Seizure history and/or potential, associated limb apraxia, presence of oral apraxia, and general knowledge of neurological functioning, may influence the overall management program for a given child and thus warrant such a referral.

Recommended Phonological Assessment Battery for DVD

1. Case history (including review of feeding history)
2. Hearing screening/testing
3. Screening of voice and fluency characteristics
4. Speech mechanism examination
   - Structure and function
   - Strength, tone, stability
   - Diadokokinetic rate
5. Connected speech sample
   - Segmental productions
   - Syllable and word shape productions
   - Phonologic patterns present and/or lacking
   - Intonation, vocal loudness, resonance

6. Segmental productions (citation form testing; independent analysis for those with a limited phonological repertoire)
   - Consonants, vowels, and diphthongs
   - Syllable shapes used in response to stimulus items
7. Phonological process review
   - Patterns used
   - Patterns missing
8. Intelligibility — how well the acoustic signal is understood with and without context
9. Stimulability testing
   - Segments
   - Syllables
   - Words with increasing number of syllables
10. Interpersonal skills
    - Social interaction
    - Behavioral interactions
    - Academic/community interactions
11. Language evaluation
    - Comprehension and production
    - Sound productions at various semantic and syntactic levels

Tests specifically designed for use with the DVD population are the *Screening Test for Developmental Apraxia of Speech* (Blakely, 2001), *The Apraxia Profile* (Hickman, 1997), and the *Kaufman Speech Praxis Test for Children* (Kaufman, 1995). Data reported by Ball, Beukelman, and Bernthal (2002) indicated that examination of the child's social and behavioral interactions, academic performance, and written language literacy were useful components when assessing a child with DVD.

Treatment

The recommended treatment of children with DVD is different from traditional motor and/or linguistic approaches to phonologic intervention. Two significant differences between what has been discussed elsewhere in this chapter and what is presented here are short-term goals of therapy and the production units focused on in therapy.

A major short-term therapy goal is to build a functional vocabulary for a client. Often DVD children have significant intelligibility problems, and efforts need to be directed toward building a core of intelligible words to facilitate the communication process. To the extent possible, the phonologic production activities suggested here should include attention to syllabic structures and combinations of these syllables so that the child will gain verbal building blocks for words.

A focus of instructional activities is on the motor-planning component of the disorder. Rather than using drill motor activities that focus on repetition of the same sounds or syllables, a variety of speech and language motor planning activities should be provided to practice transitions and timing movements required in the dynamic process of ongoing speech. Emphasis is placed on shifting the stimulus materials to incorporate a wider variety of syllable sequences. For example, one could start by having a child name a succession of animals with one-syllable names (e.g., *bat, bear, bird, bug*), then shift to animals with two-syllable names (e.g., *baboon, beaver, camel*), then increase to three-syllable names (e.g., *buffalo, butterfly, elephant*). Names could then be combined, with an emphasis on being able to do the motor planning necessary to accommodate shifts and variations in syllable sequencing that represent increasing linguistic complexity. Rosenbeck, Kent, and LaPointe (1984) also recommended continually shifting the segmental targets in a succession of syllables beginning with CV or VC, repeating the patterns, and then systematically varying the CV pattern and moving into word combinations.

Strand and Skindner (1999) recommended integral stimulation methods to include tactile and proprioceptive monitoring of articulatory configurations, movement paths, practice with movements, and to provide knowledge of results to the child. They suggested that more frequent distribution of sessions may result in better motor learning (e.g., 2 hours of therapy per week is better distributed in 4 half-hour sessions than in two 1-hour sessions). They also suggested choosing stimuli for treatment that are useful and meaningful to the child, to allow the child to experience successful communication. They emphasized the importance of stimulus selection, including length and phonetic context of the target words.

Square (1999) outlined three additional types of interventions, including tactile-kinesthetic, rhythmic and melodic facilitation, and gestural cueing. In "touch-cueing" (Bashir, Grahamjones, and Bostwick, 1984), the clinician touches a particular area of the face or neck as each sound in a sequence is produced. Children learn the sound associated with each touching cue. Thus, children can be presented with simultaneous touch, auditory, and sometimes visual cues as they produce sounds in various movement patterns. The "touch-cue" method is an example of a tactile-kinesthetic approach. Another tactile-kinesthetic approach is *Prompts for Restructuring Oral Muscular Phonetic Targets* (PROMPT) developed by Chumpelik (1984). This approach specifies jaw height, facial-labial contraction, tongue height and advancement, muscular tension, duration of contractions, and airstream management for phoneme production. An example of a rhythmic and melodic facilitation approach is known as Melodic Intonation Therapy (Helfrich-Miller, 1984). This program uses stimuli that progress over a hierarchy of difficulty while being intoned with Signed English use as a pacer.

A set of guidelines for working with DVD clients is presented in Table 7.7 (Velleman and Strand, 1994). For children who are very young or severely impaired, gestures and pantomime may be encouraged. An augmentative communication system assessment may be desired, particularly for school-age children who are unintelligible. Such assessment should target the various systems that may be appropriate for facilitating language development and written language. Facilitating communication through these techniques is often viewed as a means to develop verbal communication as well as other aspects of language. Perhaps the most comprehensive set of instructional materials for treating clients with motor planning difficulties is the *Nuffield Centre Dyspraxia Programme* (1994), which was developed at the Royal National Throat Nose and Ear Hospital in London, England. Other programs commercially available may provide assistance in organizing treatment strategies; however, it is important to remember that individualized programs designed specifically for a child based on his or her assessment performance will likely result in the most effective interventions and progress.

TABLE 7.7   Basic Principles of a Speech Production Treatment Program for Children with DVD

1. Main focus of treatment should be syllable structure control and organization within a variety of dynamic linguistic contexts.
2. A successful program is one that will facilitate correct production of varying syllable shapes and the organization of these shapes into longer and increasingly complex phonotatic patterns.
3. A sound-by-sound treatment plan that emphasizes phoneme production in isolation prior to moving to words and phrases does *not* address the hierarchical dynamic movement problem in DVD.
4. Auditory discrimination training does *not* address the problem.
5. Frequent, short sessions with breaks are most successful. Because DVD is a dynamic disorder, system fatigue is a problem.
6. Sessions should be divided into short parts:
   a. Warm-ups: Imitation of body and/or oral motor sequences.
   b. Practicing the scales: Syllable sequence drill activities. Establish consistent connected syllable productions from within the child's repertoir. Include sequences that vary articulatory positions, for example, from front to back ([bʌdʌgʌ] or "buttercup") or vice versa ([gʌ dʌ bʌ] or "go to bed").
   c. Learning the song: Meaningful single-word activities to include a core group of words that would increase overall intelligibility of speech.
   d. Changing the song: Short sentence activities starting with a key carrier phrase and changing one word, gradually increasing in length and complexity.

Source: Adapted from Velleman, S., and K. Strand, "Developmental verbal dyspraxia." In J. Bernthal, and N. Bankson (Eds.), *Child Phonology: Characteristics, Assessment, and Intervention with Special Populations* (pp. 110–139). New York, N.Y.: Thieme Publishers, 1994. Used by permission.

Case Study

Intervention Recommendations

In Chapter 5, we discussed the speech samples obtained from Kirk, with an analysis and interpretation of his test data. We now discuss how one might proceed in developing an intervention plan based on that interpretation. As you recall, Kirk is a 3-year-old child with multiple errors who is in need of phonological intervention because of poor speech intelligibility. You might wish to review the case study report at the end of Chapter 5 at this time. As you move through the discussion that follows, bear in mind that the steps involved and the variables taken into consideration are applicable with many clients with phonological impairments.

First Consideration—Do I Use a Motor or Phonological Approach to Intervention, or Both?

For most error sounds, with the exception of /ʃ/, /tʃ/, /dʒ/, /r/, and /ɝ/, Kirk is stimulable. Some of the stimulable sounds were more easily imitated than others. Because he could imitate most of his error sounds, a major goal of instruction will be to help Kirk learn to use sounds contrastively, or in other words, diminish his sound collapses, by using sounds appropriately in word contrasts. This goal is phonologically oriented, but instruction must also include teaching or stabilization of the motor production of sounds that he cannot consistently imitate on demand. Thus, therapy will include both sound contrast training and motor production activities.

Second Consideration—How Many Targets Should I Address in a Session?

Because Kirk has multiple error sounds, a focus on several targets is suggested, either within a single lesson, or across lessons within a 3–4-week time frame (cycles or horizontal approach). We have already stated that Kirk's difficulties seem to be primarily phonological: he can produce many sounds but just isn't using them appropriately. He also has a production problem with /ɝ/ and may also need motor practice with some of the other consonants. This means that in lesson planning, we will probably want to allow time for motor practice activities to teach the production of sounds as well as activities that focus on using sounds contrastively. Even though instructional activities may be considered phonological as opposed to motor oriented, they involve production practice. It is suggested that treatment sessions for Kirk should address: (1) error patterns, beginning with stopping and the sound collapses reflected in that pattern (i.e., /d/ replacing numerous other sounds); and (2) instruction and production practice for sounds that are not stimulable or readily produced on demand (e.g., /ɝ/, /ʃ/, /s/, /tʃ/).

Third Consideration—How Should I Conceptualize the Overall Treatment Program?

Because Kirk has so many sounds in error, and because some of those sounds are not stabilized at an imitative level, it is suggested that the clinician begin a session by spending about 5 minutes engaged in what has been identified as "sound stimulation/practice," an activity designed to enhance Kirk's stimulability for all error sounds. Kirk is young and still acquiring phonemes, so it seems advisable to provide him the opportunity to produce a variety of sounds that are not produced correctly in his conversational speech. Sound stimulation can include not only practice on error sounds (e.g., /ɝ/, /s/, /f/) but also sounds that he does say correctly (/p/, /h/, /f/). Successful production of such sounds may facilitate his willingness to try the more "difficult" sounds.

Kirk should make five attempts to produce each sound target during sound stimulation, using a cueing hierarchy for those in error, based on the level of support necessary to produce a sound (e.g., modeling, phonetic placement, or selected context). After five attempts, another sound is practiced. With only five attempts, the client is not overwhelmed with repeated failures if he or she cannot produce a sound. It is hoped that by briefly focusing in each session on production of a variety of sounds and levels of complexity (i.e., isolation, syllables, words), a child will acquire the skill to imitate the sound when given an auditory and/or visual model. Production in this type of activity is a building block for focusing on phonological contrasts and for facilitating generalization when a child is stimulable. Following sound stimulation/production practice, the treatment program will focus on Kirk's need to establish sound contrasts.

One treatment option for addressing Kirk's errors is to use a cycling approach, wherein one or more sounds are targeted in a given lesson to help him learn to use a particular phonological pattern (e.g., frication because he currently substitutes stops for most fricatives). In a subsequent lesson, other fricatives related to that process would be focused on, continuing until most of the fricatives have been practiced. At this point, another pattern would be targeted, including one or more sounds in a given lesson (e.g., use of final consonants). This cycling approach may employ auditory bombardment, perceptual training of minimal pairs, and sound production of minimal pairs, including drill and play activities. The linguistic complexity of activities is increased as progress is made (e.g., going from words to phrases to sentences to conversation).

An alternative treatment approach that specifically addresses sound contrasts is to teach multiple oppositions that simultaneously address the collapse of numerous sounds to /d/. Instruction might initially focus on sound collapses that include sounds in Kirk's repertoire and then, as other sounds are established, expand to other sound collapses. In the following example, solid lines indicate initial collapses to focus on because the sounds are in Kirk's repertoire; broken lines reflect targets that can be addressed as additional sounds are added to Kirk's repertoire.

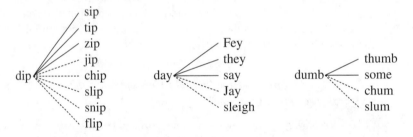

Another way to approach Kirk's stopping pattern is the use of focused minimal pairs rather than the multiple-oppositions approach. This method is a more traditional approach to using minimal pairs to establish sound contrasts; that is, focusing on a single pair and then progressing to other minimal pairs to establish other contrasts in his system. Instruction would begin with a minimal pair evidencing maximal opposition between a target sound and a contrasting sound. For example, instruction might first focus on the word pair *seal—meal*, and once Kirk can produce that pair, go to *seal—veal*, and finally *deal—seal*. The hope is that by initially contrasting /s/ with /m/ (sounds that evidence several feature differences from /d/), such practice will facilitate more rapid acquisition of other sound contrasts.

Fourth Consideration—How Do Instructional Goals Relate to the Treatment Continuum and Specific Instructional Steps?

The treatment continuum was discussed earlier, including establishment, generalization, and maintenance, with generalization being the focus of much of what we do in therapy. In the case of Kirk, the /ɝ/ or other nonstimulable sounds will require an establishment activity such as sound stimulation mentioned above. His other goals (i.e., initial consonant deletion; use of frication—to eliminate the stopping process; final consonant deletion) will fit into the generalization phase of the continuum because he is stimulable on many of the sounds required to establish sound contrasts in words. Earlier we discussed how at each stage of the treatment, continuum therapy comprises a sequence of steps and activities that include antecedent events from the clinician, responses from the client, and consequating events from the clinician based on client responses. One of the initial planning tasks is to determine how one is going to sequence antecedent events (e.g., verbal instruction, pictures, printed symbols, game activity), and consequating events (e.g., verbal reinforcement, tokens, back-up reinforcers).

Table 7.8 outlines components of therapy sessions based on the preceding considerations. Included is a possible way to construct therapy. Remember that good clinical practice involves creativity, flexibility, and letting client performance guide day-to-day therapy.

TABLE 7.8   Summary of Intervention Sequencing for Kirk

Component	Procedure	Rationale
Sound Stimulation/ Practice	Ask the client to produce a variety of sounds five times each (both incorrect and correct sounds). Provide auditory models and cueing as necessary.	Generalization has been shown to be highly influenced by a child's stimulability. Therefore, we must help children acquire all the sounds at a motor level. Brief practice periods serve to encourage continued attempts at sounds that may be particularly difficult.
Production Activities	Focus on teaching frication and final consonant usage. Focus on one or two sounds per session, moving from /f/ to /m/ to /s/, and other stimulable sounds. Use minimal pairs at a perceptual level before practice on pairs at a production level. Drill/Play games and activities are recommended. Use a listening task to introduce each sound. Consider using multiple opposition contrasts for the /d/ collapses.	Cycling across patterns and sounds is helpful for children with multiple errors. Kirk is young and still developing his sound system, and he has a good attention span. Therefore, he could benefit from shifting focus from week to week. Multiple oppositions can be helpful for phoneme collapses and are recommended because Kirk is stimulable on many of the collapses.
Increasing Linguistic Complexity	When Kirk can produce word targets accurately, including minimal pairs, shift production to phrases and then sentences. In addition, progress from targets occurring only once in a word or phrase to more complex productions involving more than one occurrence, and competing sounds.	To reach the terminal objective of spontaneous use of appropriate speech sounds and patterns, Kirk must be able to use his new speech sounds and patterns in increasingly complex linguistic units.

(continues)

TABLE 7.8 (*Continued*)

Component	Procedure	Rationale
Situational Generalization	Bring persons in the child's environment into activities to reinforce Kirk's new speech skills. Using target names, preschool vocabulary, and frequently used words as a focus may be helpful. Arrange for Kirk to "use" his new speech in the classroom and home.	Focusing on situational generalization as early as possible will help this young client generalize the new language skills to his environment. Increased intelligibility will be powerfully reinforced by the environment.

QUESTIONS FOR CHAPTER 7

1. How would one assess auditory perception in a child suspected of having difficulty with sound contrasts?

2. Outline a traditional approach to articulation therapy and specify for whom it is appropriate.

3. Outline a linguistic approach to phonological intervention and specify for whom it is appropriate.

4. What characteristics distinguish DVD children from other phonological delayed children and what distinguishes their treatment?

5. Discuss how one can use minimal pairs in phonological treatment.

6. Outline the procedures for a cycles approach to therapy.

REFERENCES

Aram, D., "Assessment and treatment of developmental apraxia." *Seminars in Speech and Language*, *5* (1984): 2.

Baker, R. D., and B. P. Ryan, *Programmed Conditioning for Articulation*. Monterey, Calif.: Monterey Learning Systems, 1971.

Ball, L., "Communication characteristics of children with developmental apraxia of speech." Unpublished Doctoral Dissertation, University of Nebraska—Lincoln, Neb., 1999.

Ball, L., D. Beukelman, and J. Bernthal, "Profiling communication characteristics of children with developmental apraxia of speech." *Medical Speech-Language Pathology*, *10* (2002): 221–229.

Bashir, A., F. Grahamjones, and R. Bostwick, "A touch-cue method of therapy for developmental apraxia." *Seminars in Speech and Language*, *5* (1984): 127–137.

Bird, A., and A. Higgins. Minimal Pair Cards. Austin, Tex. : PRO-ED, 1990.

Blache, S. E., "A distinctive feature approach." In N. Creaghead, P. Newman, and W. Secord (Eds.), *Assessment and Remediation of Articulatory and Phonological Disorders*. Columbus, Ohio: Charles E. Merrill, 1989.

Blakely, R., *Screening Test for Developmental Apraxia of Speech*. Austin, Tex.: PRO-ED, 2001.

Bleile, K. M., *Manual of Articulation and Phonological Disorders*. San Diego, Calif.: Singular Publishing Group, Inc., 1995.

Camarata, S., and R. Schwartz, "Production of object words and action words: Evidence for a relationship between phonology and semantics." *Journal of Speech and Hearing Research, 26* (1985): 50–53.

Chumpelik, D., "The prompt system of therapy: Theoretical framework and applications for developmental apraxia of speech." *Seminars in Speech and Language, 5* (1984): 139–155.

Costello, J., and J. Onstein, "The modification of multiple articulation errors based on distinctive feature theory." *Journal of Speech and Hearing Disorders, 41* (1976): 199–215.

Curtis, J. R., and J. C. Hardy, "A phonetic study of misarticulation of /r/." *Journal of Speech and Hearing Research, 2* (1959): 244–257.

Elbert, M., and J. Gierut, *Handbook of Clinical Phonology Approaches to Assessment and Treatment.* San Diego, Calif.: College Hill Press, 1986.

Ferrier, L., and M. Davis, "A lexical approach to the remediation of final sound omission." *Journal of Speech and Hearing Disorders, 38* (1973): 126–130.

Fey, M. E., "Articulation and phonology: Inextricable constructs in speech pathology." *Language, Speech, and Hearing Services in Schools, 23* (1992): 225–232.

Fey, M. E., P. L. Cleave, A. I. Ravida, S. H. Long, A. E. Dejmal, and D. L. Easton, "Effects of grammar facilitation on the phonological performance of children with speech and language impairments." *Journal of Speech and Hearing Research, 37* (1994): 594–607.

Forrest, K., "Are oral-motor exercises useful in the treatment of phonological/articulatory disorders?" *Seminars in Speech and Language, 23* (2002): 15–25.

Gierut, J., "Maximal opposition approach to phonological treatment." *Journal of Speech and Hearing Disorders, 54* (1989): 9–19.

Gierut, J. A., "Differential learning of phonological oppositions." *Journal of Speech and Hearing Research, 33* (1990): 540–549.

Gordon-Brannan, M., B. Hodson, and M. Wynne, "Remediating unintelligible utterances of a child with a mild hearing loss." *American Journal of Clinical Practice, 1* (1992): 28–38.

Gray, G., "A field study on programmed articulation therapy." *Language, Speech, and Hearing Services in Schools, 5* (1974): 119–131.

Gray, B., and B. Ryan, *A Language Program for the Non-language Child.* Champaign, Ill.: Research Press, 1973.

Green, J., C. Moore, M. Higashikawa, and R. Steeve, "The physiologic development of speech motor control: Lip and jaw coordination. *Journal of Speech, Language, and Hearing Research, 43* (2000): 239–256.

Helfrich-Miller, K., "Melodic intonation therapy with developmentally apraxic children." *Seminars in Speech and Language, 5* (1984): 19–126.

Hickman, L., *The Apraxia Profile.* San Antonio, Tex.: Psychological Corporation, 1997.

Hodson, B., "Phonological remediation: A cycles approach." In N. Creaghead, P. Newman, and W. Secord (Eds.), *Assessment and Remediation of Articulatory and Phonological Disorders.* Columbus, Ohio: Charles E. Merrill, 1989.

Hodson, B., "Helping individuals become intelligible, literate, and articulate: The role of phonology." In B. Hodson (Ed.), *From Phonology to Metaphonology: Issues, Assessment and Intervention. Topics in Language Disorders, 14* (1994): 1–16.

Hodson, B., *The Assessment of Phonological Process Patterns,* 3rd ed. Austin, Tex.: PRO-ED, 2003

Hodson, B., L. Chin, B. Redmond, and R. Simpson, "Phonological evaluation and remediation of speech deviations of a child with a repaired cleft palate: A case study." *Journal of Speech and Hearing Disorders, 48* (1983): 93–98.

Hodson, B., and E. Paden, *Targeting Intelligible Speech: A Phonological Approach to Remediation,* 2nd Ed. Austin, Tex.: PRO-ED, 1991.

Hoffman, P., J. Norris, and J. Monjure, "Comparison of process targeting and whole language treatments for phonologically delayed preschool children." *Language, Speech, and Hearing Services in Schools, 21* (1990): 102–109.

Hoffman, P., G. Schuckers, and R. Daniloff, *Children's Phonetic Disorders: Theory and Treatment.* Boston, Mass.: Little, Brown, 1989.

Howell, J., and E. Dean, *Treating Phonological Disorders in Children: Metaphon-Theory to Practice.* San Diego, Calif.: Singular, 1991.

Kamhi, A. G., R. Friemoth-Lee, and L. Nelson, "Word, syllable and sound awareness in language disordered children." *Journal of Speech and Hearing Disorders, 50* (1985): 207–212.

Kaufman, N., *Kaufman Speech Praxis Test for Children.* Detroit, Mich.: Wayne State University Press, 1995.

La Riviere, C., H. Winitz, J. Reeds, and E. Herriman, "The conceptual reality of selected distinctive features." *Journal of Speech and Hearing Research, 17* (1974): 122–133.

Locke, J. L., "The influence of speech perception in the phonologically disordered child. Part I. A rationale, some criteria, the conventional tests." *Journal of Speech and Hearing Disorders, 40* (1980): 431–444.

Marshalla, P., *Oral-Motor Techniques in Articulation Therapy.* Temecula, Calif.: Speech Dynamics, 1996.

Matheny, N., and J. Panagos, "Comparing the effects of articulation and syntax programs on syntax and articulation improvement." *Language, Speech, and Hearing Services in Schools, 9* (1978): 57–61.

McDonald, E. T., *Articulation Testing and Treatment: A*

Sensory Motor Approach. Pittsburgh, Penn.: Stanwix House, 1964.

McReynolds, L. V., and S. Bennett, "Distinctive feature generalization in articulation training." *Journal of Speech and Hearing Disorders, 37* (1972): 462–470.

Meyer, P. G., "Tongue, lip, and jaw differentiation and its relationship to orofacial myofunctional treatment." *International Journal of Orofacial Myology, 26* (2000): 44-52.

Norris, J., and P. Hoffman, "Language intervention within naturalistic environments." *Language, Speech, and Hearing Services in Schools, 2* (1990): 72–84.

Nuffield Centre Dyspraxia Programme. London, England: Royal National Throat Nose and Ear Hospital, 1994.

Palin, M. Contrast Pairs for Phonological Training. Austin, Tex. PRO-ED, 1992.

Panagos, J., and P. Prelock, "Phonological constraints on the sentence productions of language-disordered children." *Journal of Speech and Hearing Research, 24* (1982): 171–177.

Paul, R., and L. Shriberg, "Associations between phonology and syntax in speech delayed children." *Journal of Speech and Hearing Research, 25* (1982): 536–546.

Powers, M. J., "Clinical and educational procedures in functional disorders of articulation." In L. Travis (Ed.), *Handbook of Speech Pathology and Audiology*. Englewood Cliffs, N.J.: Prentice-Hall, 1971.

Price, E., and M. Scarry-Larkin. *Phonology* (CD-ROM). San Luis Obispo, Calif. LocuTour Multimedia, 1999.

Rosenbeck, J. C., R. D. Kent, and L. L. LaPointe, "Apraxia of speech: An overview and some perspectives." In J. C. Rosenbeck, M. R. McNeil, and A. E. Aronson (Eds.), *Apraxia of Speech: Physiology, Acoustics, Linguistics Management* (pp. 1–72). San Diego, Calif.: College Hill Press, 1984.

Ruscello, D., "Motor learning as a model for articulation instruction." In J. Costello (Ed.), *Speech Disorders in Children*. San Diego, Calif.: College-Hill Press, 1984.

Ruscello, D., and R. Shelton, "Planning and self-assessment in articulatory training." *Journal of Speech and Hearing Disorders, 44* (1979): 504–512.

Rvachew, S., "Speech perception training can facilitate sound production learning." *Journal of Speech and Hearing Research, 37* (1994): 347–357.

Scripture, M. K., and E. Jackson, *A Manual of Exercises for the Correction of Speech Disorders*. Philadelphia, Penn.: F.A. Davis, 1927.

Secord, W., "The traditional approach to treatment." In N. Creaghead, P. Newman, and W. Secord (Eds.), *Assessment and Remediation of Articulatory and Phonological Disorders*. Columbus, Ohio: Charles E. Merrill, 1989.

Shriberg, L., "A response evocation program for /ɝ/." *Journal of Speech and Hearing Disorders, 40* (1975): 92–105.

Shriberg, L. D., D. M. Aram, and J. Kwiatkowski. "Developmental apraxia of speech: II. Toward a diagnostic marker." *Journal of Speech, Language, and Hearing Research, 40* (1997): 286–312.

Square, P., "Treatment of developmental apraxia of speech: Tactile-kinesthetic, rhythmic, and gestural approaches." In A. Caruso and E. Strand (Eds.), *Clinical Management of Motor Speech Disorders in Children*. New York: Thieme, 1999.

Strand, E., and R. McCauley, "Assessment procedures for treatment planning in children with phonologic and motor speech disorders." In A. Caruso and E. Strand (Eds.), *Clinical Management of Motor Speech Disorders in Children*. New York: Thieme, 1999.

Strand, E., and A. Skindner, "Treatment of developmental apraxia of speech: Integral stimulation methods." In A. Caruso and E. Strand (Eds.), *Clinical Management of Motor Speech Disorders in Children*. New York: Thieme, 1999.

Tyler, A. A., K. E. Lewis, A. Haskill, and L. C. Tolbert, "Efficacy of cross-domain effects of a morphosyntax and a phonologic intervention." *Language, Speech, and Hearing Services in Schools, 33* (2002): 52–66.

Tyler, A. A., and K. T. Sandoval, "Preschoolers with phonological and language disorders: Treating different linguistic domains." *Language, Speech, and Hearing Services in Schools, 25* (1994): 215–234.

Tyler, A., and K. Watterson, "Effects of phonological versus language intervention in preschoolers with both phonological and language impairment." *Child Language Teaching and Therapy, 7* (1991): 141–160.

Van Riper, C., *Speech Correction: Principles and Methods*. Englewood Cliffs, N.J.: Prentice-Hall, 1939.

Van Riper, C. and L. Emerick, *Speech Correction: An Introduction to Speech Pathology and Audiology*. Englewood Cliffs, N.J.: Prentice-Hall, Inc., 1984.

Van Riper C., and R. Erickson, *Speech Correction: An Introduction to Speech Pathology and Audiology*, 9th ed. Englewood Cliffs, N.J.: Prentice-Hall, Inc., 1996.

Velleman, S., and K. Strand, "Developmental verbal dyspraxia." In J. Bernthal, and N. Bankson (Eds.), *Child Phonology: Characteristics, Assessment, and Intervention with Special Populations* (pp 110–139). New York, N.Y.: Thieme Publishers, 1994.

Weber, J., "Patterning of deviant articulation behavior." *Journal of Speech and Hearing Disorders, 35* (1970): 135–141.

Weiner, F., "Treatment of phonological disability using the method of meaningful minimal contrast: Two case studies." *Journal of Speech and Hearing Disorders, 46* (1981): 97–103.

Weiner, F., and N. Bankson, "Teaching features." *Language, Speech, and Hearing Services in Schools, 9* (1978): 29–34.

Williams, A. L., "Generalization patterns associated with training least phonological knowledge." *Journal of Speech and Hearing Research, 34* (1991): 722–733

Williams, A. L., "Phonological reorganization: A qualitative measure of phonological improvement." *American Journal of Speech-Language Pathology, 2* (1993): 44–51.

Williams, A. L., "Multiple oppositions: Theoretical foundations for an alternative approach. *American Journal of Speech-Language Pathology, 9* (2000a): 282–288.

Williams, A. L., "Multiple oppositions: Case studies of variables in phonological intervention." *American Journal of Speech-Language Pathology, 9* (2000b): 289–299.

Williams, A. L., *Speech Disorders Resource Guide for Preschool Children.* Clifton Park, NY.: Singular Publishing Group, 2003.

Williams, G., and L. V. McReynolds, "The relationship between discrimination and articulation training in children with misarticulation." *Journal of Speech and Hearing Research, 18* (1975): 401–412.

Winitz, H., *From Syllable to Conversation.* Baltimore, Md.: University Park Press, 1975.

Winitz, H., "Auditory considerations in articulation training." In H. Winitz (Ed.), *Treating Articulation Disorders for Clinicians by Clinicians.* Baltimore, Md.: University Park Press, 1984.

8 Language And Dialectal Variations

BRIAN GOLDSTEIN
Temple University

AQUILES IGLESIAS
Temple University

Introduction

Speech patterns used by individuals in our society vary as a function of language, age, social-economic status, and geography. Speech patterns also vary as a function of an individual's ability to acquire and produce the speech patterns of their community. As speech-language pathologists (SLPs), it is our responsibility to sort out the array of patterns that are typical of a child's speech community from those that are indicative of a phonological disorder. Information on variations in speech patterns seen within and across particular speech communities is necessary to conduct least-biased phonological assessments that reflect the characteristics of the child's speech community. For example, if members of a child's speech community consist of individuals who are bilingual (Spanish and English) and the variety of English spoken in the child's community is African American English (AAE), the child will most likely speak a variety of English that has been influenced by both AAE and Spanish. Phonological assessment of such a child must take into account the influence that AAE and Spanish might have on the child's phonological patterns. Sensitivity and knowledge of variation are also required to adequately serve individuals who elect to modify the language variety that they speak. In the following sections, we examine phonological variation within and across languages and show how this information can be used to conduct least-biased assessment and plan for intervention.

Dialect

Dialects are mutually intelligible forms of a language associated with a particular region, social class, or ethnic group. General American English (GAE), Southern White Standard, Appalachian English, Caribbean English, AAE, Eastern American English, and Spanish-influenced English are just some of the dialects spoken in the United States. No dialect of any language is superior to any other, because all thoughts can be expressed using any dialect of any language. This is not to say that all varieties of a language carry the same prestige. Some varieties of a language, specifically those used by the dominant groups in any socially stratified society, are considered to have higher prestige (Wolfram, 1986), are promulgated within the educational system (Adler, 1984), and are valued by the private sector of the society (Shuy, 1972; Terrell and Terrell, 1983).

The promulgation of General American English (GAE; the prestige dialect in the United States) within the educational system and the broadcast media to some extent has decreased differences between regional dialects (**dialect leveling**). At the same time, lack of linguistic contact among groups due to geographical or socio-economic reasons has resulted in a linguistic isolation that has increased the distance between dialects for some populations (Labov, 1991). In addition, the increased immigration and ethnic isolation that have occurred among some subgroups have further increased the number and pervasiveness of dialects. The courts' acknowledgment of the rights of linguistic minority populations has resulted in greater acceptance of varieties other than General American English. For example, *Martin Luther King Junior Elementary School Children et al. v Ann Arbor School District Board* (1978) provided for the use of children's home language, including AAE, in the educational process.

Regardless of whether dialects are becoming more or less alike, people hold many different myths about dialects. Wolfram and Schilling-Estes (1998) have indicated a number of myths held about dialects and have countered those myths with corresponding facts. (See Table 8.1.)

Speakers of a particular dialect do not always use all of the features present in their dialect. A speaker's use of particular features depends on the context and interlocutors (**register**). **Registral varieties** are dependent on the participants, setting, and topic. For example, one would typically use one register when talking to friends about an enjoyable weekend and use another when speaking to a policeman about a speeding violation. The extent to which particular individuals use the available features of their dialect (**dialect density**) may depend on factors such as socioeconomic status and geography. Sometimes the differences in dialect density are associated with socioeconomic status; a sociolinguistic phenomenon referred to by Wolfram (1986) as **social diagnosticity**. Wolfram (1986) observed the frequency of occurrence of selected AAE features among the speech of individuals representing four socioeconomic groups: upper middle class, lower middle class, upper working class, and lower working class. His research revealed that certain AAE linguistic features showed **gradient stratification** across the four groups. That is, individuals in lower socioeconomic groups used more of the available features of that dialect than individuals in higher socioeconomic groups. Washington and Craig (1998) found the same effect for 5- and 6-year-old, AAE-speaking boys. For example, the lack of realization of postvocalic *r* (e.g., /sɪstɚ/ → [sɪstə]) is an example of gradient stratification because all socioeconomic groups use this phonological feature, albeit with different levels of frequency. On the other hand, certain AAE features show a pattern of usage referred to as **sharp stratification**, which refers to linguistic features that more clearly differentiate socioeconomic groups, based upon significant differences in frequency of usage. One example of this type of stratification is the substitution of [f] for /θ/. The use of this feature

TABLE 8.1   Myths about Dialects

Myth	Fact	Example
A dialect is a variety spoken by someone else.	Everyone speaks some dialect of a language.	Although there is a dialect form often referred to as the "standard" (e.g., Standard or General American English), it is usually a form not actually spoken by anyone in an invariable form. There is variation to one extent or another used by all speakers.
Dialectal features are always distinct and noticeable.	Some dialectal features are shared by many different dialects.	The weakening of postvocalic *r* (e.g., /moɚ·ə/ → [moə]) is exhibited by speakers of African American English, Eastern American English, and Southern American English.
Dialects arise from ineffective tries at speaking the correct form of the language.	Speakers of dialects acquire those features by interacting with members of the speech community in which they live.	Some native speakers of Spanish often use characteristics of African American English because speakers of both varieties live in the same community (Poplack, 1978).
Dialects are random changes from the "standard."	Dialects are precise and show regular patterns.	In many dialects of the American South, /ɪ/ and /ɛ/ are pronounced as [ɪ] before nasals; /pɪn/; /pɛn/ → [pɪn].
Dialects are always viewed negatively.	Dialects are not inherently viewed negatively (or positively, for that matter); prestige of any dialect is derived from the social prestige of its speakers.	Ramirez and Milk (1986) found that bilingual teachers rated the local Mexican dialect of Spanish as less prestigious than the general dialect of Spanish. The dialect of English spoken by the British monarchy, however, is often perceived as prestigious.

contrasts middle-class with working-class groups, which use the feature much more frequently. Wolfram has indicated that features revealing sharp stratification are of greater social diagnosticity than those showing gradient stratification.

Geography may also play a role in the likelihood of a specific dialect feature being expressed. For example, Hinton and Pollock (1999) examined the occurrence of vocalic and postvocalic American English /ɹ/[1] in AAE speakers from two geographic regions (Davenport, Iowa, and Memphis, Tennessee). Overall, they found that speakers in Davenport were more likely than speakers in Memphis to maintain the rhotic quality of vocalic and postvocalic /ɹ/.

---

[1]The symbol /ɹ/ is used to represent the rhotic sound found in GAE and its dialects. The symbol /r/, as specified by the International Phonetic Alphabet Association, is used to designate the alveolar trill.

Characteristics of American English Dialects

In addition to GAE, a number of dialects of English are spoken in the United States. This chapter focuses on five common dialects: AAE, Southern American English, Eastern American English, Appalachian English, and Ozark English. Most of the available literature on these dialects focuses on their characteristics rather than on their development.

African American English (AAE)

AAE is a variety of American English that is spoken by many, but not all, African Americans. Other groups who have contact with AAE speakers also speak it. English-speaking Puerto Rican teenagers in East Harlem, New York, have been found to use features of AAE (Wolfram, 1974). Wolfram found that the degree of contact that the teenagers had with AAE speakers greatly influenced the number of AAE features in their speech. Individuals with the most contact showed the greatest number of features in their speech. Poplack (1978) examined the use of AAE, Puerto Rican Spanish, and Philadelphia English variants in the speech of sixth-grade Puerto Rican boys and girls. She found that the Puerto Rican boys tended to use more features of AAE and the girls used more features of Philadelphia English. Poplack concluded that the specific variants used by the children were more related to "covert prestige" than to their linguistic environment, with the boys assigning more prestige to AAE speakers and the girls assigning more to Philadelphia English. The results of both of these studies support the notions that use of dialect features is influenced by patterns in the speech community and that speech patterns are greatly affected by peer interaction.

Like all dialects, AAE is systematic, with rule-governed phonological, semantic, syntactic, pragmatic, and proxemic systems. There are two major hypotheses accounting for the origin of AAE (Poplack, 2000; Wolfram and Schilling-Estes, 1998). The Anglicist Hypothesis states that AAE is considered a dialect of English. An alternative hypothesis, the Creole Hypothesis, assumes that AAE descended from Plantation Creole (Wolfram, 1994; Wolfram and Schilling-Estes, 1998), a language that developed from a mixture of languages brought into contact during the slave trade period. Plantation Creole was commonly used by African Americans on plantations in the South but was not spoken by European Americans at the time. Over time, AAE has further spread and changed. The exodus of African Americans from the Southeast to the Northeast and other parts of the United States in the early 1900s brought AAE to the urban areas of the North (Stewart, 1971). In many cases, individuals from a particular state tended to migrate to particular cities (e.g., South Carolinians moving to Philadelphia). The restricted social environments in which many African Americans lived, in addition to the continued contact with their southern families and communities, reinforced the use of AAE. In its evolution, AAE has undergone a decreolization process, showing fewer links to its creole past and acquiring features that are not traceable to the original Creole (e.g., stopping of interdental fricatives) (Wolfram and Schilling-Estes, 1998).

A number of linguistic features distinguish AAE from GAE. The major phonological features that distinguish these two varieties are listed in Table 8.2 (compiled from Bailey and Thomas, 1998; Hyter, 1996; Pollock, Bailey, Berni, Fletcher, Hinton, Johnson, and Weaver, 1998; Rickford, 1999; Stockman, 1996a; Wolfram and Schilling-Estes, 1998).

TABLE 8.2. Major Phonological Features Distinguishing African American English and General American English

Pattern	Example(s)
Word-final consonant cluster reduction (particularly when one of the two consonants is an alveolar)	/tɛst/ → [tɛs]
Deletion of /ɹ/	/sɪstɚ/ → [sɪstə] /kærəl/ → [kæəl] /pɹʌfɛsɚ/ → [pʌfɛsə]
Deletion of /l/ in word-final abutting consonants	/hɛlp/ → [hɛp]
Deletion of nasal consonant in word-final position with nasalization of preceding vowel	/mun/ → [mũ)]
Substitution of [ɪ] for /ɛ/ before nasals	"pin" /pɪn/ and "pen" /pɛn/ pronounced as [pɪn]
Substitution of [k] for /t/ in initial /stɹ/ clusters	/stɹit/ → [skɹit]
Realization of /θɹ/ as [θ]	/θɹo/ → [θo]
Substitution of f/θ and v/ð in intervocalic position	/nʌθiŋ/ → [nʌfiŋ] /beðiŋ/ → [beviŋ]
Substitution of f/θ in word-final position	/sɑʊθ/ → [sɑʊf]
Realization of /v/ as [b] and /z/ as [d], in word-internal position before syllabic nasals	/sɛvən/ → [sɛbən]
Stopping of word-initial interdentals	/ðe/ → [de] /θɑt/ → [tɑt]
Metathesis	/æsk/ → [æks]

These features are always optional, are not used in each possible phonetic context, and are not produced by all AAE speakers. For example, the simplification of word-final clusters tends to occur when one of the consonants is an alveolar and the other (i.e., the deleted consonant) is a morphological marker (Stockman, 1996a). Hence, some AAE speakers may not differentiate between the present and past tense of the same verb (e.g., *miss* and *missed* are pronounced as /mɪs/), but would retain the cluster in a word such as *mist*.

Features of AAE extend to suprasegmental phenomena as well (Hyter, 1996; Stockman, 1996a). For example, AAE speakers may place stress on the first rather than second syllable (Detróit → Détroit), use a wide range of intonation contours and vowel elongations, and produce more level and falling final contours than rising contours.

Phonological Development in AAE

Surprisingly little information exists on the development of AAE phonology. Existing studies have examined phonological development in typically developing AAE-speaking children and AAE-speaking children with phonological disorders. Major findings indicate that

AAE-speaking children tend to produce the same phonetic inventory as speakers of GAE (Stockman, 1996a); show great intersubject variability; exhibit systematic error patterns; and demonstrate differences in both the type and quantity of speech errors exhibited by typically developing speakers and those with phonological disorders.

AAE- and GAE-speaking preschool children often exhibit similar phonological patterns, although with different frequencies. Seymour and Seymour (1981) compared the performance of 4- and 5-year-old African-American and white children. They reported that both groups evidenced phonological variations typically associated with AAE (e.g., f/θ in medial and final positions; d/ð in initial and medial positions; b/v in initial and medial positions). The AAE features, however, occurred more frequently in the productions of the African-American children. Thus, both groups produced the same type of substitutions, but the frequency of their use differed between the two groups. These results suggested that for the children they studied, the contrast between AAE and GAE was *qualitatively* undifferentiated at this age. The same result has also been demonstrated for phonological processes (Haynes and Moran, 1989).

Variability across children has been found to be a hallmark of AAE phonological development. Seymour and Seymour (1981) reported considerable intersubject variability among AAE speakers. Not all of the target features were present in each AAE speaker, nor were they equally distributed among the speakers. They inferred that African-American children from AAE-speaking communities would likely show developmental patterns similar to those exhibited by GAE-speaking children.

Although there is variability in phonological development between AAE-speaking children, the context for error patterns exhibited by these children has been found to be systematic. For example, although AAE-speaking children delete final consonants, they do not do so arbitrarily. Stockman (1996a) noted that alveolar consonants were more likely than labials to be deleted; oral stops and nasals were more likely than fricatives to be deleted; and final consonants preceding a consonant were more likely to be deleted. In addition, the absence of final consonants may be marked by lengthening or nasalizing the vowel that preceded the absent consonant (Moran, 1993). Bryant, Velleman, Abdualkarim, and Seymour (2001) found that AAE-speaking children were more likely to delete one element of a word-final cluster if a more sonorous element preceded a less sonorous element. For example, words ending in /sk/ clusters (more sonorous element preceding less sonorous element) were more likely to undergo deletion than were /ks/ clusters (less sonorous element preceding more sonorous element). In addition, their results indicated that in the clusters in which a more sonorous element preceded a less sonorous one, the most sonorous element was preserved. For example, AAE-speaking children would produce "desk" /dɛsk/ as [dɛs] and not [dɛk].

Developmental differences between typically developing AAE speakers and those with phonological disorders have been found to be quantitatively and qualitatively different. Bleile and Wallach (1992) compared the articulation of nonspeech-delayed and speech-delayed AAE-speaking children ranging in age from 3;6 to 5;5. Head Start teachers who shared the same racial and linguistic background as the children differentiated the two groups of children. Data analysis was based on non-AAE phonological patterns exhibited by the children in a picture-identification, single-word test. The delayed and nondelayed groups demonstrated differences in the type and quantity of their speech errors. Speech-delayed children had a larger number of (1) stop errors (especially velars), (2) fricative errors in all positions (especially fricatives other than /θ/), and (3) affricate errors in all positions. Nonspeech-delayed subjects evidenced greater devoicing of final /d/, sonorant errors, and errors related to /ɹ/. Both groups of children produced a large number of consonant cluster errors, with the speech-delayed children exhibiting a larger number of cluster errors. Bleile and Wallach (1992) concluded that a combination of characteristics, rather than a single indicator, appears to be the most reliable index of speech delay in AAE speakers, just as it is with children who do not speak AAE.

Eastern American English and Southern American English

Eastern American English and Southern American English, described by Labov (1991) as Northern and Southern dialects, are two geographical variations of GAE. The Eastern American dialect runs generally from the New England states to the north, and south to New Jersey (Wolfram and Schilling-Estes, 1998). The Southern American dialect runs generally from Maryland south to Florida and to parts of Texas to the west (Wolfram and Schilling-Estes, 1998). Although these two dialects share many of the same features, they can also be differentiated from each other through differences in the production of both vowels and consonants (Table 8.3) (compiled from Parker and Riley, 2000; Small, 1999; Wolfram and Schilling-Estes, 1998).

TABLE 8.3   Common Dialectal Variations in English

Pattern	Example		Dialect
Vowels			
Tense → Lax	/i/ → [ɪ]	/rili/ → [rɪlɪ]	SAE
	/u/ → [ʊ]	/rut/ → [rʊt]	EAE
Lax → Tense	/ɪ/ → [i]	/fɪʃ/ → [fiʃ]	SAE
	/ɛ/ → [e]	/ɛg/ → [eg]	SAE
	/æ/ → [ɑ]	/hæf/ → [hɑf]	EAE
Vowel Neutralization	/ɪ/; /ɛ/ → [ɪ]	/pɪn/; /pɛn/ → [pɪn]	SAE
Diphthong Reduction	/ɑɪ/ → [ɑ]	/pɑɪ/ → [pɑ]	SAE
a/ɔ		[fɔt] → [fɑt]	SAE, EAE
Lowering	/ɔ/ → [ɑ]	/fɔɚ/ → [fɑɚ]	SAE, EAE
Derhoticization	/ɚ,ɝ/ → [ə]	/fɔɚ/ → [fɔə]	SAE, EAE
		/kɝv/ → [kəv]	SAE, EAE
"r" Deletion		/kɑɚ/ → [kɑ]	SAE, EAE
"r" Addition	/ə/ → [ɚ]	/lɪndə/ → [lɪndɚ]	EAE
Consonants			
Velar Fronting	/ŋ/ → [n]	/ɹʌnɪŋ/ → [ɹʌnɪn]	SAE
/j/ Addition		/nu/ → [nju]	SAE, EAE
Voicing Assimilation	/s/ → [z]	/gɹisi/ → [gɹizi]	SAE
Glottalization	/t/; /d/ → [ʔ]	/batəl/ → [baʔəl]	EAE
[t]; [d] for /θ/; /ð/	/θ/ → [t]	/θɪŋk/ → [tɪŋk]	EAE
	/ð/ → [d]	/ðɪs/ → [dɪs]	EAE

Key: SAE = Southern American English; EAE = Eastern American English

Appalachian English and Ozark English

Two other common geographical dialects of English are Appalachian English (AE) and Ozark English (OE). Christian, Wolfram, and Nube (1988) indicate that AE and OE are related linguistically, showing many similar features. Given the phonological similarities of these two dialects, they will be discussed together. AE is spoken generally in parts of Kentucky, Tennessee, Virginia, North Carolina, and West Virginia (parts of the Carolinas, Georgia, and Alabama may also be included). OE is spoken in an area encompassing northern Arkansas, southern Missouri, and northwestern Oklahoma.

Christian and colleagues (1988, pp. 153–159) have outlined the following characteristics of AE and OE, Table 8.4. Only the most common features are outlined here (see Christian, et al., 1988 for more details).

As was the case for AAE in African-American speakers, not all features of AE/OE will be utilized by every speaker, used in every situation, or produced in every context. For example, the rule noted as *intrusive t*, in which [t] may be added to words ending in /s/ or /f/, is usually limited to a small set of words. Most commonly, the rule takes effect on the words *once* and *twice*. In addition, the number of words exhibiting this rule seems to be more extensive in AE than OE.

TABLE 8.4   Characteristics of Appalachian English and Ozark English

Rule	Example
Epenthesis Following Clusters CCC# → CCəC#	/gosts/ → [gostəs]
Intrusive *t* (more common in AE) /s/# → [st] /f/# → [ft]	/wʌns/ → [wʌnst] /klɪf/ → [klɪft]
Stopping of Fricatives /θ/ → [t] /ð/ → [d]	/θɑt/ → [tɑt] /ðe/ → [de]
Initial *w* Reduction /w/ → ø	/wɪl/ → [ɪl]
Initial Unstressed Syllables IUS → ø	/əlaʊd/ → [laʊd]
h Retention ø → [h]	/ɪt/ → [hɪt]
Retroflex *r* /ɹ/ → ø, postconsonantal /ɹ/ → ø, intervocalic	/θɹo/ → [θo] /kæɹi/ → [kæi]
Lateral *l* /l/ → ø before labials	/wʊlf/ → [wʊf]

Phonology in Speakers of Language Varieties other than English

Prior to the arrival of Europeans, what is now the continental United States was a polyglot area with over 200 languages or dialects spoken (Leap, 1981). Over the past 600 years, immigrants to this area have brought their culture and language. Historically, the general trend for most immigrants to the United States was to use their home language as their primary language of communication. By the third generation, though, immigrants tended to lose their language of origin (Veltman, 1988). Some immigrant groups, however, have maintained the use of their home language (first language) from generation to generation, with reinforcement from new immigrants and travel to their country of origin. In total, there are more than 43 million individuals older than 5 years in the United States who speak a language other than or in addition to English, almost 45 percent of whom speak English less than "very well" (U.S. Bureau of the Census, 2000). The number of individuals speaking a language variety other than English in the United States is likely to increase in the coming years. It is estimated that by the year 2050 (U.S. Department of Commerce, Bureau of the Census, 1995), if birth rates and current immigration trends continue, the percentage of individuals of Asian descent will almost triple, the percentage of individuals of Hispanic/Latino descent will almost double, and the percentage of Native Americans will increase to about 1 percent (for information on Native American languages, see Goldstein, 2000). The percentage of whites will decrease to slightly over one-half the population.

There has been a realization that, although English is the most common and dominant language spoken in the United States, other languages have a right to co-exist in our linguistically plural society. For example, *Lau v Nichols* (1974) and the *Lau* Remedies (1975) mandated that federally funded schools must eliminate language barriers in school programs that exclude nonnative English speakers. The *Individuals with Disabilities Education Act Amendments* (IDEA, 1997) required that the native language commonly used in the home or learning environment be utilized in all contact for a child with a disability.

The current number and future increase of individuals from culturally and linguistically diverse populations mean that SLPs will likely encounter speakers of language varieties other than English. To complete appropriate phonological assessments that guide the intervention process for children whose home language is not English, SLPs need to gather segmental, prosodic, syllabic, and developmental information. In this section, the characteristics of pidgins, creoles, and Spanish and Asian languages, along with information about phonological acquisition and development in speakers of Spanish and Asian languages, are described.

Pidgins and Creoles

Language is always changing. This change is represented in all areas of language—phonology, syntax, semantics, lexicon, and pragmatics. This change may take place because of a number of factors such as geography, social prestige, and the introduction of new vocabulary (Crystal, 1987). Pidgins and creoles are two examples of language change.

A **pidgin** is a communication system used by groups of people who wish and need to communicate with each other but have no means to do so. They use a limited vocabulary and "simplified" syntactic structure compared with their two native languages (Crystal, 1987). Pidgins are not simply degraded natural languages but come to have rules all their own. In fact, some pidgins, for example, Tok Pisin in Papua New Guinea, have become the most widely used linguistic variety in the country. Crystal notes, however, that a pidgin often has a short life (perhaps a few years) and disappears when the need for a common communication system ceases to exist. He also suggests that a pidgin may develop into a creole.

A **creóle** is "a pidgin language which has become the mother tongue of a community—a definition which emphasizes that pidgins and creoles are two stages in a single process of linguistic development" (Crystal, 1987; p. 336). In essence, a creole is a pidgin that serves as primary input to the next generation of speakers. That is, a pidgin becomes a creole when it is passed on to child speakers. Compared with pidgins, creoles show increased complexity in syntax, phonology, lexicon, semantics, and pragmatics (Muyksen and Smith, 1995). Creoles tend to show rules that were not exhibited in their pidgin ancestor (Holm, 1988).

Common Creoles in the United States

There are four main creoles that SLPs may encounter: Gullah, Hawaiian Creole, Louisiana French Creole, and Haitian Creole. In this section, we briefly outline their phonological characteristics.

Gullah (or Geechee or Sea Island Creole as it is sometimes called) is spoken by approximately 250,000–300,000 speakers, mainly on the barrier islands off the coasts off South Carolina and Georgia (Holm, 1989). This English creole is closely related to other creoles such as Sierra Leone Krio, Cameroons Creole, Jamaican Creole, the Creole of British Guiana, and the Creoles of Surinam (Cunningham, 1992). The origin of this creole is debated. Some believe that Gullah arrived in the American colonies from the West Coast of Africa as a fully developed creole (Nichols, 1981). Others link its development to a complex interaction of white British settlers, Africans, and Caribbeans (Holm, 1989). Some phonological features of Gullah (compared with GAE) include the use of [a] for /æ/, [t] for /θ/, [d] for /ð/, [dʒ] for /z/, and deletion of postvocalic /ɹ/.

Hawaiian Creole arose in the 19th century and culminates from the influence of many sources such as Polynesian, European, Asian, and pidgin languages (Holm, 1989). Some phonological features of Hawaiian Creole (compared with GAE) include [t] for /θ/, [d] for /ð/, backing in the environment of [ɹ] (/θɹ/ → [tʃɹ]; /tɹ/ → [tʃɹ]; /stɹ/ → [ʃɹ]), deletion of postvocalic /ɹ/, and deletion of the second member of word-final abutting consonants, for example, /nɛst/ → [nɛs] (Bleile, 1996).

Louisiana French Creole evolved as the native language of descendants of West African slaves brought to southern Louisiana by French colonists (Nichols, 1981). The creole has also been influenced by features of Cajun, a variety of regional French brought from Canada (Holm, 1989). It is estimated that there are 60,000-80,000 speakers of this creole. The vowel system consists of four front vowels, /i, e, ɛ, a/, four back vowels, /u, o, ɔ, a/, schwa /ə/, and three nasalized vowels /ɛ̃, ɔ̃, ã/ (Morgan, 1959; Nichols, 1981). The consonant system contains six oral stops /b, d, g, p, t, k/, three nasal stops /m, n, ɲ/, seven fricatives /f, s, ʃ, v, z, ʒ, h/, two liquids /l, ɹ/, and one glide /j/. There are four common phonological patterns noted by Nichols (1981). First, abutting consonants across word boundaries are often assimilated to the voicing of the second member of the consonant pair; for example, /pæsði/ → [pæzði]. Second, word-final consonants may be deleted. Third, word-final unstressed syllables are often weakened or deleted. Finally, vowel raising may take place in which [i] is substituted for /ɛ/.

Speech-language pathologists might also encounter speakers of Haitian Creole. This Caribbean Creole, spoken in Haiti, has approximately 6 million speakers (Muyksen and Veenstra, 1995). There are three dialects of Haitian Creole: northern, central (including the capital, Port-au-Prince), and southern. The Haitian Creole vowel system contains seven segments, /i, u, e, o, a/ and two front rounded vowels /ø/ and /œ/. It also contains 17 consonants, six stops /b, d, g, p, t, k/, six fricatives /f, s, ʃ v, z, ʒ/, three nasals /m, n, ɲ/, and two liquids /l/ and /r/.

Spanish

Spanish has become the second most common language spoken in the United States, with approximately 27 million speakers, or 10.5 percent of the population (U.S. Bureau of the Census, 2000). According to Dalbor (1980), there are six major dialects of American Spanish: Mexican and Southwestern United States; Central American; Caribbean; Highlandian; Chilean; and Southern Paraguayan, Uruguayan and Argentinean. The principal differences among these dialects are in vocabulary and phonology. Although all of these dialects are spoken in the mainland United States, the two most prevalent dialects are Southwestern United States (e.g., speakers of Mexican/Mexican-American Spanish) and Caribbean (e.g., speakers of Puerto Rican and Cuban Spanish). In the following sections, we review Spanish phonology and phonological development in Spanish speakers.

Spanish Phonology

A brief overview of the Spanish consonant and vowel system is presented here (for a more complete description, see Goldstein, 1995). There are five primary vowels in Spanish. The two front vowels are /i/ and /e/, and the three back vowels are /u/, /o/, and /a/. There are 18 phonemes in General Spanish (Núñez-Cedeño and Morales-Front, 1999): the voiceless unaspirated stops, /p/, /t/, and /k/; the voiced stops, /b/, /d/, and /g/; the voiceless fricatives, /f/, /x/, and /s/; the affricate, /tʃ/; the glides, /w/ and /j/; the lateral, /l/; the flap /ɾ/ and trill /r/; and the nasals, /m/, /n/, and /ɲ/.

The existence of differences between Spanish dialects further complicates the process of characterizing phonological patterns in Spanish-speaking children. Unlike English, in which dialectal variations are generally defined by variations in vowels, Spanish dialectal differences primarily affect consonant sound classes rather than vowels or a few specific phonemes. The dialect differences affect certain sound classes over others. Fricatives and liquids (in particular /s/, flap /ɾ/, and trill /r/) tend to show more variation than stops, glides, or the affricate. The differences between Spanish dialects make it paramount that SLPs be aware of the dialect the children are speaking. Otherwise, the likelihood of misdiagnosis increases.

Phonological Development in Spanish-Speaking Children

Normative data (summarized in detail in Goldstein, 1995; 2000) show that typically developing Spanish-speaking infants tend to produce CV syllables containing oral and nasal stops with front vowels (e.g., Oller and Eilers, 1982). It is likely that by the time Spanish-speaking children reach 3 years of age, they will use the dialect features of the community and will have mastered the vowel system and most of the consonant system (e.g., Anderson and Smith, 1987; Goldstein and Cintron, 2001; Pandolfi and Herrera, 1990). In terms of vowel development in Spanish-speaking children, Oller and Eilers (1982) found that the mean proportion occurrence of vowel-like productions in 12–14-month-old English- and Spanish-speaking children was remarkably similar. In general, they noted that the children were likely to produce more anteriorlike vowels than posteriorlike ones. The rank order of the first 10 vowels in Spanish-speaking infants was: (1) [ɛ]; (2) [æ]; (3) [e]; (4) [i]; (5) [a]; (6) [ʌ]; (7) [ʊ]; (8) [u]; (9) [ɪ]; (10) [o] (p. 573). Maez (1981) indicated that by 18 months, the three children in the study had mastered (i.e., produced correctly at least 90 percent of the time) the five basic Spanish vowels, [i], [e], [u], [o], and [a]. Maez's study, however, focused on consonant development and did not indicate whether vowel errors occurred.

Goldstein and Pollock (2000) examined vowel productions in 23 Spanish-speaking children (ten 3-year-olds and thirteen 4-year-olds) with phonological disorders. Fourteen of the 23 children in the study exhibited vowel errors. Only one child exhibited more than one vowel error; that subject evidenced five errors. The other 13 children each exhibited only one vowel error. Across all children, the results indicated that there were only 18 total vowel errors, almost half of which were on the vowel /o/.

In terms of consonant production, children continue to exhibit some difficulty at the end of preschool with consonant clusters and a few phones, specifically, [ð], [x], [s], [ɲ], [tʃ], [ɾ], [r], and [l] (e.g., Acevedo, 1991; Jimenez, 1987). These children may exhibit some of the following phonological processes: cluster reduction, unstressed syllable deletion, stridency deletion, and tap/trill deviation, but will likely have suppressed phonological processes such as velar and palatal fronting, prevocalic singleton omission, stopping, and assimilation (e.g., Goldstein and Iglesias, 1996a; Stepanof, 1990). For some Spanish-speaking children, phonetic mastery will continue into the early elementary school years when they continue to show some, although infrequent, errors on the fricatives [x] and [s], the affricate [tʃ], the flap [ɾ], the trill [r], the lateral [l], and consonant clusters (e.g., Bailey, 1982; De la Fuente, 1985).

Although quite a number of studies describe phonological patterns in typically developing children, the data remain scarce for Spanish-speaking children with phonological disorders. Data indicate that the percentage of Spanish-speaking children with phonological disorders who exhibit specific processes is similar across studies (e.g., Bichotte, Dunn, Gonzalez, Orpi, and Nye, 1993; Goldstein and Iglesias, 1996b; Meza, 1983). Phonological processes exhibited by a large percentage of children (>40 percent) included cluster reduction, unstressed syllable deletion, stopping, liquid simplification, and assimilation, in findings not unlike that observed in American English-speaking children.

Asian Languages

In the year 2000, there were approximately 7 million speakers of Asian languages in the United States, 2.7 percent of the total U.S. population (U.S. Bureau of the Census, 2000). Three main families of languages are spoken in Asia (Crystal, 1987). The first includes 100 Austro-Asiatic languages, most of the languages spoken in Southeast Asia (the countries between China and Indonesia) including Khmer, Hmong, and Vietnamese. The second is the Tai family, centered on Thailand and extending into Laos, North Vietnam, and parts of China. The third branch is Sino-Tibetan, comprising the languages of China, Tibet, and Burma, including Mandarin (also termed Putonghua) and Cantonese. Combined, these families contain more than 440 languages spoken by more than 1 billion people. Two other families, Austronesian and Papuan, contain languages spoken in the Pacific Islands (Cheng, 1993). Austronesian comprises languages such as Hawaiian, Chamorro, Ilocano, and Tagalog. The Papuan family includes New Guinean.

There are a number of dialectal variations in Asian languages just as there are within English (e.g., Wang, 1990). For example, two main dialects of Chinese are spoken in the United States, Mandarin and Cantonese (Cheng, 1987). There are also a number of subdialects within those two main dialects. Japanese has a few dialects, but they are mutually unintelligible; however, Khmer's four dialects are mutually intelligible (Cheng, 1993). In the next two sections, Asian language phonology and phonological development in children speaking Asian languages are described.

Asian Language Phonology

The phonological structure of Asian languages varies greatly. In general, there are few syllable-final segments and few consonant clusters. For example: (1) the only syllable final consonants in Mandarin Chinese are /n/ and /ŋ/, (2) there are no labiodental, interdental, or palatal fricatives in Korean, and (3) Hawaiian contains only five vowels and eight consonants. There are, however, segmental systems in Asian languages that are relatively complex. For example, Hmong (the language spoken by dwellers in mountainous areas of Indochina) contains 56 initial consonants, 13 or 14 vowels (depending on dialect), seven tones, and one final consonant /ŋ/ (Cheng, 1993). For segmental information on specific languages and dialects, readers might consult the following sources: Cheng (1987; 1993), Tipton (1975) and Wang (1989).

Syllable structure in Asian languages also shows considerable variation. For example, Laotian contains three syllable types (CVC, CVVC, and CVV). Khmer exhibits eight syllable types (CVC, CCVC, CCCVC, CVVC, CCVVC, CCCVVC, CVV, CCVV) but few polysyllabic words (Cheng, 1987). Many Asian languages also show restrictions on the types of segments that may appear in certain syllable positions. Vietnamese has a limited number of final consonants (voiceless stops and nasals), the only final consonant in Hmong is /ŋ/, and Korean has no fricatives or affricates in word-final position. Stress also may be different in Asian languages compared with English. For example, there is no tonic word stress in Korean so native speakers of Korean may sound somewhat "monotone" to native English-speakers when speaking English (Cheng, 1993).

Many, but not all, Asian languages are tone languages. For example, Cantonese is a tone language, but Japanese is not. In **tone languages** differences in word meaning are signified by differences in pitch. Tone languages are generally composed of *register tones* (typically two or three in a language) and *contour tones* (usually two or three per language) (O'Grady, Dobrovolsky, and Aranoff, 1993). Register tones are level tones, usually signaled by high, mid, and low tones. Contour tones are a combination of register tones over a single syllable. For example, in Mandarin Chinese, the phonetic string [ma] takes on different meanings depending on the tone or tone sequence that is applied (O'Grady, Dobrovolsky, and Aranoff, 1993). If produced with a high, level tone, [ma] means "mother," but if the same phonetic form is produced with a high-fall, register tone (i.e., a high then low tone), it means "scold."

There have been few studies on tone acquisition in Asian languages. Four studies have examined tone acquisition in typically developing children speaking Chinese languages, illustrating the developmental process of tone (Li and Thompson, 1977; So and Dodd, 1995; Tse, 1978; Zhu and Dodd, 2000a). Tse (1978) found that perceptual discrimination of tone began as early as 10 months. The results from all four studies found that (1) children acquired the correct tone system relatively quickly (in about eight months), (2) mastery of tone occurred before segmental mastery, (3) high and falling tones were acquired earlier and more easily than rising and contour tones, and (4) substitution errors often exist for rising and contour tones during the two- and three-word stages.

Phonological Development in Speakers of Asian Languages

Few studies have investigated phonological patterns in children speaking Asian languages, and those have investigated development in children speaking Mandarin (Putonghua) and Cantonese. Zhu and Dodd (2000a) examined the phonological skills of 129 typically developing speakers of Putonghua, aged 1;6-4;6. Their results indicated that tone was acquired first, followed by syllable-final consonants and vowels, and finally syllable-initial consonants. By age 4;6, 90 percent of the children accurately produced all syllable-initial consonants. Similar to typically developing children acquiring other languages, the Putonghua-speaking children exhibited syllabic and substitution phonological processes such as unstressed syllable deletion, fronting, and gliding. The children also showed language-specific patterns such as deaspiration and triphthong reduction of vowels. So and Dodd (1994; 1995) investigated phonological development in typically developing Cantonese-speaking children and noted phoneme acquisition similar to English but at a more rapid rate. In general, anterior consonants were acquired before posterior ones, and oral and nasal stops and glides were acquired before fricatives and affricates. They also noted the presence of phonological processes and found that by age 4, no process was exhibited more than 15 percent of the time. Between the ages of 2;0–4;0, these children showed processes similar in quantity (greater than 15 percent) and type to English-speaking children: assimilation, cluster reduction, stopping, fronting, affrication, and final consonant deletion.

Two studies have also investigated Mandarin- (Putonghua) and Cantonese-speaking children with phonological disorders. Zhu and Dodd (2000b) assessed 33 children aged 2;8–7;6 with "atypical speech development" (p. 170). The largest subgroup of speakers (18 of 33 children) was characterized with delayed phonological development ("use of non-age-appropriate processes and/or restricted phonetic or phonemic inventory," p. 168). Phonological processes exhibited most commonly included fronting and stopping. These children had less difficulty with syllable components described as having more "phonological saliency" (p. 180). Phonological saliency, according to the authors, is based on syllable structure and is specific to each ambient language. In the case of Putonghua, tones, vowels, and syllable-final consonants are more salient, and syllable-initial consonants are less salient. As predicted, children with disorders had the most difficulty with less salient features (i.e., syllable-initial consonants). So and Dodd (1994, pp. 238–240) outlined and defined four subgroups of English-speaking children with phonological disorders: delayed phonological development ("rules or processes used by more than 10 percent of children acquiring phonology normally"), consistent use of one or more unusual rules ("rules not used by more than 10 percent of children acquiring phonology normally"), articulation disorder ("consistent distortion of a phoneme"), and children who make inconsistent errors ("production of specific words or particular phonological segments"). They applied these categories to 17 Cantonese-speaking children with phonological disorders, aged 3;6–6;4. Their results revealed that 8 of 17 subjects (47 percent) displayed delayed phonological development, 5 of 17 (30 percent) were categorized as consistent users of one or more unusual rules, 2 of 17 (12 percent) had an articulation disorder, and another 2 of 17 (12 percent) were defined as making inconsistent errors.

They further provided increased detail on the phonological patterns exhibited by the 13 subjects labeled as "delayed phonological development" or "consistently disordered." Children with phonological development tended to exhibit assimilation, cluster reduction, stopping, fronting, deaspiration, affrication, and final consonant deletion. Children with consistent phonological errors tended to exhibit final consonant deletion, aspiration, gliding, vowel substitution errors, initial consonant deletion, and backing.

Phonological Development in Bilingual Children

Although there is no doubt that SLPs will be assessing and providing intervention services to monolingual speakers of Spanish and Asian languages, it is more likely that SLPs will be delivering clinical services to children acquiring both their home language and English. Studies of Spanish-English and Cantonese-English bilingual children indicate that phonological development in these bilingual children is somewhat different than that for monolingual speakers of either language.

Dodd, So, and Li (1996) examined the phonology of 16 typically developing, Cantonese-speaking children who were acquiring English in preschool. The results indicated that the children differentiated the phonology of each language. They also found that the children's error patterns were atypical for monolingual speakers of either language. However, bilingual children produced a higher number of atypical error patterns (e.g., initial consonant deletion) a problem usually associated with children evidencing phonological disorders.

Gildersleeve, Davis, and Stubbe (1996) examined the English phonological skills of typically developing, bilingual (English-Spanish) 3-year-olds. Their results showed that bilingual children showed an overall lower intelligibility rating, made more consonant and vowel errors, distorted more sounds, and produced more uncommon error patterns than either monolingual English or monolingual Spanish speakers. Gildersleeve-Neumann and Davis (1998), however, demonstrated that although bilingual speakers exhibited different developmental patterns than their monolingual peers and exhibited more errors initially than monolingual speakers, these differences faded over time. The differences between monolingual and bilingual speakers are also supported by the work off Goldstein and Washington (2001), who examined the Spanish and English phonological skills in typically developing 4-year-old bilingual (Spanish-English) children and found marked differences in the accuracy of production of sounds in specific sound classes, especially in Spanish. Spirants, flap, and trill in Spanish were produced much less accurately in bilingual children than in monolingual Spanish-speaking children (Goldstein, 1988). Accuracy rates of sounds in other sound classes, however, were similar to those for monolingual children.

The Influence of One Language on Another

When there is contact between speakers of two or more languages, a tendency exists for one language to influence the other. This influence is bidirectional with L_1 influencing L_2 and L_2 influencing L_1. For example, a native Spanish speaker acquiring English exhibits characteristics of Spanish-influenced English and English-influenced Spanish. In a group of bilingual (Spanish-English) children, Goldstein and Iglesias (1999) found that a few children substituted [tʃ] for /ʃ/; /ʃʌvəl/ ("shovel") was produced as [tʃʌvəl] (Spanish-influenced English). The children also used the postvocalic "r" of GAE for the Spanish flap; /floɾ/ (flower) was produced as [floɹ] (English-influenced Spanish).

For speakers acquiring more than one language, the phonology of one language may have many effects on the phonology of another language. First, the specific phonemes and allophones in the inventories of each language are not the same. For example, the alveo-palatal affricate [tʃ] found in English is not in the inventory of Cantonese (Cheng, 1993). A native Cantonese-speaking individual acquiring English might substitute [ts] for the alveo-palatal affricate because [ts] exists in the inventory of Cantonese and is close to the place of articulation of the English affricate. Second, differences in the distribution of sounds exist across languages. For example, [ŋ] might be the only word-final sound realized in English by a native Hmong speaker because it is the only word-final sound in Hmong (Cheng, 1993). Third, consonants may have different places of articulation in each language. For example, Spanish speakers acquiring English may produce /d/ with a dental place of articulation, as is common in Spanish, rather than an alveolar place of articulation, which is typical in English (Perez, 1994). Fourth, phonological rules may be different in each language. For example, the phrase *cómo se llama su niño?* (what is your child's name?), produced as [*komo se jama su niɲo*], in Spanish might be realized as [koʊmoʊ se jama su niɲoʊ] in English-influenced Spanish because the speaker is diphthongizing vowels, as is common in English. Finally, how and when pronunciation is acquired may contribute to the influence of one language on another. For some individuals learning English as a second language, their major exposure might be in school, where written language is being introduced. The lack of one-to-one correspondence between grapheme and phoneme in English may influence pronunciation. For example, the grapheme "s" in English is produced as [s] in *basin* and as [ʒ] in *measure* causing a speaker of Spanish-influenced English to produce both as [s].

Assessment Considerations for Children from Culturally and Linguistically Diverse Populations

In assessing the speech and language skills of children from culturally and linguistically diverse populations, the same types of information are gathered as for all children: case history, oral-peripheral examination, hearing screening, language (e.g., syntax, semantics, etc.), voice, fluency, and phonological patterns. The analysis of phonological patterns in children from culturally and linguistically diverse populations requires a determination of whether their phonological systems are within normal limits for their linguistic communities. Thus, the assessment must be approached with an understanding of the social, cultural, and linguistic characteristics of that community, always guarding against stereotyping (Taylor, Payne, and Anderson, 1987). One cannot assume that any individual from any geographical area or ethnic/racial group is a speaker of a particular dialect. For example, while one African American's production of f/θ in the word *mouth* may be regarded as a dialect feature of AAE, it would be inappropriate to make the same clinical judgment for another African American who also produces f/θ. The first speaker may be an AAE speaker, but the second speaker may not; therefore, the production would be considered a true error.

Speech-language pathologists must also differentiate dialect differences from phonological disorders. ASHA's position papers on social dialects, communication disorders, and variations officially acknowledge the distinction between a speech-language difference and a speech-language disorder (ASHA, 1993; 1983). A few investigators have attempted to determine whether scoring dialectal features as "errors" would penalize children for patterns that are, in effect, dialect features, thus artificially inflating their severity ratings. Four studies have specifically investigated the effect of dialect on the diagnosis of phonological disorders in children. In their examination of 10 AAE-speaking children aged 5;11–6;11, Cole and Taylor (1990) found that not taking dialect into account resulted in the misdiagnosis of phonological disorder for half the children, on average, across three phonological assessments. Two other studies, while advocating that dialect should be accounted for in phonological assessment, did not show results similar to those reported by Cole and Taylor. Fleming and Hartman (1989) examined seventy-two 4-year-old AAE speakers using the *Computer Assessment of Phonological Processes* (CAPP) (Hodson, 1985). They determined that although some test items are influenced by "Black English phonological rules," the assessment as a whole is not invalidated (p. 28). Moreover, they indicated that no typically developing child was labeled as having a disorder based solely on the factor of dialect. Washington and Craig (1992) examined 28 preschool AAE-speaking children aged 4;6–5;3. Their results indicated that dialect scoring changes did "not seem to penalize the

BE-speaking preschooler to a degree that is clinically significant" (p. 203). Washington and Craig attributed the differences in their results when compared to those of Cole and Taylor to geographical location. The subjects in Cole and Taylor's study were from Mississippi, and the children in Washington and Craig's study resided in Detroit. Goldstein and Iglesias (2001) examined 54 typically developing Spanish-speaking children and 54 Spanish-speaking children with phonological disorders to determine whether taking or not taking into account Puerto Rican Spanish dialect features altered the results of phonological analyses. The results indicated that if dialect features had not been considered, almost 75 percent of typically developing children might have been erroneously characterized as phonologically disordered. In addition, not considering dialect might have resulted in unnecessarily targeting for intervention phonological processes whose percentages-of-occurrence were inflated because of dialectical differences.

Although the results of the studies cited above came to somewhat different conclusions as to whether or not scoring dialectal features as "errors" affected severity ratings, these researchers all agreed that accounting for dialect features is a prime consideration in the assessment of children from culturally and linguistically diverse populations. Analysis of phonological information must be made, taking the child's dialect into account. Sound differences are errors only when they are in conflict with the child's dialect. For example, in the Puerto Rican dialect of Spanish, the production of /dos/ ("two") as [do:] would not be scored as an error because syllable-final /s/ is often deleted. The production of /floɾ/ ("flower") as [flo] would be scored as an error because syllable-final deletion of /ɾ/ is not a typical feature of the dialect.

To minimize the possibility of misdiagnosis, all phonological analyses must take into account the features of a particular dialect. Dialectical differences are not errors. To account for dialect features in any particular linguistic group, SLPs should (1) sample the adult speakers in the child's linguistic community, (2) obtain information from interpreters/support personnel, and (3) become thoroughly familiar with features of the dialects and language.

To minimize the effect of not accounting for dialect features on the phonological analysis of speakers from culturally and linguistically diverse populations, Stockman (1996b) has suggested assessing a "minimal competency core" (MCC), developed to decrease bias in the assessment of AAE-speaking children" (p. 358). MCC is defined as "the *least* amount of knowledge that one must exhibit to be judged as normal in a given age range" (p. 358, emphasis original). Stockman noted that MCC may best be used as a screening tool focused on a core subgroup of specific sounds. The phonological features core includes the following word/syllable initial sounds that are invariable in GAE and AAE: /m, n, p, b, t, d, k, g, f, s, h, w, j, l, ɹ/. Wilcox and Anderson (1998) found that assessing these sounds along with clusters provided enough information to differentiate typical from atypical speech sound development in a group of AAE speakers.

Goldstein, Iglesias, and Rojas (2001) adopted Stockman's notion of MCC to examine how typically developing bilingual (Spanish-English) children and bilingual children with phonological disorders produced consonants that were shared by the two languages (e.g., /b/ and /k/) and consonants that were not shared (e.g., /ɲ/ and /r/ [voiced alveolar trill] exist in Spanish but not in English; /θ/ and /ʒ/ exist in English but not in Spanish). The results indicated that bilingual children tend to be more accurate in producing sounds that are found in both languages. This pattern was consistent across both groups. Children in both groups exhibited a higher accuracy on consonants shared by the two languages than on those not shared. In addition, both typically developing children and those with phonological disorders exhibited a higher accuracy on manner of articulation categories in which there were more shared consonants than unshared consonants and a lower accuracy on manner categories in which there were more unshared consonants than shared consonants.

Examiners must be aware of their own dialects and their effect on the assessment process. Seymour and Seymour (1977) noted that the client's perception of the formality of the situation affects dialect density. Casual speaking settings may increase dialect density by encouraging more frequent use of AAE, while a more formal setting may result in a decrease by inhibiting and stigmatizing speech forms other than GAE. A similar issue may be encountered when a clinician uses Castillian Spanish (i.e., the standard dialect of Spanish spoken in Spain and taught in most educational systems in the United States) when conversing to a speaker of any of the other major Spanish dialects. This is not to say that one must use the client's dialect. One must realize, however, the potential effect that a particular dialect may have on a client and family.

The assessment of individuals who speak a language other than or in addition to English presents a challenge to the SLP. The SLP must determine the language or languages of assessment and then choose appropriate assessment tools. Assuming that the individual speaks two languages, the clinician could assess in: (1) their home language (L_1) only, (2) their second language (L_2) only, or (3) L_1 and L_2. Even if the child seems to be a "dominant" English speaker, it is common practice to assess phonological skills in both languages (Goldstein, 2001). Analyses then should be completed in L_1 and L_2. The speech-language pathologist must then differentiate speech sound differences that result from the influences that one language has on the other.

A detailed phonological assessment includes both formal measures (instruments standardized on speakers from a particular language group) and informal measures (such as a spontaneous language sample). The formal assessment tool should be designed specifically to assess phonological patterns in that language. Unfortunately, few formal measures covering a variety of languages exist. Using an assessment tool designed for any linguistic group other than the one for which it was intended will likely increase bias and lead to over-referral. In the absence of formal measures, the SLP might utilize informal client observations with siblings, peers, and/or parent(s), asking a series of questions designed to determine the adequacy of the child's phonological system (Yavas and Goldstein, 1998): Does the child sound like other children in his or her peer group (i.e., like other members of their speech community)? What consonants does the child produce (front versus back, syllable-initial versus syllable-final)? Does the child make any vowel errors? Does the child use tone accurately? Is the child understood by parents, family members, teachers, and friends—all, some, or none of the time?

Role of the Monolingual Speech-Language Pathologist

Speech-language pathologists may have difficulty assessing children who speak more than one language (Goldstein, 2001). Those who do not speak the language of the individuals they are assessing might consider alternatives such as hiring a bilingual consultant or bilingual diagnostician, training bilingual aides, or using interpreters/translators (I/Ts). If I/Ts are used, SLPs should be sure the I/Ts are trained, have exemplary bilingual/bidialectal communication skills, understand their responsibilities, act professionally, and can relate to members of the cultural group (Kayser, 1995). They should assist the SLP in completing the assessment but not conduct the assessment themselves. SLPs may be tempted to use family members as I/Ts. Lynch (1992) advises against this practice because acting in this role may be burdensome to the family member, and family members may be reticent in discussing emotional matters, uncomfortable providing information to older or younger family members or to members of the opposite gender, and leave out information provided by the SLP.

In the absence of a bilingual SLP at the site, monolingual SLPs may also play a role in the assessment of non-English-speaking children. If they have knowledge, skills, competencies, and/or training in providing services to individuals with limited- or non-English proficiency, monolingual SLPs may assess in English, administer an oral-peripheral examination, conduct a hearing screening, and administer nonverbal assessments (ASHA, 1985).

Intervention for Phonological Disorders in Children from Culturally and Linguistically Diverse Populations

After the results of an assessment have been gathered, SLPs must decide whether intervention is warranted. The traditional role of the SLP has been to provide clinical services for communication disorders but not for dialectal differences. However, ASHA's position paper on social dialects identifies the following expanded role for SLPs (ASHA, 1983):

> Aside from the traditionally recognized role, the speech-language pathologist may also be available to provide *elective* clinical services to nonstandard English speakers who do not present a disorder. The role of the speech-language pathologist for these individuals is to prepare the desired competency in Standard English without jeopardizing the integrity of the individual's first dialect. The approach must be functional and based on context-specific appropriateness of the given dialect. (p. 24)

If elective services are indicated, it is important to remember that elective therapy does not necessarily mean that the client wants to eliminate the first dialect (D_1). More often the client prefers to be bidialectal. Taylor (1986) suggested a number of principles designed for SLP's who seek to guide speakers who want to acquire a second dialect: (1) develop a positive attitude toward the home dialect, (2) compare the features of the home dialect to the one being acquired, (3) select targets based on language acquisition norms and frequency of occurrence of the features, (4) know the speaker's attitude towards the features, (5) know the rules of the speaker's home dialect and the ones to be acquired, (6) take the speaker's learning style into account, and (7) integrate language issues into the larger culture of the speaker. Taylor also proposed a series of steps for maintaining both dialects. First, a positive attitude toward D_1 must be established. Second, the client must learn to contrast the features of the first dialect and second dialect (D_2). Finally, the client should use D_2 in controlled, structured, and eventually spontaneous situations, with a focus on form, content, and use.

Modifying someone's dialect involves more than simply having them produce consonants and vowels as a native speaker would pronounce them. Learning nonsegmental aspects of speech production such as stress, pitch, and intonation are equally important. There are likely to be differences between the person's home language/dialect and the variety being acquired as a second language/dialect. For example, stress in English is relatively more complicated than in other languages. Placement of stress depends on a number of factors, including syntactic category and weight of the syllable (i.e., whether or not the vowel is long or short and the number of consonants that follow the vowel) (Goodluck, 1991). Pitch also differs as a function of language. For example, pitch modulates less in Spanish than it does in English (Hadlich, Holton, and Montes, 1968). Finally, intonational contours for statements, questions, and exclamations may be different in English than in other languages. For example, in English, utterances (statements, questions, and exclamations) may begin at an overall higher pitch than in other languages.

Speech-language pathologists must also recognize how dialectal variation and phonological disorder interact (Wolfram, 1994). Wolfram has suggested the following guiding principles. He divided impairments into three types. **Type I** impairments are judged to be atypical patterns regardless of the speaker's dialect, (for example, initial consonant deletion (e.g., [it] for /mit/) or velar fronting (e.g., [dot] for /got/). **Type II** impairments show a cross-dialectal difference in the normative (or underlying) form. For example, the normative form for the word *bathing* would be [beðɪŋ] for speakers of GAE but [beviŋ] for AAE speakers, even though speakers from both dialect groups might misarticulate that word as [beziŋ]. **Type III** impairments influence forms shared across dialects but applied with different frequency. For example, syllable-final cluster reduction is exhibited in many dialects, but more frequently in AAE than in other dialects. Wolfram noted that treating a Type I impairment does not necessitate gathering different norms across dialect groups. The treatment of Type II and Type III impairments, however, involves taking into account both qualitative and quantitative differences between dialect groups.

Intervention for Individuals Speaking a Language in Addition to or Other than English

Little information is available to direct intervention for individuals with phonological disorders who speak a language other than or in addition to English. There is no reason to suspect that the principles guiding intervention choices for bilingual children would differ from those designed for children from culturally and linguistically diverse populations, though data to support this statement does not exist. There are, however, a number of guidelines that SLPs might follow (Beaumont, 1992; Goldstein, 2000; Langdon, 1995; Yavas and Goldstein, 1998). The clinical management process should begin with an appropriate and least-biased assessment. SLPs should:

1. take a person's cultural values and learning style into account;
2. ask for help from colleagues, parents, teachers, and others, if necessary;
3. enter the classroom to view children in a naturalistic context;
4. possess knowledge of the community's dialectal features;
5. take the child's dialect into account;

6. use least-biased assessment tools; and
7. complete phonological analyses in both L_1 and L_2.

Speech-language pathologists should remember neither to use normative phonological data gathered from English-speaking children to assess children who speak a language other than or in addition to English, nor to generalize developmental phonological data from one dialect group to another. Second, they should apply sensitive intervention techniques. That is, the remediation approach may need to vary depending on a number of factors, including the child's age, language status (monolingual L_1, bilingual, etc.), length of exposure to L_1/L_2, and dialect (Perez, 1994). Third, SLPs must decide in which language (or languages) to treat the phonological disorder.

It is often difficult to determine in which language to intervene. There are little data to indicate when intervention for a phonological disorder should be conducted in L_1 versus L_2. Much of our knowledge in this area comes from information on treating language disorders in children from culturally and linguistically diverse populations. A number of factors might be taken into account when deciding in which language to treat (Beaumont, 1992). These include: length of residency, motivation, age, length of exposure to L_1 and L_2, family's goals, and language of the child's peers. For language disorders, Beaumont (1992) has indicated that intervention in L_1 is warranted if it is the "dominant" language, it is used for several aspects of communication, more concepts are known in L_1, background and past experiences are coded in L_1, and L_1 reflects the cultural environment of the child. Roseberry-McKibbin (1995) has suggested that SLPs attempt to answer the following questions to help determine language of intervention:

■ What is the child's proficiency in L_1 and in English?
■ What means are available for conducting intervention in L_1?
■ What language is spoken in the home? By whom? In what situations? With whom does the individual need to communicate in L_1 and in English?
■ Do the parents want L_1 to be maintained?
■ Does the individual want to use and maintain L_1?
■ What support is there from the school system to use L_1 at school?

Given that these suggestions and questions are designed to guide intervention for *language* disorders, they must be interpreted cautiously in their application to the management of children with phonological disorders.

In choosing specific phonological targets for bilingual speakers, Yavas and Goldstein (1998) suggested that for a bilingual child with at least a moderate phonological disorder, SLPs should choose intervention targets based on the error rates in both languages. Initially, error patterns exhibited with similar rates in both languages should be targeted. For example, in bilingual children with phonological disorders, a pattern such as unstressed syllable deletion would affect intelligibility greatly in both languages and is likely to show similar error rates in both L_1 and L_2. Second, treat error patterns that were exhibited in both languages with unequal frequency. For example, final consonant deletion is a phonological pattern that is likely to be exhibited with a percentage of occurrence that is high in English but low in Spanish. Finally, phonological patterns exhibited in only one language should be targeted. For example, final consonant devoicing may be exhibited in English but not in Spanish.

Monolingual SLPs may also have a role to play in helping classroom teachers provide appropriate support to children acquiring English proficiency. Langdon (1995) indicates that if the classroom teacher speaks the children's L_1, the SLP can collaborate with the classroom teacher, observe and confer with the teacher and family members, and outline goals to develop specific concepts and communication skills. If the classroom teacher does not speak the children's L_1, however, the SLP can seek collaboration from an L_1-speaking aide and/or other support personnel and suggest techniques to aid in English language development.

Adapting Intervention Approaches to Individuals from Culturally and Linguistically Diverse Populations

Although there is little specific information to guide the intervention of phonological disorders in speakers of languages other than or in addition to English, specific intervention approaches developed for English-speaking children can be adapted for use with those from culturally and linguistically diverse populations. Clinicians will use a combination of motor- and linguistically-based treatment methods for such clients.

Certain aspects of treatment should be kept in mind with linguistically diverse populations. First, the SLP must be able to carry out the perceptual training phase of treatment, which includes the ability to produce an auditory model for the child potentially evolving sounds from L_1. Second, the clinician must be aware of the segments in the child's home language, the segments in the child's repertoire, and must prioritize treatment targets (order of acquisition of the sounds, ease of production for the sounds, frequency of occurrence of each phone in the language, and phonetic contexts that may facilitate production of the target sound).

Treatment will have to be adapted to the child's language and dialect. A number of approaches advocate the use of contrastive word pairs (i.e., minimal opposition pairs, *so/toe*, or maximal opposition pairs, *beet/seat*). Contrastive word pairs, however, may be difficult to adapt to speakers of languages other than English, which, unlike other languages, is replete with minimal pairs words. It may be more difficult to apply this methodology to languages other than English if those languages lack a significant number of contrastive word pairs.

Summary

To provide adequate and appropriate speech and language services to linguistically diverse individuals, SLPs should be knowledgeable about the dialects of their clients. Furthermore, clinicians must be aware that not all speakers of a particular dialect show or use every characteristic of it. It is common knowledge that the next 15 to 20 years will bring an increase in the number of individuals who speak a language other than or in addition to English. Regardless of whether or not services are provided in the individual speaker's first or second language, it is incumbent upon clinicians to become knowledgeable regarding the phonological rules of the first language and its dialectal variations.

QUESTIONS FOR CHAPTER 4

1. How would you determine whether or not the phonological patterns exhibited by someone were characteristic of true errors or dialect features?

2. Define pidgin, Creole, and dialect as they relate to language. What are the similarities and differences between these language varieties?

3. Create a quick reference guide for phonological development in AAE, Spanish, Cantonese, and Mandarin. You might list sounds in each of their inventories, age of acquisition for segments and tones (if appropriate), and age of suppression for phonological processes. Create a reference guide for a language/dialect not listed here.

4. Design a protocol for modifying the dialect of a native Spanish-speaking woman who wishes to sound "more like a native English speaker." List at least 10 questions you would ask her during the case history, enumerate the ways in which you would assess her speech, and outline your short-term and long-term goals, providing a rationale for each of those goals. What aspects of her speech do you think will be less difficult and more difficult to modify? Why?

5. Do you think newcomers to the United States who do not speak English should maintain their home language? Provide a rationale for your response. What are the advantages and disadvantages for immigrants to the United States who maintain/lose their native language?

6. Do you think all children should be given treatment so that they speak one dialect? Justify your answer.

7. Based on the following productions from a 4-year, 5-month-old African American-speaking child, place a check mark in the appropriate column, indicating whether the child's production is a dialect feature of AAE or a true error.

	Gloss	*Child's Production*	*AAE Feature*	*True Error*
example:	soap	[top]		✓
	mother	[mʌðə]		
	mouth	[maʊf]		
	tell	[tɪl]		
	self	[sɛf]		
	cool	[ku]		
	bell	[bɛ]		
	cool	[kũ]		
	playing	[pejiŋ]		
	fast	[fæs]		
	stool	[tul]		

REFERENCES

Acevedo, M., "Spanish consonants among two groups of Head Start children." Paper presented at the convention of the American Speech-Language-Hearing Association, Atlanta, Georgia, November 1991.

Adler, S., *Cultural Language Differences: Their Educational and Clinical-Professional Implications.* Springfield, Ill.: Charles C. Thomas, 1984.

American Speech-Language-Hearing Association, "Social dialects: A position paper." *ASHA* (1983): 23–27.

American Speech-Language-Hearing Association, "Clinical

management of communicatively handicapped minority language populations." *ASHA*, (1985): 29–32.

American Speech-Language-Hearing Association, "Definitions of communication disorders and variations." *ASHA, Suppl., 10* (1993): 40–41.

Anderson, R., and B. Smith., "Phonological development of two-year-old monolingual Puerto Rican Spanish-speaking children." *Journal of Child Language, 14* (1987): 57–78.

Bailey, G., and E. Thomas, "Some aspects of African-American Vernacular English phonology." In S. Mufwene, J. Rickford, G. Bailey, and J. Baugh (Eds.), *African American English: History and Use* (pp. 85–109). London: Routledge, 1998.

Bailey, S., "Normative data for Spanish articulatory skills of Mexican children between the ages of six and seven." Master's thesis, San Diego State University, 1982.

Beaumont, C., "Service delivery issues." In H. Langdon (Ed.), *Hispanic Children and Adults with Communication Disorders: Assessment and Intervention* (pp. 343–372). Gaithersburg, Md.: Aspen Publishers, 1992.

Bichotte, M., B. Dunn, L. Gonzalez, J. Orpi, and C. Nye, "Assessing phonological performance of bilingual school-age Puerto Rican children." Paper presented at the convention of the American Speech-Language-Hearing Association, Anaheim, Calif., November 1993.

Bleile, K., *Articulation and Phonological Disorders: A Book of Exercises* (2nd ed.). San Diego, Calif.: Singular Publishing Group, 1996.

Bleile, K., and H. Wallach, "A sociolinguistic investigation of the speech of African-American preschoolers." *American Journal of Speech-Language Pathology, 1* (1992): 44–52.

Bryant, T., S. Velleman, L. Abdualkarim, and H. Seymour, "A sonority account of consonant cluster reduction in AAE." Paper presented at the Child Phonology Conference, Boston, Mass., 2001.

Cheng, L. R. L., *Assessing Asian Language Performance: Guidelines for Evaluating Limited-English-Proficient Students*. Rockville, Md.: Aspen Publishers, 1987.

Cheng, L. R. L., "Asian-American cultures." In D. Battle (Ed.), *Communication Disorders in Multicultural Populations* (pp. 38–77). Boston, Mass.: Andover Medical Publishers, 1993.

Christian, D., W. Wolfram, and N. Nube, *Variation and Change in Geographically Isolated Communities: Appalachian English and Ozark English*. Tuscaloosa, Ala.: University of Alabama Press, 1988.

Cole, P., and O. Taylor, "Performance of working class African-American children on three tests of articulation." *Language, Speech, and Hearing Services in Schools, 21* (1990): 171–176.

Crystal, D., *The Cambridge Encyclopedia of Language*. Cambridge: Cambridge University Press, 1987.

Cunningham, I., *A Syntactic Analysis of Sea Island Creole*. Tuscaloosa, Ala.: University of Alabama Press, 1992.

Dalbor, J., *Spanish Pronunciation: Theory and Practice* (2nd ed.). New York: Holt, Rinehart and Winston, 1980.

De la Fuente, M. T., "The order of acquisition of Spanish consonant phonemes by monolingual Spanish-speaking children between the ages of 2.0 and 6.5." Unpublished doctoral dissertation, Georgetown University, Washington, D.C., 1985.

Dodd, B., L. So, and W. Li, "Symptoms of disorder without impairment: The written and spoken errors of bilinguals." In B. Dodd, R. Campbell, and L. Worrall (Eds.), *Evaluating Theories of Language: Evidence Form Disorder* (pp. 119–136). London: Whurr Publishers, 1996.

Fleming, K., and J. Hartman, "Establishing cultural validity of the computer analysis of phonological processes." *Florida Educational Research Council Bulletin, 22* (1989): 8–32.

Gildersleeve, C., B. Davis, and E. Stubbe, "When monolingual rules don't apply: Speech development in a bilingual environment." Paper presented at the convention of the American Speech-Language-Hearing Association, Seattle, Wash., November 1996.

Gildersleeve-Newmann, C., and B. Davis, "Learning English in a bilingual preschool environment: Change over time." Paper presented at the convention of the American Speech-Language-Hearing Association, San Antonio, Tex., November 1998.

Goldstein, B., "The evidence phonological processes of 3- and 4-year-old Spanish speakers." Unpublished master's thesis, Temple University, Philadelphia, Penn., 1988.

Goldstein, B., "Spanish phonological development." In H. Kayser (Ed.), *Bilingual Speech-Language Pathology: An Hispanic Focus* (pp. 17–38). San Diego, Calif.: Singular Publishing Co., 1995.

Goldstein, B., *Cultural and Linguistic Diversity Resource Guide for Speech-Language Pathology*. San Diego, Calif.: Singular Publishing Group, 2000.

Goldstein, B., "Assessing phonological skills in Hispanic/Latino children." *Seminars in Speech and Language, 22* (2001): 39–49.

Goldstein, B., and P. Cintron, "An investigation of phonological skills in Puerto Rican Spanish-speaking 2-year-olds." *Clinical Linguistics and Phonetics, 15* (2001): 343–361.

Goldstein, B., and A. Iglesias, "Phonological patterns in normally developing Spanish-speaking 3- and 4-year-olds of Puerto Rican descent." *Language, Speech, and Hearing Services in Schools, 27*(1) (1996a): 82–90.

Goldstein, B., and A. Iglesias, "Phonological patterns in Puerto Rican Spanish-speaking children with phonological disorders." *Journal of Communication Disorders, 29*(5) (1996b): 367–387.

Goldstein, B., and A. Iglesias, "Phonological patterns in bilingual (Spanish-English) children." Seminar presented at the 1999 Texas Research Symposium on Language Diversity, Austin, Tex., 1999.

Goldstein, B., and A. Iglesias, "The effect of dialect on phonological analysis: Evidence from Spanish-speaking children." *American Journal of Speech-Language Pathology*, (2001): 394–406.

Goldstein, B., A. Iglesias, and R. Rojas, "Shared and unshared consonants in Spanish-English bilingual children." Seminar presented at the convention of the American Speech-Language-Hearing Association, New Orleans, La., November 2001.

Goldstein, B., and K. Pollock, "Vowel errors in Spanish-speaking children with phonological disorders: A retrospective, comparative study." *Clinical Linguistics and Phonetics*, 14(3) (2000): 217–234.

Goldstein, B., and P. Washington, "An initial investigation of phonological patterns in 4-year-old typically developing Spanish-English bilingual children." *Language, Speech, and Hearing Services in Schools*, 10 (2001): 153–164.

Goodluck, H., *Language Acquisition: A Linguistic Introduction*. Oxford: Blackwell, 1991.

Hadlich, R., J. Holton, and M. Montes, *A Drillbook of Spanish Pronunciation*. New York: Harper & Row, 1968.

Haynes, W., and M. Moran, "A cross-sectional developmental study of final consonant production in Southern Black children from preschool through third grade. *Language, Speech, and Hearing Services in Schools*, 20 (1989): 400–406.

Hinton, L., and K. Pollock, "Regional variations in the phonological characteristics of African American Vernacular English (AAVE) speakers." Paper presented at the Texas Research Symposium on Language Diversity, Austin, Tex., 1999.

Hodson, B., *Computer Assessment of Phonological Processes*. Danville, Ill.: Interstate Printers and Publishers, 1985.

Holm, J., *Pidgins and Creoles, Volume I: Theory and Structure*. Cambridge: Cambridge University Press, 1988.

Holm, J., *Pidgins and Creoles, Volume II: Reference Survey*. Cambridge: Cambridge University Press, 1989.

Hyter, Y., "Ties that bind: The sounds of African American English." *ASLHA Special Interest Division 14 Newsletter*, 2 (1996): 3–6.

Individuals with Disabilities Education Act Amendments of 1997, PL No. 105–17, 20 U.S.C. Section 1400 et seq., 1997.

Jimenez, B. C., "Acquisition of Spanish consonants in children aged 3–5 years, 7 months." *Language, Speech, and Hearing Services in Schools*, 18(4) (1987): 357–363.

Kayser, H., "Interpreters." In H. Kayser (Ed.), *Bilingual Speech-Language Pathology: An Hispanic Focus* (pp. 207–221). San Diego, Calif.: Singular Publishing Group, 1995.

Labov, W., "The three dialects of English." In P. Eckert (Ed.), *New Ways of Analyzing Sound Change* (pp. 1–44). New York: Academic Press, 1991.

Langdon, H.,"Meeting the needs of culturally and linguistically diverse students who might have language-learning disabilities." Seminar presented at the First Annual Multicultural Symposium, Salem, Ore., April 1995.

Lau v Nichols, 414 U.S. 563,1974.

Lau Remedies, Office of Civil Rights, Task Force findings specifying remedies available for eliminating past educational practices rules unlawful under *Lau v Nicholas*, IX, pt. 5, 1975.

Leap, W., "American Indian languages." In C. Ferguson and S. Heath (Eds.), *Language in the USA* (pp. 116–144). Cambridge: Cambridge University Press, 1981.

Li, C., and S. Thompson, "The acquisition of tone in Mandarin-speaking children." *Journal of Child Language*, 4 (1977): 185–199.

Lynch, E., "Developing cross-cultural competence." In E. Lynch and M. Hanson (Eds.), *Developing Cross-Cultural Competence* (pp. 35–62). Baltimore, Md.: Paul H. Brookes Publishing, 1992.

Maez, L., "Spanish as a first language." Unpublished doctoral dissertation, University of California, Santa Barbara, 1981.

Martin Luther King Junior Elementary School Children, et al. v Ann Arbor School District Board, Civil Action No. 7-71861, 451 F. Supp. 1324, 1978.

Meza, P., "Phonological analysis of Spanish utterances of highly unintelligible Mexican-American children." Unpublished master's thesis, San Diego State University, 1983.

Moran, M., "Final consonant deletion in African American English: A closer look." *Language, Speech, and Hearing Services in Schools*, 24 (1993): 161–166.

Morgan, R., "Structural sketch of Saint Martin Creole." *Anthropological Linguistics*, 1(8) (1959): 20–24.

Muyksen, P., and N. Smith, "The study of pidgin and creole languages." In J. Arends, P. Muyksen, and N. Smith (Eds.), *Pidgins and Creoles: An Introduction* (pp. 3–14). Amsterdam: John Benjamins Publishing Company, 1995.

Muyksen, P., and T. Veenstra, "Haitian." In J. Arends, P. Muyksen, and N. Smith (Eds.), *Pidgins and Creoles: An Introduction* (pp. 153–164). Amsterdam: John Benjamins Publishing Company, 1995.

Nichols, P., "Creoles of the USA." In C. Ferguson and S. Heath (Eds.), *Language in the USA* (pp. 69–91). Cambridge: Cambridge University Press, 1981.

Núñez-Cedeño, R., and A. Morales-Front, *Fonología Generative Contemporánea de la Lengua Española* (Contemporary Generative Phonology of the Spanish Language). Washington, D.C.: Georgetown University Press, 1999.

O'Grady, W., M. Dobrovolsky, and M. Aranoff, *Contemporary Linguistics: An Introduction* (2nd ed.). New York: St. Martin's Press, 1993.

Oller, D. K., and R. Eilers, "Similarity of babbling in Spanish- and English-learning babies." *Child Language, 9* (1982): 565–577.

Pandolfi, A. M., and M. O. Herrera, "Producción fonologica distratica de niños menores de tres de tres años (Phonological production in children less than three-years-old)." *Revista Teorica y Aplicada, 28* (1990): 101–122.

Parker, F., and K. Riley, *Linguistics for Non-Linguists: A Primer with Exercises* (3rd ed.). Needham Heights, Mass.: Allyn & Bacon, 2000.

Perez, E., "Phonological differences among speakers of Spanish-influenced English." In J. Bernthal and N. Bankson (Eds.), *Child Phonology: Characteristics, Assessment, and Intervention with Special Populations* (pp. 245–254). New York: Thieme Medical Publishers, 1994.

Pollock, K., G. Bailey, M. Berni, D. Fletcher, L. Hinton, I. Johnson, and R. Weaver, "Phonological characteristics of African American English Vernacular English (AAVE): An updated feature list." Seminar presented at the convention of the American Speech-Language-Hearing Association, San Antonio, Tex., November 1998.

Poplack, S., "Dialect acquisition among Puerto Rican bilinguals." *Language in Society, 7* (1978): 89–103.

Poplack, S., "Introduction" In S. Poplack (Ed.), *The English History of African American English* (pp. 1–32). Oxford, England: Blackwell, 2000.

Ramirez, A., and R. Milk, "Notions of grammaticality among teachers of bilingual pupils." *TESOL Quarterly, 20* (1986): 495–513.

Rickford, J., *African American Vernacular English: Features, Evolution, Educational Implications.* Oxford, England: Blackwell, 1999.

Roseberry-McKibbin, C., *Multicultural Students with Special Language Needs.* Oceanside, Calif.: Academic Communication Associates, 1995.

Seymour, H., and C. Seymour, "Black English and Standard American English contrasts in consonantal development of four- and five-year-old children." *Journal of Speech and Hearing Disorders, 46* (1981): 274–280.

Shuy, R., "Social dialect and employability: Some pitfalls of good intentions." In L. Davis (Ed.), *Studies in Linguistics.* Birmingham, Ala.: University of Alabama Press, 1972.

Small, L., *Fundamentals of Phonetics: A Practical Guide for Students.* Needham Heights, Mass.: Allyn & Bacon, 1999.

So, L., and B. Dodd, "Phonologically disordered Cantonese-speaking children." *Clinical Linguistics and Phonetics, 8* (1994): 235–255.

So, L., and B. Dodd, "The acquisition of phonology by Cantonese-speaking children." *Journal of Child Language, 22* (1995): 473–495.

Stepanof, E.R., "Procesos phonologicos de niños Puertorriqueños de 3 y 4 años evidenciado en la prueba APP-Spanish (Phonological processes evidenced on the APP-Spanish by 3- and 4-year-old Puerto Rican children)." *Opphla, 8*(2) (1990): 15–20.

Stewart, W., "Continuity and change in American Negro dialects." In W. Wolfram and N. Clarke (Eds.), *Black-White Speech Relationships* (pp. 51–73). Washington, D.C.: Center for Applied Linguistics, 1971.

Stockman, I., "Phonological development and disorders in African American children." In A. Kamhi, K. Pollock, and J. Harris (Eds.), *Communication Development and Disorders in African American Children* (pp. 117–154). Baltimore, Md.: Paul H. Brookes Publishing, 1996a.

Stockman, I., "The promises and pitfalls of language sample analysis as an assessment tool for linguistic minority children." *Language, Speech, and Hearing Services in Schools, 27* (1996b): 355–366.

Taylor, O., "Teaching standard English as a second dialect." In O. Taylor (Ed., *Treatment of Communication Disorders in Culturally and Linguistically Diverse Populations* pp. 153–178). San Diego, Calif.: College-Hill Press, 1986.

Taylor, O., K. Payne, and N. Anderson, "Distinguishing between communication disorders and differences." *Seminars in Speech and Language, 8* (1987): 415–427.

Terrell, S., and F. Terrell, "Effects of speaking Black English upon employment opportunities." *ASHA, 25* (1983): 27–29.

Tipton, G., "Non-cognate consonants of Mandarin and Cantonese." *Journal of the Chinese Language Teachers Association, 10*(1) (1975): 1–13.

Tse, J., "Tone acquisition in Cantonese: A longitudinal case study." *Journal of Child Language, 5* (1978): 191–204.

U.S. Bureau of the Census, "Age by language spoken at home by ability to speak English for the population 5 years and over." Retrieved August 8, 2001, from http://www.census.gov/, 2000.

U.S. Department of Commerce, Bureau of the Census, *National Data Books and Guides to Resources: Statistical Abstract of the U.S.* (115th ed.). Washington, D.C.: U.S. Government Printing Office, 1995.

Veltman, C., *The Future of the Spanish Language in the United States.* Washington, D.C.: Hispanic Policy Development Project, 1988.

Wang, W., *Languages and Dialects of Chinese.* Palo Alto, Calif.: Stanford University Press, 1989.

Wang, W., "Theoretical issues in studying Chinese dialects." *Journal of the Chinese Language Teachers Association*, *25* (1990): 1–34.

Washington, J., and H. Craig, "Articulation test performances of low-income African American preschoolers with communication impairments." *Language, Speech, and Hearing Services in Schools*, *23* (1992): 201–207.

Washington, J., and H. Craig, "Socioeconomic status and gender influences on children's dialectal variations." *Journal of Speech, Language, and Hearing Research*, *41* (1998): 618–626.

Wilcox, L., and R. Anderson, "Distinguishing between phonological difference and disorder in children who speak African-American Vernacular English: An experimental testing instrument." *Journal of Communication Disorders*, *31* (1998): 315–335.

Wolfram, W., *Sociolinguistic Aspects of Assimilation: Puerto Rican English in New York City*. Arlington, Va.: Center for Applied Linguistics, 1974.

Wolfram, W., "Language variation in the United States." In O. Taylor (Ed.), *Treatment of Communication Disorders in Culturally and Linguistically Diverse Populations* (pp. 73–116). San Diego, Calif.: College-Hill Press, 1986.

Wolfram, W., "The phonology of a sociocultural variety: The case of African American Vernacular English." In J. Bernthal and N. Bankson (Eds.), *Child Phonology: Characteristics, Assessment, and Intervention with Special Populations* (pp. 227–244). New York: Thieme Medical Publishers, 1994.

Wolfram, W., and N. Schilling-Estes, *American English: Dialects and Variation*. Oxford: Blackwell, 1998.

Yavas, M., and B. Goldstein, "Phonological assessment and treatment of bilingual speakers." *American Journal of Speech-Language Pathology*, *7* (1998): 49–60.

Zhu, H., and B. Dodd, "The phonological acquisition of Putonghua (Modern Standard Chinese)." *Journal of Child Language*, *27* (2000a): 3–42.

Zhu, H., and B. Dodd, "Putonghua (Modern Standard Chinese)-speaking children with speech disorder." *Clinical Linguistics and Phonetics*, *14* (2000b): 165–191.

Phonological Awareness: Description, Assessment, and Intervention

LAURA M. JUSTICE
University of Virginia

C. MELANIE SCHUELE
Vanderbilt University

Introduction

Running speech consists of varying types of linguistic units that range in size from larger (sentences, words, syllables) to smaller (morphemes, phonemes). Most adult speakers of a language can readily and consciously recognize that the speech stream consists of sentences, words, syllables, morphonemes, and phonemes, and that these units are separate, recurring elements of language (Content, Kolinsky, Morais, and Bertelson, 1986). Young children, in contrast, have considerable difficulty recognizing that the speech stream can be segmented into words, syllables, and phonemes. For instance, 4-year-old children are seldom able to identify the number of words comprising a short sentence (e.g., asked how many words are in the sentence "Spot walks," children at this age are unlikely to respond correctly). Four-year-old children appear unable to recognize that the speech stream can be divided into smaller discrete and recurrent elements (Justice and Ezell, 2001). This linguistic awareness—referred to as phonological awareness—develops over time during the course of childhood.

What Is Phonological Awareness?

Phonological awareness is an umbrella term that refers to one's ability to identify the discrete linguistic units (e.g., words, syllables, phonemes) that the speech signal comprises. This awareness is **sublexical**, meaning that representation of these units occurs at a level distinct from meaning. This awareness is also viewed as being **metalinguistic** in nature, in that it involves the ability to focus on language as an object of thought. Children exhibiting phonological awareness consciously recognize (or at least are sensitive to) the variety of sublexical linguistic segments—including words, syllables, and phonemes—that serve as the building blocks of running speech. This type of metalinguistic awareness is contingent upon and mediated by one's access to the phonology of his or her language (Wagner and Torgesen, 1987).

Other terms, such as *phonological processing, phonemic awareness, phonological sensitivity, phonemic analysis, phonetic awareness,* and *linguistic awareness,* have been used more or less interchangeably with phonological awareness. Some scholars use the term phonological awareness only in reference to awareness at the level of the phoneme. Ball and Blachman (1991), for instance, specify that phonological awareness describes one's ability to represent spoken words and syllables as discrete sequences of individual sound segments at the level of the phoneme. This restricted use of the term phonological awareness, in emphasizing only that level at which conscious, explicit awareness of phonemes is fully realized, does not encompass more implicit levels of sensitivity to the phonological structure of language (e.g., sensitivity to syllables and words). A more encompassing perspective of phonological awareness includes reference to skills ranging along a continuum of **shallow** to **deep** levels of awareness (Stanovich, 1992).

Shallow Levels of Awareness

At more shallow levels, children show sensitivity to the sound patterns that recur across and within words. At these levels, children may recognize, for instance, that the words *ball* and *mall* demonstrate certain phonological similarities (i.e., these words rhyme). Likewise, children may recognize that *me* and *moon* also share phonological similarities (i.e., that these words share a phoneme in the word-initial position). With only shallow or implicit levels of phonological awareness, however, children would be unable to explain or otherwise account for the perceived similarities across such word pairs (i.e., they would not explicitly recognize that these two words share a common phoneme). In other words, the children are sensitive to the fact that the pairs *ball* and *mall* or *me* and *moon* share common phonological elements but are as of yet unable to consciously represent or reflect upon the discrete phonemic elements of these words, a level of skill that would be required to explicitly test such hypotheses.

Deep Levels of Awareness

At the opposite end of the continuum, representing deeper levels of sensitivity, children demonstrate more conscious levels of awareness regarding the phonological structure of words and syllables. With access to deeper levels of sensitivity, children are able to compare, contrast, and even manipulate phonological segments within and across syllables and words. Children with deep levels of awareness can compare the phonemic composition of *me* and *moon,* thereby recognizing that these two words share a common phoneme. Deeper levels of sensitivity also provide children the requisite skills for consciously manipulating words on the basis of phonological structure, such as modifying the word *baby* using Pig Latin conventions (resulting in *abyba*), or deleting the first sound in *track* to get *rack.* At the most sophisticated level of skill, children are able to analyze and segment words or syllables into their phonological segments (e.g., the child recognizes that *hot* comprises three

phonemes: /h/, /a/, /t/). The term **phonemic awareness** has been used by a number of scholars in reference to this most sophisticated level of awareness, the point at which children are
able to represent and successfully navigate words and syllables at the level of the phoneme.
Phonemic awareness is fully realized when children recognize that each word or syllable
consists of a series of discrete phonemic segments.

A Developmental Perspective

Recognizing that the development of phonological awareness occurs along a continuum
reflecting the transition from shallow to deep levels, with phonemic awareness representing the most sophisticated level of skill, is consistent with the perspective that children's
attainment of phonological awareness is developmental in nature (Stanovich, 1992). A
considerable body of research supports a developmental trajectory in the growth of phonological awareness, such that awareness of the phonological structure of oral language gradually increases over the course of early and middle childhood. Moreover, children's growth
in phonological awareness is highly mediated by both linguistic experience and language
abilities (Lonigan, Burgess, Anthony, and Barker, 1998; Stahl and Murray, 1994).

Phonological Awareness as Literacy Development

Phonological awareness has often been framed within the context of children's **literacy
development**. Although children's ability to represent and manipulate the phonological
structure of language consciously is highly mediated by linguistic influences and experiences, the fundamental role that phonological awareness plays in reading development has
encouraged many scientists and practitioners to study phonological awareness within the
framework of literacy development. The term *literacy* is used here in a general sense to
describe children's attainment of both emergent and conventional literacy skills; **emergent
literacy** refers to skills and knowledge serving as prerequisites to reading and writing,
whereas **conventional literacy** refers to actual skills in reading and writing.

More specifically, emergent literacy describes literacy skills that are acquired by most
children within the preschool and kindergarten period. This "range of skills developed by the
preliterate child lays the foundation for eventual print [or conventional] literacy" (van
Kleeck, 1998, p. 33). The two primary domains of development within this preliterate period
are **written language awareness** (knowledge about forms and functions of written language) and **phonological awareness** (knowledge about the phonological structure of oral
language). Children's development of both written language and phonological awareness are
viewed as legitimate and critical elements of literacy development (Whitehurst and Lonigan,
1998) and provide the foundation for their eventual attainment of conventional literacy. To
this end, preschool children with sophisticated levels of written language awareness and
phonological awareness are more likely to develop into proficient conventional readers and
writers as compared to preschoolers with low levels of awareness (Badian, 2000; Christensen, 2000; Stuart, 1995). Conventional literacy is typically acquired within the context of
formal instruction, usually beginning in first grade, or at about 6 to 7 years of age.

Historical perspectives of literacy development took the viewpoint—in both theoretical and practical terms—that children's acquisition of literacy skills began only within the

context of formal literacy instruction. Recently scientists began to study literacy in very young children and found that preschool children, as young as 2 and 3 years of age, possess knowledge about reading and writing. A substantial number of researchers in the last two decades have described what young children know about literacy, as well as determining how this knowledge is mediated by linguistic, cognitive, and environmental influences (for review, see Snow, Burns, and Griffin, 1998). Across numerous studies of literacy development in young children, a single set of variables—those representing phonological awareness—has stood out in terms of its robust value in predicting both early and later reading achievement.

The Development of Phonological Awareness

Serendipitously, the following conversation between a father and his son (who appeared to be about 4 years old) was overheard by the first author during the preparation of this chapter. The conversation took place in a local bookstore, where father and son were looking at the cover of a magazine.

SON: Is that a butterfly?
DAD: Yes, that's a butterfly.
SON: But-ter-fly. Hey Dad, is *but* a word?
DAD: Yes, *but* is a word.
SON: Is *ter* a word?
DAD: No, *ter* is not a word.
SON: Is *fly* a word?
DAD: Yes, *fly* is a word.
SON: Dad, is *ter* a word?
DAD: Didn't we just go through this?

This dialogue provides a perfect preface to discussion of how young children gradually acquire the ability to break the speech stream (in this case, a multisyllabic word, *butterfly*) into its discrete component parts (e.g., syllables, phonemes). In this particular instance, the child decomposed a multisyllabic word at the level of the syllable; the conversation suggests that the child was trying to make sense of how these smaller units (i.e., the syllables) fit into his existing knowledge of language structure (e.g., are these smaller units words? Do these smaller units carry meaning?).

Development of phonological awareness occurs on a continuum representing a hierarchy of sensitivity to the linguistic units that compose the speech signal (Hempenstall, 1997): (1) **awareness of words**, (2) **awareness of syllables**, and (3) **awareness of phonemes**. The order of the linguistic units to which children become increasingly sensitive appears to be based on the size of the unit, with words representing larger units and phonemes representing the smallest units (Treiman and Zukowski, 1996). Children's early sensitivity to larger units, such as words and syllables, represents shallow levels of awareness, whereas later sensitivity to phonemes represents deep or higher levels of awareness (Burgess and Lonigan, 1998). Evidence for this developmental continuum comes from a substantial literature base indicating that sensitivity to word and syllable structure occurs considerably earlier than sensitivity to phonemes (e.g., Fox and Routh, 1975; Lonigan et al., 1998).

Awareness of Words

Phonological awareness develops gradually in young children, with implicit levels of awareness (often referred to as *phonological sensitivity*) emerging between 2 and 3 years of age for most children (van Kleeck and Schuele, 1987). The earliest levels of awareness emerge as children begin to attend to the phonological structure of words as separate from meaning. At these early stages, they attend to phonological structure at the whole-word level by displaying sensitivity to phonological similarities shared by two words in terms of rhyme and alliteration. Sensitivity to rhyme and alliteration (the latter term referring to the sharing of a phoneme across two words, such as *b*ad and *b*ig) are viewed as the earliest benchmarks in the growth of phonological awareness, given that awareness of rhyme and alliteration are contingent upon one's ability to represent words as discrete units that can be analyzed on a distinctly phonological basis (Bryant, MacLean, and Bradley, 1990).

Awareness of Rhyme

The ability to detect and produce patterns of rhyme across words, observed in children as young as 2 years of age, has been viewed as a critical entry point in the development of phonological awareness (Hempenstall, 1997). Apparently, sensitivity to rhyme begins to emerge not long after children exhibit productive use of oral language. By 2 years of age, for example, children perform at levels greater than chance on rhyme detection tasks. Lonigan et al. (1998) administered a rhyme oddity task to 356 children, ages 2–5, in which children were asked to identify one word from a set of three that did not rhyme with the others (e.g., *fish, dish, book*). At 2 years of age, children performed with 41 percent accuracy. Moreover, there was little change in performance when comparing 2- and 3-year-old children, suggesting a period of relative stability in rhyme detection within this age range. By 5 years of age, performance on such tasks reached about 50 percent accuracy.

Other studies employing different methods for examining rhyme awareness in young children have reported similar findings. Chaney (1992), for instance, studied awareness of rhyme in 3-year-old children, using a judgment task. Children were asked to determine whether two words did or did not rhyme. Overall performance was 61 percent, surpassing that which would be expected by chance (i.e., chance alone would result in 50 percent accuracy). In the same study, children were also administered a rhyme production task, in which they were asked to generate words rhyming with a target word. Thirty-five (35) percent of the 3-year-old children were able to generate at least one rhyming word. Positive, significant intercorrelations between rhyme detection and production tasks suggested that both measures tapped similar underlying abilities.

These laboratory findings suggesting an early proficiency in rhyming ability have been supported by more naturalistic observations of spontaneous use of rhyme by preschool children. Dowker (1989) elicited poems from 133 children, ages 2–6. Many of the children's poems exhibited rhyme, even those of the youngest children: 32 percent of the poems produced by children under 3 years of age exhibited rhyming patterns, as compared to 46 percent of 6-year-old children.

In sum, rhyme awareness is viewed as one of the earliest indicators that children are able to consider the phonological structure of oral language at the level of the word. Sensitivity to rhyme can be measured in children as young as 2 years of age. The ability to detect and produce rhymes gradually increases in the preschool period; by 5 years of age, children often generate rhymes spontaneously during play (and on demand in language games or other literacy activities) and show general proficiency in rhyme detection tasks.

Awareness of Alliteration

Sensitivity to alliteration is also an early indicator of the advent of phonological awareness. Alliteration refers to the sharing of a phoneme (initial, medial, or final position) across two syllables or words. Each of the following word pairs exhibits alliteration: *mag/mop*, *tin/pick*, *rip/nap*. Sensitivity to alliteration, like rhyme awareness, reflects phonological awareness at the whole-word level. Such sensitivity is not viewed as phonemic in nature, given that children's recognition of phonological similarities across words does not appear to occur at the level of the phoneme. That is, presented with two words sharing a common sound (e.g., *pill* and *pan*), young children may be able to recognize a phonological similarity between the two words but would not be aware that the similarity occurs on the basis of a single shared phoneme.

By age 3, many children show sensitivity to alliteration across words. However, this awareness lags behind their awareness of rhyme. In the study cited previously, Lonigan and colleagues (1998) also examined alliteration awareness in 2- to 5-year-old children. Using an alliteration oddity task, in which children were asked to identify which of three words did not start with the same sound as the others (e.g., *bed*, *hair*, *bell*), children at 2 years of age performed with only 27 percent accuracy (a figure similar to that which would be expected by chance). By 3 years of age, performance increased only slightly, to 32 percent, although by four years of age, children performed with 43 percent accuracy. At 5 years of age, children were able to perform such tasks with greater than 50 percent accuracy.

Production tasks have also been used to investigate young children's awareness of alliteration. Chaney (1992) asked 3-year-old children to produce words starting with the same sound as a target word: 30 percent of 3-year-old children were able to generate at least one word beginning with the target initial phoneme. This propensity toward alliteration by very young children was also described by Dowker (1989). Examining the elicited poems of children ranging from 2 to 6 years of age, Dowker found that even 2-year-old children used alliteration with some frequency in their poems (27 percent of her 2-year-old sample used alliterative devices). In fact, children who were 2 years of age used alliteration with the same frequency as older subjects.

Awareness of Syllables

Soon after children demonstrate sensitivity to phonological structure at the level of the word, increased awareness of the internal elements of word structure occurs. Initially, children begin to recognize that multisyllabic words can be segmented at the level of the syllable (e.g., that *butterfly* can be broken into three parts). Subsequently, they show increased sensitivity to distinctions within intrasyllabic units, that is, the linguistic units of syllables. The structure of the syllable in the English language can be distinguished on the basis of a naturally occurring onset-rime distinction (Treiman, Fowler, Gross, Berch, and Weatherston, 1995). *Onset* refers to the consonant or consonant cluster that precedes the vowel in a syllable, whereas the *rime* encompasses the vowel and any subsequent consonants. For example, the onset of the word *hog* is "h" and the rime is "og." Likewise, the onset of *stripe* is "str" and the rime is "ipe." Studies have shown that the onset and rime compose natural boundaries governing the internal structure of the syllabic unit (Treiman and Zukowski, 1990).

Usually around 4 years of age, children begin to exhibit explicit awareness of syllabic distinctions within multisyllabic words (i.e., that *hotdog* can be readily divided into *hot* and *dog*, or that *baby* can be segmented into *ba - by*). Moats's (2000) review of a number of studies of phonological awareness in young children indicated that 50 percent of 4-year-olds and 90 percent of 5-year-olds can count the number of syllables in a word. During the same period, children also begin to display intrasyllabic representations coinciding with the onset-rime distinction governing the internal structure of syllables (Treiman, 1983, 1985). The primacy of the onset-rime distinction in children's growth of phonological awareness is suggested by studies showing greater facility in isolating initial phonemes as compared to final phonemes (Kirtley, Bryant, MacLean, and Bradley, 1989; Treiman, 1983). That is, children initially represent syllables as comprising only two elements—the onset and the rime—in which the rime is perceived as a single structure rather than a unit consisting of a series of phonemes (i.e., the vowel and all following consonants). Likewise, onsets comprising more than a single phoneme (e.g., the onset in *splat* consists of three phonemes) are viewed as a single unit.

Specific patterns govern children's growth in sensitivity to intrasyllabic units. In the early stages of sensitivity to syllable structure (when children are not yet perceiving phonemes as the basic linguistic unit), children show greater facility at segmenting syllables into onsets and rimes when onsets occur as singleton consonants rather than consonant clusters (Treiman, 1983). For instance, children are more likely to be able to segment *tar* into an onset and rime as compared to *star*. They are also more proficient at comparing and contrasting initial phonemes across two words if the words share a common vowel, such as *cup/cut* versus *cup/cat*; the identification of a similarity across the latter pair would be more difficult (Kirtley et al., 1989). In addition, children show substantially greater performance at comparing and contrasting final phonemes across syllables or monosyllabic words if the two words share a common vowel (in other words, the two words share a rime or rhyme: Kirtley et al., 1989). For instance, children are much better at identifying a final phoneme commonality for *map* and *tap* than for *map* and *tip*.

To summarize, children are able to represent and manipulate syllables on the basis of onset-rime distinctions by about 4 and 5 years of age (Fox and Routh, 1980; Treiman and Baron, 1981). The ability to represent syllables as comprising smaller units (onsets and rimes) appears after children first demonstrate sensitivity to phonological structure at the word level. Pursuant to developmental trends showing that sensitivity to word structure precedes sensitivity to syllable structure, performance on rhyming and alliteration tasks at this time tends to be superior to performance on tasks requiring syllable manipulation (Fox and Routh, 1975). To some extent, children's facility with onset-rime distinctions may be explained by their skills in rhyme analysis, although some authors contend that the reverse is true (see Treiman, 1983). Sensitivity to the onset-rime distinction appears to facilitate children's phonological awareness, providing the framework for analysis at the level of the phoneme.

Awareness of Phonemes

True phonemic awareness—the ability to identify phonemes as the units comprising syllables and words—is typically not seen in children until about 6 or 7 years of age (Ball, 1993). Phonemic awareness can be viewed as the most sophisticated level of phonological awareness. There is considerable overlap between children's development of phonemic awareness and learning to read. Consequently, there is controversy regarding the relationship between reading instruction and phonemic awareness (Johnston, Anderson, and Holligan, 1996; Morais, Cary, Alegria, and Bertelson, 1979; Vandervelden and Siegel, 1995; Wagner and Torgesen, 1987). Some researchers contend that reading development is driven by phonemic awareness, a view that asserts a causal relationship between phonemic awareness and reading ability. Such perspectives argue that at least some level of phonemic awareness is required for reading. Other researchers assert that phonemic awareness and reading skill develop in a reciprocal, rather than causal, manner. Evidence showing that phonemic awareness skills increase reciprocally and concomitantly with reading proficiency provides support for this argument. A position representing both perspectives is that a certain level of phonemic awareness is required for the development of reading skill, but that subsequently phonemic awareness and reading ability develop in a reciprocal and interrelated manner.

Phonemic Analysis and Synthesis

Phonemic awareness comprises two areas of growth: phonemic analysis and phonemic synthesis (Torgesen, Morgan, and Davis, 1992). Both areas of skill represent an explicit awareness of the relationship between phonemes and syllables or words; that is, the accurate representation of phonemes as the building blocks of these larger linguistic units. *Phonemic analysis*, also referred to as *phoneme segmentation*, is the ability to sequentially isolate all of the individual sounds in a syllable or word. *Phonemic synthesis* is the ability to take a sequence of phonemes and build them into a larger linguistic unit.

Using the word *pond*, for example, a phonemic analysis task requires that a child break the word into its component phonemes and express those four phonemes in sequence: /p/ . . . /a/ . . . /n/ . . . /d/. In contrast, a phonemic synthesis task involves presenting a series of four phonemes to the child (in this case, /p/, /a/, /n/, and /d/) and asking the child to combine the sounds into a word. Skills in both phonemic analysis and synthesis are critical requisites for learning to read.

There is a developmental trend in children's performance on phonemic analysis and synthesis tasks, such that their ability to analyze and synthesize phonemic segments within syllables and words increases gradually from about 6 to 10 years of age. In general, performance on phonemic synthesis tasks is superior to that on analysis tasks. Laboratory studies of phonemic synthesis have shown that kindergarten children perform these tasks with about 32 percent accuracy, whereas first graders demonstrate about 74 percent accuracy (Vandervelden and Siegel, 1995). By second grade, children perform such tasks with nearly 100 percent accuracy.

In contrast, phonemic analysis skills develop much more gradually and performance is highly mediated by the complexity of the linguistic units being analyzed. Nation and Hulme (1997) asked first, second, and third graders to segment 12 spoken nonsense words (e.g., /san/, /gat/) into their component phonemes. First-grade children performed nonsense words with 20 percent accuracy, second graders with 22 percent accuracy, and third graders with 25 percent accuracy. Although these figures suggest overall low levels of performance on analysis tasks, the nonsense words varied considerably in terms of phonemic complexity. Item analyses indicated that third-grade children performed with 100 percent accuracy in analyzing CVC words (consonant-vowel-consonant), about 80 percent for CCVC words, 65 percent for CCVCC words, and approximately 60 percent for CCCVCC words. Thus, although children clearly demonstrate phonemic analysis skills by the end of first grade, performance is influenced by the phonemic complexity of individual words. Skills in phonemic analysis continue to improve over the next several years of literacy exposure, with children showing gradually increasing proficiency in analyzing the phonemic structure of more complex words. Children who are unable to perform such synthesis and analysis tasks typically show difficulty on more conventional reading tasks.

Phonemic analysis and synthesis tasks examine the extent to which children have acquired adequate representations of phonemes as the discrete elements of syllables and words. After children have these representations in place, they also acquire skills in manipulating phonemes. Examining children's abilities to manipulate phonemes demonstrates the depth and robustness of their phonemic representations. Calfee, Lindamood, and Lindamood (1973), in a seminal work, examined the attainment of these more sophisticated levels of phonemic awareness in a study of 660 children from kindergarten through 12th grade. These researchers asked children to manipulate colored blocks representing the phonemic arrangements of nonsense syllables. In one set of tasks, representing phonemic analysis, children were presented with a sequence of two or three phonemes and were instructed to represent them in a linear sequence, using the colored blocks. In another set of tasks, representing phonemic manipulation, children were instructed to manipulate phonemes (using blocks) to represent various arrangements of a series of phonemes (e.g., changing /pl/ to /lp/ and /lps/ to /lsp/). Kindergarten children performed proficiently on the phonemic analysis tasks (with performance averaging about 50 percent), and by sixth grade, most children showed mastery of these tasks. In contrast, children's performance on phoneme manipulation tasks indicated marked difficulties, with performance approximating about 18 percent accuracy for the kindergarteners. Although children showed gradual improvement on phoneme manipulation across the grades, 12th grade students showed only about 60 percent accuracy.

Such findings indicate that although young children gradually increase in their ability to represent words as discrete phonemic segments, the ability to manipulate words at the level of the phoneme requires more advanced representational abilities. Some children never acquire full proficiency on phonemic manipulation tasks. Such circumstances have very practical implications: children's performance on higher-level phonemic representation and manipulation tasks is critically related to reading ability.

Phonological Awareness and Reading

As has been noted, young children gradually gain key insights into the way in which recurrent and discrete phonological elements compose the speech signal. Children first develop sensitivity to phonological structure at the level of the word and subsequently refine their representations to coincide with intrasyllabic (onset and rime) and phonemic boundaries.

Phonological awareness has been shown to be a good predictor of children's reading achievement.

To illustrate, in a particularly important work, Bradley and Bryant (1983) tested 403 children ages 4 and 5 in their ability to categorize sounds, that is, their skills in determining which word, of three or four words presented, did not share a common phoneme with the other words (e.g., *hill, pig, pen*). This measure of children's sensitivity to alliteration accounted for a significant and substantial proportion of variance in their reading skills three years later. Similar findings were also reported by O'Connor and Jenkins (1999). In this study, measures of phonological awareness (e.g., initial sound identification, rhyme production, phoneme segmentation) collected at kindergarten predicted differences in reading achievement at the end of first grade and identified children who would later have a reading disability.

The relationship between phonological awareness and reading is understood by considering the skills that are most critical for the beginning reader. Two areas of knowledge appearing most critical include letter name knowledge and phonemic awareness (Lomax and McGee, 1987). Faced with the task of decoding a novel word, the novice reader must know the distinctive features and names of alphabet letters in the word and must know its phonemic structure. In addition, and most importantly, the novice reader must bridge these two areas of knowledge by recognizing the systematic relationships between letters and phonemes (Vandervelden and Siegel, 1995). Skill in recognizing and using the systematic correspondence between letters and phonemes is usually referred to as *phonological recoding* (Vandervelden and Siegel, 1995) or *phonological recoding in lexical access* (Wagner and Torgesen, 1987). The successful integration of these two areas of knowledge allows the child to decode novel words. Children with limited awareness of letter names and/or deficits in phonemic awareness are prone to difficulties in reading (Stanovich, 1986).

Stahl and Murray (1994) sought to determine the amount of phonological awareness necessary for a beginning reader to negotiate novel words. These researchers found that the ability to represent syllables as onset-rime distinctions and to isolate phonemes at the beginning and end of words were prerequisites for beginning reading. In other words, children without these requisite abilities were unable to achieve or surpass preprimer instructional levels.

For children who are already readers, abilities in phonemic awareness continue to distinguish reliably between children who are proficient at reading and those who are struggling. Calfee and colleagues (1973) found that many older and struggling readers show consistent deficits in their ability to represent and manipulate words at the phonemic level. For instance, fifth-grade students who were struggling readers performed phoneme manipulation tasks with about 37 percent accuracy, as compared to about 80 percent accuracy for peers who were above average readers. Stanovich (1986) referred to this phenomenon as the Matthew Effect (that is, "the poor get poorer and the rich get richer"), in that the gap separating children who are proficient readers from those who are failing steadily gets larger over time.

This contention was supported by Juel (1988), who followed a group of 54 children from first through fourth grade. Juel found remarkable stability in reading achievement across these grades, such that "the probability that a child would remain a poor reader at the end of fourth grade, if the child was a poor reader at the end of first grade, was .88" (p. 440). In other words, children who experienced reading failure in first grade continued to experience failure in the next three grades. Deficits in phonemic awareness were important explanatory variables in distinguishing children who failed at reading from those who experienced success. At entry to first grade, children who subsequently experienced reading failure showed no skills in segmenting words into phonemes and analyzing words on the basis of phonemic properties. Such findings implicate the strong and reciprocal relationship between deficits in phonological awareness and the circumstances surrounding reading failure.

Phonological Awareness and Disorders of Speech Production

As a group, children exhibiting speech production impairment are at risk for experiencing difficulty in phonological awareness. This does not mean that all children exhibiting speech production problems will have difficulties with phonological awareness. Children with speech production problems specific to deficits in phonological rules are prone to experiencing difficulties with phonological awareness (Bird, Bishop, and Freeman, 1995; Webster and Plante, 1992, 1995). Children with phonologic disorders and concomitant language difficulties are at greater risk for difficulties in phonological awareness than those with phonologic impairment alone (Bird et al., 1995; Larrivee and Catts, 1999). Children with speech production problems that are articulatory rather than phonologic in nature do not generally display difficulties in attaining phonological awareness (Bishop and Adams, 1990; Catts, 1993; Levi, Capozzi, Fabrizi, and Sechi, 1982). Catts (1993), for instance, found that first graders with disorders of articulation performed similarly to a comparison group of typically developing peers on a variety of phonological awareness tasks.

Studies that have examined phonological awareness in groups of children exhibiting language impairment, many displaying concomitant phonologic impairment (e.g., Bird et al., 1995; Lewis, O'Donnell, Freebairn, and Taylor, 1998; Magnusson and Naucler, 1993), have shown that these children display less skill on a wide range of phonological awareness tasks than do typically developing children, including measures of rhyme and alliteration detection and syllable and phoneme segmentation. In general, the developmental trajectory of growth in phonological awareness for children with oral language impairment (phonologic or otherwise) appears to lag behind that of typically developing children.

The relationship of phonological awareness development and difficulties in children with phonologic impairment was studied by Bird and colleagues (1995). In this investigation, phonological awareness and reading abilities of thirty-one 5- to 7-year-old children with phonologic impairment were followed for a two-year period and compared to same-age peers matched on nonverbal intelligence. Children with phonologic impairment scored below the 10th percentile on analysis of expressive phonology attained from a continuous speech sample. Based on Shriberg and Kwiatkowski's (1982) criteria for identifying the severity of impairment, 23 percent of the children displayed a mild to moderate disorder, whereas 77 percent displayed a moderate to severe or severe disorder of phonology. Of the

31 participants, 12 had phonologic impairment alone and 19 had phonologic impairment in tandem with language problems.

Phonological awareness measures utilized in Bird and colleagues' study (1995) included rhyme detection (identifying the word from an array of four rhyming with a target word) and alliteration detection (identifying the word from an array of four starting with the same sound as a target word). In addition, measures of letter names, letter sounds, spelling, and reading ability were also collected on two occasions of follow-up testing (approximately one and two years following initial testing). At the time of initial testing, children with phonologic impairment demonstrated deficits in phonological awareness as compared to unimpaired peers. Children with phonologic impairment also demonstrated longitudinal deficits in sound-letter knowledge, spelling, and reading. More children with phonologic impairment exhibited such literacy difficulties as compared to the control group. The children with concomitant phonologic and language impairment were even more likely to exhibit widespread literacy difficulties than were children with phonologic impairment alone. These findings are consistent with reports by Lewis and colleagues (1998) and Larrivee and Catts (1999), which have shown that children with phonologic impairment and concomitant language difficulties are likely to have difficulties with phonological awareness (and literacy in general) and that such difficulties are more pronounced than those in children with phonologic impairment alone.

Bird and colleagues (1995) assert that problems in phonological awareness for children with phonologic impairment can be attributed to their inability to master the phonological system, which translates into difficulties representing the phonological structure of language. These children have particular difficulties perceiving phonemes as the basic phonological building blocks of syllables and are therefore unable to break syllables into phonemic elements (Bird and Bishop, 1992). In other words, "at an age when most children are discovering that letters can represent individual phonemes, children with phonological impairment are still unable to match words that share a common onset or rime" (Bird et al., 1995, p. 460).

Collectively, the research on phonological awareness for children with phonological disorders suggests several tentative conclusions, although further research on this population is warranted to better understand the impact of speech production difficulties on phonological awareness and literacy.

1. Children with phonologic impairment are more likely than unimpaired peers to experience difficulties with phonological awareness and literacy achievement. Children who are most at risk for such problems are those whose speech difficulties are still pronounced at the onset of literacy instruction (e.g., kindergarten and first grade). That is, those whose speech difficulties are largely resolved at school entry are at the least risk.

2. Children with phonologic impairment who have concomitant receptive and/or expressive language difficulties are at greater risk than those with phonologic impairment alone. These children are more likely to experience subsequent reading difficulties than are children with phonologic impairment alone (Bird, et al., 1995; Larrivee and Catts, 1999; Lewis et al., 1998).

3. Some children with phonologic impairment may evidence problems in acquiring phonological awareness, but these problems do not necessarily impact early reading development. That is, these children may not exhibit obvious difficulties in the early stages of literacy instruction. However, as demands in the curriculum increase over the elementary period, difficulties may become evident or more pronounced. Phonological awareness deficits may have their greatest impact on spelling, particularly around third grade and beyond (Clark-Klein and Hodson, 1995).

The Role of the Speech-Language Pathologist

Speech-language pathologists can and should play a critical role in promoting phonological awareness (and literacy skills in general) in preschool and school-age children exhibiting communication disorders (American Speech-Language-Hearing Association [ASHA], 2001). A guiding principle for doing so is the need for speech-language services to promote children's general academic performance and accordingly, to encourage children's successful transition to later and more sophisticated levels of educational endeavor (Fey, Catts, and Larrivee, 1995).

There is evidence that many young children comprising the speech-language pathologist's caseload are at risk for problems in educational achievement (e.g., Aram and Nation, 1980; Bird et al., 1995). Such problems may interfere with the attainment of critical literacy skills, given the important contribution of early literacy skills to children's later success in the academic curriculum. For this reason, it is imperative that speech-language pathologists make concerted efforts to promote children's skills in areas most related to both short- and long-term educational achievement.

The evidence presented previously in this chapter has made clear the very important contribution of phonological awareness to literacy and educational achievement in general. To this end, speech-language pathologists have been encouraged by ASHA (2001) to play a "critical and direct role in the development of literacy for children and adolescents with communication disorders" (p. 3). Primary roles and responsibilities include: (a) prevention, (b) identification, (c) assessment, and (d) intervention. An overview of these roles and responsibilities with respect to phonological awareness specifically is presented in Table 9.1.

Assessment

Two principles guide phonological awareness assessment and intervention with children with speech production disorders. First, all children should be engaged in experiences that sensitize them to language structure, with a focus on promoting sensitivity at the phonemic level. Second, children who lag behind their peers in phonological awareness attainment may need explicit phonological awareness intervention.

Implementation of the first principle suggests that assessment of phonological awareness is not always a prerequisite to addressing these skills in therapy. Young children develop phonological awareness through frequent and natural participation in literacy activities (Snow et al., 1998), and such knowledge is critically related to reading and academic

TABLE 9.1   Roles and Responsibilities of Speech-Language Pathologists: Phonological Awareness

Role	Responsibility
Prevention	Encourage development of phonological awareness in young children at risk. Prevention activities focus on preventing problems with phonological awareness before they occur, so necessarily focus on younger children. Primary focus is on high frequency engagement of children in naturalistic exposure to phonological properties of oral language (e.g., listening to nursery rhymes).
Identification	Locate children who are experiencing difficulties in phonological awareness attainment by: (a) observing children in phonological awareness activities, and (b) educating other professionals on strategies for identifying early problems with phonological awareness.
Assessment	Adopt a speech-language evaluation protocol that includes assessment of phonological awareness. Preschool assessment includes rhyme and alliteration awareness and emphasizes informal observation; school-age assessment includes syllable and phonemic awareness and can be accomplished using standardized or criterion-based measures.
Intervention	Implement curriculum-relevant and collaborative interventions that are individualized to target those aspects of phonological awareness that require attention for particular children. Intervention activities are developmentally appropriate, following the normal developmental sequence for phonological awareness (e.g., for preschool and kindergarten children, focus first on awareness of rhyme and alliteration, and only later target analysis at the level of the syllable and phoneme). For elementary students, training in phonological awareness should be combined with explicit alphabetic principle instruction.

Source: American Speech-Language-Hearing Association, *Roles and Responsibilities of Speech-Language Pathologists with Respect to Reading and Writing in Children and Adolescents*. Rockville, Md.: Author, 2001.

achievement. Thus, any educator working with young children should engage in "best practice" by involving *all* children in literacy experiences that facilitate phonological awareness. Thus, experiences that facilitate phonological awareness should be woven into therapeutic activities targeting the primary goal of improving speech production. Ultimately, the infusion of such literacy experiences should encourage a phonological awareness foundation so as to optimize children's later success at formal literacy instruction. In contrast, implementation of the second principle suggests several circumstances in which formal explicit assessment of phonological awareness might be undertaken for children with speech production impairment. First, some children may appear to lag behind their peers in general literacy performance, as indicated through informal observations by the speech-language pathologist, parent, or other educators. Poor phonological awareness may be at the root of poor literacy achievement. In such cases, formal assessment of phonological awareness is warranted.

Second, phonological awareness assessment is often conducted at transition points when it is expected that because of maturational development or instructional experiences, children will have acquired particular competencies. For example, many kindergarten programs explicitly target development of phonological awareness through such activities as recognizing rhyming words and identifying words beginning with a given sound. If in the latter half of kindergarten, a child appears to be struggling in such activities, formal assessment is warranted to whether an intervention program for phonological awareness is needed.

Third, phonological awareness assessment should be conducted for school-age children who exhibit any difficulty in written language, including spelling. Children with a history of phonologic impairment often demonstrate particular difficulties with spelling; such difficulties may be indicative of a linguistic vulnerability at the level of analyzing the sound structure of language (Clark-Klein and Hodson, 1995; Dayton, Mross, Keesey, and Schuele, 1997). For these children, a comprehensive assessment focused on determining the extent to which phonological awareness problems are contributing to such difficulties is recommended.

Lastly, phonological awareness assessment may be undertaken before and following a course of instruction or intervention so as to document progress and to determine the need for further intervention. Assessment options for this or any other purpose described previously include norm-referenced, standardized measures as well as criterion-referenced and dynamic assessment measures.

Norm-Referenced Procedures

Norm-referenced testing is used to establish whether school-age children exhibit adequate literacy skills for their age. Administration of norm-referenced measures also may establish a child's eligibility for special education services. However, for children already receiving special education services, norm-referenced testing typically is not necessary to document a need for phonological awareness instruction.

Norm-Referenced Measures: Preschool and Kindergarten.   The use of norm-referenced instruments is generally not recommended for evaluating phonological awareness in kindergarten children (or those who are even younger). The problem with using such measures at these ages is that children's scores are compared to those of peers in a normative sample on the basis of age rather than grade (ASHA, 2001). The school experiences of kindergarten children vary substantially across and even within school divisions, and to a large extent phonological awareness development is influenced by such experiences. In some kindergarten classrooms, for instance, children may receive extensive and explicit guidance in sound-symbol correspondence (e.g., the sound /g/ goes with the letter G), whereas in other classrooms, activities focus on rhyme and letter naming. It would obviously be unfair to compare phonological awareness performance of a child in the latter kindergarten program to one in the former because performance would likely have been influenced by instructional experiences. Children's phonological awareness skills should be based on local norms in lieu of national norms, or on alternative measurement strategies. In first grade and beyond, this concern is reduced because literacy-based expectations and experiences across schools tend to converge and be more similar.

Norm-Referenced Measures: Elementary and Beyond.   Several norm-referenced instruments for evaluating phonological awareness in school-age children have been developed in recent years. These measures provide norms for children's performance across age. Common tasks on such measures include syllable or phoneme deletion (e.g., *Say baseball without the ball*; *Say pat without the /p/*) and forced-choice tasks (e.g., *I'll say three words and you tell me which two start with the same sound.*). Although such tasks differentiate children with adequate phonological awareness from those who are deficient, it should be pointed out that such information is not designed to prescribe the direction for intervention planning.

In selecting a norm-referenced instrument, clinicians must consider the scope of behaviors that are evaluated. Tasks that evaluate exclusively phonological awareness involve the analysis or synthesis of the phonemes in syllables or words (e.g., *Tell me the sounds in* hot; *Put these sounds together to make a word: /h/, /a/, /t/*), and print is *not* involved. Although it may be desirable to evaluate phonological awareness in conjunction with written language or phonics skills (e.g., knowledge of sound-symbol correspondence, skills in decoding simple words), such tasks do not evaluate phonological awareness per se, but rather examine more broad-based literacy skills that may require phonological awareness abilities. To this end, some tests designed to measure phonological awareness go beyond it and measure other areas of knowledge and literacy development.

Table 9.2 provides a summary of three instruments widely used to assess phonological awareness in school-age children. These three measures use age norms rather than grade norms; thus one should be cautious when applying these norms to children who are young or old for their grade (i.e., their experiences may not be similar to that of their age-matched peers). The *Test of Phonological Awareness* (TOPA) (Torgesen and Bryant, 1994) and the *Comprehensive Test of Phonological Processing* (CTOPP) (Wagner, Torgesen, and Rashotte, 1999) were both developed from a research-derived model of phonological

TABLE 9.2   Overview of Three Norm-Referenced Phonological Awareness Tests

Test (Author)	Age (Years)	Tasks
Comprehensive Test of Phonological Processing (Wagner, Torgesen, and Rashotte, 1999)	5 to 24	Alliteration detection (initial and final sounds), phoneme blending, phoneme deletion (also includes measures of phonological memory and rapid naming)
The Phonological Awareness Test (Robertson and Salter, 1997)	5 to 9	Rhyme detection/production, sentence/ word/phoneme segmentation, phoneme isolation (initial, final, medial position), syllable/word/phoneme deletion, and syllable/phoneme blending
Test of Phonological Awareness (Torgeson and Bryant, 1994)	5 to 8	Alliteration detection (initial and final sounds)

awareness (or more broadly, phonological processing with the CTOPP) and tap only phonological awareness. *The Phonological Awareness Test* (Robertson and Salter, 1997) is also a commonly used measure of phonological awareness and is a more comprehensive measure, which includes subtests evaluating phonics knowledge (e.g., decoding simple and more complex printed nonsense words).

Such norm-referenced measures may prove useful in delineating the extent to which a child exhibits phonological awareness difficulties, compared to a cohort of age-matched peers. Intervention targets should not only be based on test results but should also be educationally relevant and developmentally appropriate.

Criterion-Referenced Procedures

Criterion-referenced measures are used "to determine whether the child can attain a certain level of performance" (Paul, 2001, p. 44); the child's performance is not compared to a cohort of age-matched peers, but rather to a particular local or curriculum-based standard. Several criterion-referenced instruments are available commercially for evaluating phonological awareness (e.g., Lindamood and Lindamood, 1971; Sawyer, 1987). In addition, the research literature also contains several descriptions of useful criterion-referenced tools (e.g., Ball, 1993; Ball and Blachman, 1991; Murray, Smith, and Murray, 2000; Swank and Catts, 1994; Yopp, 1988). One example of a commercially available instrument is the *Phonological Awareness Literacy Screening* (PALS) (Invernizzi, Meier, Swank, and Juel, 1998). This test includes both a kindergarten and an early elementary version and is used statewide in Virginia to evaluate the early literacy abilities of children in public schools. Phonological awareness tasks examine rhyme, alliteration (initial phoneme only) detection, and phoneme blending. Additional tasks examine invented spelling, word awareness, letter name and letter sound knowledge, and word reading. Children in particular grades who do not meet established performance benchmarks (e.g., at least 20 percent accuracy on phoneme blending tasks at the start of first grade) are identified as being at risk (i.e., needing additional literacy instruction). Field-testing of PALS has indicated that this test is helpful in the identification of children who are in need of additional instruction (Invernizzi, Robey, and Moon, 2000).

The goal of criterion-referenced measures is to determine children's competency in a specific area of phonological awareness, and clinicians can devise their own criterion-referenced tasks. Common tasks employed for such purposes are presented in Table 9.3. These more informal tasks can be used to identify children who are deficient relative to an established criterion, describe children's current level of performance (strengths and needs), delineate intervention goals, document treatment progress, and determine when intervention is no longer warranted.

The following presents several guidelines for evaluating children's performance on informal criterion-based tasks (Dayton and Schuele, 1997; Moats, 2000):

1. At the start of kindergarten, children should be able to perform rhyme and initial-sound alliteration detection and production tasks with at least 50 percent accuracy, and should be able to count syllables in words with nearly 100 percent accuracy.

TABLE 9.3   Common Criterion-Referenced Tasks of Phonological Awareness

Task	Competency	Example
Rhyme detection	Matching words on the basis of rhyme	*Which words rhyme: fish, hat, dish?*
Rhyme production	Producing words that share rhyme	Tell me a word that rhymes with <u>fish</u>.
Alliteration detection	Matching words on the basis of common phoneme	*Which words start the same: fish, fan, car?*
Alliteration production	Producing words that share common phoneme	*Tell me a word starting with the same sound as fish.*
Initial sound isolation	Identifying the initial phoneme in a word	*What is the first sound in fish?*
Middle sound isolation	Identifying the medial phoneme in a word	*What is the middle sound in fish?*
Final sound isolation	Identifying the final phoneme in a word	*What is the last sound in fish?*
Phoneme segmentation	Segmenting words into component phonemes	*Tell me the three sounds in fish.*
Phoneme blending	Blending isolated sounds into word	*What word is this? /f/ /I/ /sh/?*
Phoneme counting	Identifying the number of phonemes in a word	*How many sounds are in fish?*
Phoneme manipulation	Deleting or substituting target phoneme in a word	*Tell me fish without the /f/.*

2. By the end of kindergarten, children should be able to perform final-sound alliteration detection and production tasks with at least 50 percent accuracy. Children should be able to complete some basic phonemic analysis tasks, such as segmenting the initial phoneme from a simple word (e.g., saying "pig" without the /p/). Many children are successful at segmenting three-phoneme simple monosyllabic words by the end of kindergarten and generally children should be able to do this task in the early part of first grade.

3. Early first-grade children should show emerging skill in segmenting words that include consonant clusters (e.g., CCVC, CVCC), blending words consisting of two or three phonemes, and deleting initial and final phonemes from words. First-grade instructional activities (e.g., sounding out words, spelling) presume this level of phonological awareness ability.

Dynamic Assessment

The norm- and criterion-referenced assessment procedures described above can be classified as static assessment tools. That is, children's abilities are measured based on the number of correct responses on a particular set of tasks. Many clinical researchers have argued that static assessment provides only a limited view of children's capabilities (e.g., Bain and

Olswang, 1995; Olswang, Bain, and Johnson, 1992; Schneider and Watkins, 1996). In fact, two children who perform similarly on static assessments may have very different underlying capabilities. Dynamic assessment provides the means for obtaining a clearer picture of children's underlying competencies as well as their potential for learning new skills (Bain and Olswang, 1995).

Dynamic assessment examines children's performance in response to varying types of cues or prompts provided by the clinician. The goal is to determine how much and what type of assistance is required to encourage higher levels of performance by the child (Justice and Ezell, 1999). Knowledge gained from such dynamic assessments can identify children's underlying competencies and their short- and long-term propensity for change.

Spector (1992) described the use of dynamic assessment to determine how much assistance children required to segment words consisting of two or three phonemes. The dynamic assessment procedure was reported as more useful for predicting children's later phonological awareness and reading skills than were static measures. Table 9.4 provides an overview of this procedure. Lower levels of prompts (i.e., beginning with Prompt 1) are provided first to determine the extent to which children can do the phoneme segmentation task with only minimal assistance. Children who are unable to complete the task are gradually given more support by the examiner (e.g., Prompt 6 employs hand-over-hand modeling), until they are successful. Use of such a procedure stipulates careful attention to recording the level of assistance required (see Figure 9.1), so that the level of assistance can be gradually reduced as the clinician facilitates the child's movement from dependent to independent levels of performance.

Spector's (1992) prompting procedure can be adapted to assess other aspects of phonological awareness, such as rhyme production or alliteration detection. In addition, children's responses to the various prompts may provide insights into teaching strategies for therapy. Dynamic assessment can be used in conjunction with more static evaluation

TABLE 9.4   **Dynamic Assessment of Phoneme Segmentation**

Prompt	Instructions to Child
1	Tell me each sound in <u>fish</u>.
2	What's the first sound you hear in <u>fish</u>? (If incorrect, go to Prompt 6.)
3	/f/ is the first sound in <u>fish</u>. What sound comes next?
4	There are 3 sounds in <u>fish</u>. What are they?
5	Watch me. (Model segmentation of word using tokens as visual prompts.) Try to do what I just did.
6	Let's try together. (Work hand-over-hand with child using tokens to represent sounds.) Now try it yourself. Do what we just did.
7	(Model segmentation of word again.) Now try again to do it yourself.

Source: Spector, J., "Predicting progress in beginning reading: Dynamic assessment of phonemic awareness." *Journal of Educational Psychology*, 84 (1992): 353–363.

FIGURE 9.1 Record-Keeping in Dynamic Assessment

Segmentation Task		Trial	Level of Assistance Provided (Prompt Type)						
			1	2	3	4	5	6	7
moo	cv	1 2 3							
egg	vc	1 2 3							
hat	cvc	1 2 3							
high	cv	1 2 3							
ache	vc	1 2 3							
rack	cvc	1 2 3							
so	cv	1 2 3							
eat	vc	1 2 3							
mug	cvc	1 2 3							
toe	cv	1 2 3							
us	vc	1 2 3							
teen	cvc	1 2 3							

Source: Adapted from Spector, J., "Predicting progress in beginning reading: Dynamic assessment of phonemic awareness." *Journal of Educational Psychology, 84* (1992): 353–363.

strategies to derive more sensitive profiles of children's skills and to determine therapy goals and strategies.

Intervention

Several best practice guidelines for phonological awareness instruction can be gleaned from research over the last two decades (Torgesen and Mathes, 2000). First, phonological awareness activities should be provided in all early childhood instructional settings. Clinicians should provide phonological awareness experiences (and literacy development in general) as an integral part of therapy. Attention to phonological awareness can be embedded within all speech production activities, and clinicians should work collaboratively with classroom teachers and reading specialists to ensure that classroom curricula provide adequate classroom-based phonological awareness experiences. Second, children who have not attained adequate levels of performance at the end of kindergarten or the beginning of first grade should be provided small-group intensive intervention (Torgesen, 1999). For children exhibiting speech production problems, intensive phonological awareness intervention may be delivered by the speech-language pathologist. Third, for those children for whom small-group instructional intervention is not sufficient, intensive one-on-one instruction should be provided. Reading researchers have argued that if typical practice reflected what we know to be best practice, only a small percentage of children (less than 5 percent) would need intensive one-on-one instruction (e.g., Moats, 2000). The speech-language pathologist should play an integral role in promoting best practice by collaborating with other specialists, including classroom teachers.

Phonological Awareness Experiences Embedded into Therapy

Phonological awareness activities should be integrated into therapy for preschool and kindergarten children who exhibit speech and language difficulties. Phonological awareness is best provided as an integrated component of speech production tasks rather than as separate therapy activities. Speech-language pathologists can identify opportunities for targeting phonological awareness within the therapy sessions.

Some suggestions for including phonological awareness/literacy into speech sessions include:

- Write labels on pictures, and have children underline target sounds.
- Help children write stories that feature target sounds.
- Use an alphabet chart to practice target sounds.
- Play games and use books that feature rhyme and alliteration patterns.
- Use vocabulary that promotes attention to phonological structure (e.g., *rhyme, beginning sound, end sound*).

Opportunities to respond to and interact with the phonological structure of language should be provided as a matter of routine clinical practice for preschool and kindergarten children. Such instruction should *not* be contingent on the child's demonstrating deficits in phonological awareness. Phonological awareness experiences should be provided as embedded, implicit instruction aimed at the emergence of knowledge (in contrast to intervention that is focused, explicit, and aimed at mastery). The choice of activities should be guided by children's developmental age, current capabilities, and interests. Following are three types of phonological awareness/literacy experiences that might be provided:

1. *Opportunities to learn alphabet letter names and corresponding sounds.* Although learning letters and their corresponding sounds is not strictly a phonological awareness skill, to learn the alphabetic principle, children must coordinate knowledge about print form with that of phonological structure. Learning letter names and their corresponding sounds is an important step in literacy development. In addition, learning letter names for speech sounds is no less difficult or functionally and educationally relevant than learning to associate "the angry cat sound" with /f/.

   Some practical suggestions for promoting children's knowledge of letter names and corresponding phonemes include the following: First, when phonemes are targeted in isolation, pair letters with sound targets. Second, when targeting sound productions at the word or phrase level, use written words to accompany pictures or other, more functional stimuli. Written letters and words can serve as visual prompts or reminders of particular speech targets. For example, if the child is attempting to say sun and says tun, the clinician can point to the written word and the underlined target (i.e., *sun*) and use it to cue the child: "Oops. You forgot your sound. Put the /s/ at the beginning, not /t/. Here is the letter S to remind you." Such activities do not require that the child understand the alphabetic references in order to produce accurate speech. Rather, the comments clinicians make with reference to print and sound structure are provided alongside the typical cues and prompts used to elicit accurate speech production (e.g., target models, phonetic placement cues). The pairing of letters with their corresponding sounds can provide children extra exposure to the phonological structure of language.

2. *Opportunities to learn that sentences are composed of words.* When speech sounds are targeted at the phrase or sentence level, clinicians can provide many opportunities for children to experience words (both oral and written) as discrete units. Rather than practicing sentences as only spoken units, clinicians can use written sentences as stimuli (words can be paired with pictures) and assist children as they "read" their sentences. As the child "reads" each sentence, the clinician points to each word as it is said. The pointing emphasizes that one spoken word corresponds to one printed work and highlights the boundaries between words—both in written form and in terms of phonological or sound features. A recent study by Justice and Ezell (2000) suggested that parents' pointing to individual words while reading storybooks with their preschool children increased children's ability to recognize orally presented words as discrete phonological segments. Clinicians can readily embed similar strategies within the intervention context.

3. *Opportunities to learn that words consist of sounds.* Segmentation of language at the phoneme level is the most sophisticated level of phonological awareness, and it is highly related to reading success. Children enrolled in speech therapy may acquire some phonemic awareness as a natural by-product of participation in therapy, given that speech production activities, by their very nature, often provide opportunities to focus explicitly on the sound structure of language. However, clinicians can maximize the opportunities for children to analyze sound structure by deliberately exploiting opportunities in therapy sessions.

Simply modeling phonemic awareness behaviors can be beneficial for children. Clinicians can demonstrate the segmenting of words into sounds or sound sequences and the blending of sounds into words while simultaneously talking about the location of speech sounds in target words. Imitation of words divided into smaller segmented units may help children produce speech targets. For example, when targeting velar fronting, children may produce the much coveted velar in tandem with the alveolar, such that *comb* is produced as /k-tom/. Clinicians can respond with "Let's break that word into parts: /kom/ . . . /k/ . . . /o/ . . . /m/. Now you say it just the way I did /k/ . . . /o/ . . . /m/. Now let's push all those sounds back together."

The purpose of exploiting such opportunities during intervention is to provide repeated opportunities that might facilitate the child's phonological awareness. Astute clinicians take advantage of teachable moments to scaffold children's attainment of higher levels of phonological awareness.

Classroom-Based Phonological Awareness Instruction

Increasingly, explicit phonological awareness activities are found in the daily activities of preschool, kindergarten, and first grade classrooms. Providing phonological awareness intervention within the classroom can be an efficient and effective means for promoting these skills in all children, including those with speech production impairments. Service delivery in the classroom is consistent with providing intervention in the least restrictive and most naturalistic environment. Therefore, clinicians should review the school's curriculum to familiarize themselves with how phonological awareness is targeted. They may find that some curricula provide adequate instruction, whereas supplemental activities may be needed with others. Clinicians must work collaboratively with other educators to encourage children's frequent interactions with the sound structure of language.

An example of a successful classroom-based phonological awareness training program was described by Brady, Fowler, Stone, and Winbury (1994). Participants included 96 inner-city kindergarten children enrolled in four classrooms (two intervention, two control). Children in the intervention classrooms participated in an 18-week training program (three 20-minute sessions per week) conducted by classroom teachers (the two other classrooms followed the typical curriculum). The first four weeks of the program focused on training phonological awareness at the word and syllable level (i.e., rhyme production, rhyme detection, syllable counting); weeks five through eight focused on training awareness of phonemes in isolation; and the last ten weeks focused on phoneme analysis (e.g., blending, segmenting). An overview of the training program is provided in Table 9.5. Children in the intervention classrooms made substantially greater gains than their control group peers on an array of phonological awareness measures, including the ability to generate rhymes and to segment words into phonemes. Follow-up testing at the end of first grade found that children who had received the kindergarten phonological awareness intervention outperformed their peers on a set of early reading measures. Speech-language pathologists can partner with classroom teachers to implement this or other classroom-based programs (Hadley, Simmerman, Long, and Luna, 2000). These partnerships can be particularly effective in that they combine the speech-language pathologists' strength in knowledge of phonology and teachers' strength in early reading instruction.

Of interest to speech-language pathologists is the extent to which phonological awareness can be encouraged through classroom-based instruction for children with speech and/or language disorders. In one recent study, van Kleeck, Gillam, and McFadden (1998) evaluated the effectiveness of a nine-month classroom-based phonological awareness training program for preschool children. Of the 16 children participating in the experimental classrooms, 11 exhibited speech production impairment (nine of these children also exhibited language impairment). Over the course of intervention, children participated in approximately 45 minutes of phonological awareness activities daily; for the first 12 weeks of the program, rhyming skills were targeted, and in the final 12 weeks, initial and final sound awareness within and across words was targeted. The children in the intervention classrooms made significant gains when compared to a control group over the nine-month period on measures of phonological awareness (e.g., test scores on rhyme detection and production tasks nearly doubled).

Small-Group Intensive Phonological Awareness Intervention

Perhaps 20 percent of all children do not develop adequate phonological awareness by the end of kindergarten or the beginning of first grade. Children with phonologic impairment, especially those experiencing concomitant language problems, may be more likely to be in

TABLE 9.5   Sequence for Kindergarten Classroom-Based Phonological Awareness Training

Phase (Weeks)	Major Activities (Example)
I (1-4)	Rhyme awareness (listening to nursery rhymes)
	Rhyme production (generating words rhyming with a target)
	Rhyme detection (selecting words not rhyming with others)
	Word segmentation (dividing words into syllable components)
	Syllable deletion (deleting a syllable from a multisyllable word)
II (5–10)	Phoneme isolation (describing articulatory movements associated with each phoneme: e.g., /p/ is a "lip popper")
	Alliteration detection (selecting words not sharing a target phoneme with others)
	Phoneme deletion (producing words minus a target phoneme)
III (11–18)	Phoneme analysis and synthesis (identifying and manipulating the phonemes comprising words)

Source: Adapted from Brady, S., A. Fowler, B. Stone, and N. Winbury, "Training phonological awareness: A study with inner-city kindergarten children." *Annals of Dyslexia, 44* (1994): 26–59.

this 20 percent than children who have normal speech and language skills (e.g., Bird et al., 1995; Larrivee and Catts, 1999; Lewis et al., 1998). Children who are deficient in phonological awareness tasks in first grade rarely "catch up" to their peers without explicit, systematic, intensive phonological awareness instruction (Torgesen, Wagner, and Rashotte, 1994). It is important to identify children with speech production impairments who show substantial limitations in phonological awareness at the end of kindergarten and beginning of first grade, or older children with a history of speech impairment whose phonological awareness is below expectations. For both groups of children, phonological awareness training may be required. An efficient and effective model for delivering phonological awareness training is through small-group instruction (Gillon and Dodd, 1995).

The typical goal of small-group phonological awareness intervention is to provide children with a foundation of phonological awareness ability that can be built upon in formal literacy instruction. Phonological awareness abilities continue to develop and become increasingly complex as children become more proficient readers. A foundation of phonological awareness seems prerequisite to learning to read, but learning to read broadens and strengthens children's phonological awareness (Perfetti, Beck, Bell, and Hughes, 1987).

Numerous studies indicate that intensive small-group phonological awareness training results in improved phonological awareness and improved reading ability (e.g., Ball and Blachman, 1991; Byrne and Fielding-Barnsley, 1991, 1993, 1995; Dayton and Schuele, 1997; Gillon and Dodd, 1995; Gillon, 2000; Lundberg, Frost, and Peterson, 1988; Schuele, Paul, and Mazzaferri, 1998; van Kleeck et al., 1998; Warrick and Rubin, 1992; Warrick, Rubin, and Rowe-Walsh, 1993). In a study conducted in New Zealand by Gillon and Dodd (1995), ten 10- to 12-year-old children with previously diagnosed speech impairments received 12 hours of intensive phonological awareness training over a six-week period. Training activities focused on phoneme segmenting, manipulating, and blending, and employed Lindamood and Lindamood's (1975) *Auditory Discrimination in Depth Program—Revised*. Children made significant gains in phonemic awareness (e.g., 70 percent of the children showed mastery on phoneme analysis and synthesis tasks following training), and significantly improved their spelling abilities. Gillon (2000) expanded on this study in an investigation of the efficacy of an "integrated phonological awareness intervention approach" with children who demonstrated phonological and, in some cases, language impairment in addition to reading delay. She compared three groups of 5- to 7-year-old children, each of which received one of the following types of instruction:

1. Integrated phonological awareness training, which focused on phonological awareness (PA) but included sound contrast training and sound production practice on the child's speech sound errors as part of the PA activities
2. Traditional motor-oriented articulation therapy
3. Consultation of the speech-language pathologist with a child's teacher or parent (no more than once a month) regarding speech sound improvement activities (minimal instruction)

Gillon (2000) reported that the group receiving PA instruction made greater gains in phonological awareness ability and reading than did the children in either of the other groups. Although all three groups improved in phonology, the greatest gains were achieved by the PA group, followed by the articulation instruction group, with the least improvement in the consultation group. This study supports the concept of integrating phonological awareness activities and speech sound remediation.

A number of available curricula exist for organizing small-group intensive phonological awareness programs. One option is to adopt a general instructional sequence (e.g., Brady et al.'s [1994] program for classroom-based instruction, as described in Table 9.5), but to increase the frequency and intensity of instruction within the highly individualized context provided by small-group instruction. Two commercially available small-group intensive intervention programs that provide explicit guidelines for implementation, and thus can be easily and efficiently implemented, are the following: *Road to the Code* (Blachman, Ball, Black, and Tangel, 2000) and the *Intensive Phonological Awareness Program* (Schuele and Dayton, 2000). (See Torgesen and Mathes [2000] for a description and critique of additional programs.) These programs are recommended for use in the latter half of kindergarten or beginning of first grade. Small groups of about six children are provided instruction several times weekly for an extended period of time (e.g., four or five months). Instruction can be provided by speech-language pathologists, reading specialists, and regular or special educators.

The program *Road to the Code* (Blachman et al., 2000) provides a detailed curriculum for intensive phonological awareness instruction. Lessons are delivered four times weekly in 15-minute sessions for an 11-week period. The program was designed for children who are generally at risk for difficulties in early literacy achievement. The program consists of 44 detailed lesson plans, with scripts to guide implementation. Each lesson includes a phonological awareness (e.g. rhyme production), phonemic segmentation, and letter-sound correspondence activity. Investigators reported on the effectiveness of this program with kindergarten children (e.g., Ball and Blachman, 1988, 1991). They indicated that phonological awareness and word decoding skills improved significantly.

The *Intensive Phonological Awareness Program* (Schuele and Dayton, 2000) was designed to meet the needs of children with language impairments. Intervention sessions are three times a week (30-minute sessions) for a 12-week period. Skills are targeted in three-week blocks, and include rhyme, initial sounds, final sounds, and phonemic analysis and synthesis. Thirty-six lesson plans describe activities and provide detailed guidance on teaching strategies. Pilot studies (Dayton and Schuele, 1997; Schuele, 2001) have suggested that the program is effective in increasing phonological awareness and word decoding skills in children with language impairment. However, the efficacy of this program must be established by comparing a treatment group to a control group.

The extent to which such programs would be appropriate for children with speech production impairments has not yet been established. That is, the unique instructional needs of children with speech production impairments with respect to phonological awareness intervention are currently unknown. For example, in these programs it is suggested that children be guided to produce the instructional stimuli themselves so as to use articulatory feedback as well as auditory feedback in acquiring phonological awareness. However, children with speech production problems may be unable to produce particular targets correctly or may have faulty perception. At present, we do not know the impact of a phonological problem, and it is possible that a different model of intervention may be required to be maximally effective.

Intervention with Older Children

Research suggests that older children can increase their phonological awareness abilities with direct instruction in phonological awareness (Torgesen, Wagner, Rashotte, Alexander, and Conway, 1997). Thus, children in second grade and beyond who are struggling with reading and writing may benefit from explicit phonological awareness intervention; indeed, deficits in phonological awareness may be contributing substantially to many of these children's problems with reading and writing. In addition, some children who have moved beyond the early elementary grades may never have developed an adequate phonological awareness foundation. Other children may have rudimentary skills but fail to develop more complex phonological awareness skills (e.g., phoneme analysis and synthesis). For some children who have histories of phonologic impairment, this weakness may be most evident in poor spelling ability (Clark-Klein and Hodson, 1995). A thorough multidisciplinary evaluation of reading, writing, and phonological awareness will clarify children's needs (Gentry, 1988; Masterson and Crede, 1999). Subsequently, systematic instruction can be provided by clinicians, with specific goals and activities designed to meet these children's individual needs.

We can expect that explicit phonological awareness training will lead to improved phonological awareness for many struggling school-age children. However, how speech and/or language difficulties may impact upon the success of such intervention is not known. Current unanswered questions include: Are children with speech production difficulties hampered by their inability to produce words accurately in practicing phonological awareness activities? Will some children never develop adequate phonological awareness, to the extent that alternate reading instruction should be pursued? Research efforts in the years ahead will have to address these and related issues.

QUESTIONS FOR CHAPTER 9

1. What are some key indicators of phonological awareness in the preschool period?

2. What is the relationship between phonological awareness and reading ability?

3. Why are children with speech production problems at risk for problems with phonological awareness?

4. What is the speech-language pathologist's role with respect to phonological awareness?

5. What are specific strategies that the speech-language pathologist can use to promote phonological awareness during therapy?

6. What might a classroom-based or intensive small-group phonological awareness intervention program look like?

REFERENCES

American Speech-Language-Hearing Association, *Roles and responsibilities of speech-language pathologists with respect to reading and writing in children and adolescents* (position statement, executive summary of guidelines, technical report). *ASHA Supplement, 21,* 17–27. Rockville, Md.: Author, 2000.

Aram, D. M., and J. E. Nation, "Preschool language disorders and subsequent language and academic difficulties." *Journal of Communication Disorders, 13* (1980): 159–179.

Badian, N. A., "Do preschool orthographic skills contribute to prediction of reading?" In N. A. Badian (Ed.), *Prediction and Prevention of Reading Failure* (pp. 31–56). Timonium, Md.: York Press, 2000.

Bain, B., and L. Olswang, "Examining readiness for learning two-word utterances by children with specific expressive language impairment: Dynamic assessment validation." *American Journal of Speech-Language Pathology, 4*(1) (1995): 81–91.

Ball, E., "Assessing phoneme awareness." *Language, Speech, and Hearing Services in Schools, 24* (1993): 130–139.

Ball, E., and B. Blachman, "Phoneme segmentation training: Effect on reading readiness." *Annals of Dyslexia, 38* (1988): 208–225.

Ball, E., and B. Blachman, "Does phoneme awareness training in kindergarten make a difference in early word recognition and developmental spelling?" *Reading Research Quarterly, 26* (1991): 49–66.

Bird, J., and D. Bishop, "Perception and awareness of phonemes in phonologically impaired children." *European Journal of Disorders of Communication, 27* (1992): 289–311.

Bird, J., D. Bishop, and N. H. Freeman, "Phonological awareness and literacy development in children with excessive phonological impairments." *Journal of Speech and Hearing Research, 38* (1995): 446–462.

Bishop, D., and C. Adams, "A prospective study of the relationship between specific language impairment, phonological disorders and reading retardation." *Journal of Child Psychology and Psychiatry, 31* (1990): 1027–1050.

Blachman, B., E. Ball, R. Black, and D. Tangel, *Road to the Code: A Phonological Awareness Program for Young Children.* Baltimore, Md.: Brookes, 2000.

Bradley, L., and P. E. Bryant, "Categorizing sounds and learning to read—a causal connection." *Nature, 301* (1983): 419–421.

Brady, S., A. Fowler, B. Stone, and N. Winbury, "Training phonological awareness: A study with inner-city kindergarten children." *Annals of Dyslexia, 44* (1994): 26–59.

Bryant, P., M. MacLean, and L. Bradley, "Rhyme, language, and children's reading." *Applied Psycholinguistics, 11* (1990): 237–252.

Bryne, B., and R. Fielding-Barnsley, "Evaluation of a program to teach phonemic awareness to young children." *Journal of Educational Psychology, 83* (1991): 451–455.

Bryne, B., and R. Fielding-Barnsley, "Evaluation of a program to teach phonemic awareness to young children: A 1-year follow-up." *Journal of Educational Psychology, 85* (1993): 104–111.

Bryne, B., and R. Fielding-Barnsley, "Evaluation of a program to teach phonemic awareness to young children: A 2- and 3-year follow-up and a new preschool trial." *Journal of Educational Psychology, 87* (1995): 488–503.

Burgess, S. R., and C. J. Lonigan, "Bidirectional relations of phonological sensitivity and prereading abilities: Evidence from a preschool sample." *Journal of Experimental Child Psychology, 70* (1998): 117–141.

Calfee, R. C., P. Lindamood, and C. Lindamood, "Acoustic-phonetic skills and reading—kindergarten through twelfth grade." *Journal of Educational Psychology, 64* (1973): 293–298.

Catts, H. W., "The relationship between speech-language impairments and reading disabilities." *Journal of Speech and Hearing Research, 36* (1993): 948–958.

Chaney, C., "Language development, metalinguistic skills, and print awareness in 3-year-old children." *Applied Psycholinguistics, 13* (1992): 485–514.

Christensen, C. A., "Preschool phonological awareness and success in reading." In N. A. Badian (Ed.), *Prediction and Prevention of Reading Failure* (pp. 153–178). Timonium, Md.: York Press, 2000.

Clark-Klein, S., and B. Hodson, "A phonologically based analysis of misspellings by third graders with disordered-phonology histories." *Journal of Speech and Hearing Research, 38* (1995): 839–849.

Content, A., R. Kolinsky, J. Morais, and P. Bertelson, "Phonetic segmentation in prereaders: Effect of corrective information." *Journal of Experimental Child Psychology, 42* (1986): 49–72.

Dayton, N., T. Mross, S. Keesey, and C. Schuele, "Written language disability: The speech-language pathologist's role." Poster Session presented at the annual conference of the Nevada Speech-Language-Hearing Association, Reno, Nev., 1997.

Dayton, N., and C. Schuele, "Effects of phonological awareness training on young children with specific language impairment." Paper presented at the annual convention of the American Speech-Language-Hearing Association, Boston, Mass., 1997.

Dowker, A., "Rhyme and alliteration in poems elicited from young children." *Journal of Child Language, 16* (1989): 181–202.

Fey, M. E., H. W. Catts, and L. S. Larrivee, "Preparing preschoolers for the academic and social challenges of school." In M. E. Fey, J. Windsor, and S. F. Warren (Eds.), *Language Intervention: Preschool Through the Elementary Years* (pp. 3–38). Baltimore, Md.: Paul H. Brookes, 1995.

Fox, B., and D. K. Routh, "Analyzing spoken language into words, syllables, and phonemes: A developmental study." *Journal of Psycholinguistic Research, 4* (1975): 331–342.

Fox, B., and D. K. Routh, "Phonemic analysis and severe reading disability in children." *Journal of Psycholinguistic Research, 9* (1980): 115–119.

Gentry, J., "Developmental spelling and the speech-language pathologist." *National Student Speech-Language-Hearing Association, XX* (1988): 50–60.

Gillon, G. T., "The efficacy of phonological awareness intervention for children with spoken language impairment." *Language, Speech, and Hearing Services in Schools, 31* (2000): 126–141.

Gillon, G., and B. Dodd, "The effects of training phonological, semantic, and syntactic processing skills in spoken language on reading ability." *Language, Speech, and Hearing Services in Schools, 26* (1995): 58–68.

Hadley, P., A. Simmerman, M. Long, and M. Luna, "Facilitating language development for inner-city children: Experimental evaluation of a collaborative, classroom-based intervention." *Language, Speech, and Hearing Services in Schools, 31* (2000): 280–295.

Hempenstall, K., "The role of phonemic awareness in beginning reading: A review." *Behavior Change, 14* (1997): 201–214.

Invernizzi, M., J. Meier, L. Swank, and C. Juel, *Phonological Awareness Literacy Screening.* Charlottesville, Va.: University of Virginia, 1998.

Invernizzi, M., R. R. Robey, and T. R. Moon. *Phonological Awareness Literacy Screening: Technical Manual and Report.* Charlottesville, Va.: University of Virginia, 2000.

Johnston, R. S., M. Anderson, and C. Holligan, "Knowledge of the alphabet and explicit awareness of phonemes in pre-readers: The nature of the relationship." *Reading and Writing: An Interdisciplinary Journal, 8* (1996): 217–234.

Juel, C., "Learning to read and write: A longitudinal study of 54 children from first through fourth grades." *Journal of Educational Psychology, 80* (1988): 437–447.

Justice, L. M., and H. K. Ezell, "Vygotskian theory and its application to language assessment: An overview for speech-language pathologists." *Contemporary Issues in Communication Science and Disorders, 26* (1999): 111–118.

Justice, L. M., and H. K. Ezell, "Enhancing children's print and word awareness through home-based parent intervention." *American Journal of Speech-Language Pathology, 9* (2000): 257–269.

Justice, L. M., and H. K. Ezell, "Word and print awareness in four-year-old children." *Child Language and Teaching and Therapy, 17* (2002): 207–225.

Kirtley, C., P. Bryant, M. MacLean, and L. Bradley, "Rhyme, rime, and the onset of reading." *Journal of Experimental Child Psychology, 48* (1989): 224–245.

Larrivee, L., and H. Catts, "Early reading achievement in children with expressive phonological disorders." *American Journal of Speech-Language Pathology, 8*(2) (1999): 118–128.

Levi, G., F. Capozzi, A. Fabrizi, and E. Sechi, "Language disorders and prognosis for reading disabilities in developmental age." *Perceptual and Motor Skills, 54* (1982): 1119–1122.

Lewis, B., B. O'Donnell, L. Freebairn, and H. Taylor, "Spoken language and written expression-interplay of delays." *American Journal of Speech-Language Pathology, 7*(3) (1998): 77–84.

Lindamood, C., and P. Lindamood, *Lindamood Auditory Conceptualization Test.* Boston, Mass.: Teaching Resources Corporation, 1971.

Lindamood, C., and P. Lindamood, *Auditory Discrimination in Depth Program-Revised.* Allen, Tex.: DLM Teaching Resources, 1975.

Lomax, R. G., and L. M. McGee, "Young children's concepts about print and reading: Toward a model of word reading acquisition." *Reading Research Quarterly, 22* (1987): 237–256.

Lonigan, C. J., S. R. Burgess, J. S. Anthony, and T. A. Barker, "Development of phonological sensitivity in 2- to 5-year old children." *Journal of Educational Psychology, 90* (1998): 294–311.

Lundberg, I., J. Frost, and O. Peterson, "Effects of an extensive program for stimulating phonological awareness in preschool children." *Reading Research Quarterly, 23* (1988): 263–284.

Magnusson, E., and K. Naucler, "The development of linguistic awareness in language-disordered children." *First Language, 13* (1993): 93–111.

Masterson, J., and L. Crede, "Learning to spell: Implications for assessment and intervention." *Language, Speech, and Hearing Services in Schools, 30* (1999): 243–254.

Moats, L., *Speech to Print.* Baltimore, Md.: Brookes, 2000.

Morais, J., L. Cary, J. Alegria, and P. Bertelson, "Does awareness of speech as a sequence of phones arise spontaneously?" *Cognition, 7* (1979): 323–331.

Murray, B. A., K. A. Smith, and G. G. Murray, "The test of phoneme identities: Predicting alphabetic insight in prealphabetic readers." *Journal of Literacy Research, 32* (2000): 421–447.

Nation, K., and C. Hulme, "Phonemic segmentation, not onset-rime segmentation, predicts early reading and spelling skills." *Reading Research Quarterly, 32* (1997): 154–167.

O'Connor, R. E., and J. R. Jenkins, "Prediction of reading disabilities in kindergarten and first grade." *Scientific Studies of Reading, 3* (1999): 159–197.

Olswang, L., B. Bain, and G. Johnson, "Using dynamic assessment with children with language disorders." In S. Warren and J. Reichle (Eds.), *Causes and Effects in Communication and Language Intervention* (pp. 187–216). Baltimore, Md.: Brookes, 1992.

Paul, R., *Language Disorders from Infancy Through Adolescence* (2nd edition). Philadelphia, Penn.: Mosby, 2001.

Perfetti, C. A., I. Beck, L. C. Bell, and C. Hughes, "Phonemic knowledge and learning to read are reciprocal: A longitudinal study of first grade children." *Merrill-Palmer Quarterly, 33* (1987): 283–319.

Robertson, C., and W. Salter, *The Phonological Awareness Test.* East Moline, Ill.: Linguisystems, 1997.

Sawyer, D., *Test of Awareness of Language Segments.* Austin, Tex.: PRO-ED, 1987.

Schneider, P., and R. Watkins, "Applying Vygotskian developmental theory to language intervention." *Language, Speech, and Hearing Services in Schools, 27* (1996): 157–170.

Schuele, C. M., Unpublished data, 2001.

Schuele, C. M., and N. D. Dayton, *Intensive Phonological Awareness Program.* Cleveland, Ohio: Authors, 2000.

Schuele, C. M., K. Paul, and K. Mazzaferri, "Phonological awareness training: Is it worth the time?" Paper presented at the annual convention of the American Speech-Language-Hearing Association, San Antonio, Tex., 1998.

Shriberg, L. D., and J. Kwiatkowski, "Phonological disorders III: A procedure for assessing severity of involvement." *Journal of Speech and Hearing Disorders, 47* (1982): 256–270.

Snow, C., M. Burns, and P. Griffin, *Preventing Reading Difficulties in Young Children.* Washington, D.C.: National Research Council, 1998.

Spector, J., "Predicting progress in beginning reading: Dynamic assessment of phonemic awareness." *Journal of Educational Psychology, 84* (1992): 353–363.

Stahl, S. A., and B. A. Murray, "Defining phonological awareness and its relationship to early reading." *Journal of Educational Psychology, 86* (1994): 221–234.

Stanovich, K. E., "Matthew effects in reading: Some consequences of individual differences in the acquisition of literacy." *Reading Research Quarterly, 21* (1986): 360–407.

Stanovich, K. E., "Speculations on the causes and consequences of individual differences in early reading acquisition." In P. B. Gough, L. C. Ehri, and R.

Treiman (Eds.), *Reading Acquisition* (pp. 307–342). Hillsdale, N.J.: Erlbaum, 1992.

Swank, L., and H. Catts, "Phonological awareness and written word decoding." *Language, Speech, and Hearing Services in Schools, 25* (1994): 9–14.

Stuart, M., "Prediction and qualitative assessment of five- and six-year old children's reading: A longitudinal study." *British Journal of Educational Psychology, 65* (1995): 287–296.

Torgesen, J., "Assessment and instruction for phonemic awareness and word recognition skills." In H. Catts and A. Kamhi (Eds.), *Language and Reading Disabilities* (pp 128–153). Boston, Mass.: Allyn & Bacon, 1999.

Torgesen, J., and B. Bryant, *Test of Phonological Awareness*. Austin, Tex.: PRO-ED, 1994.

Torgesen, J., and P. Mathes, *A Basic Guide to Understanding, Assessing, and Teaching Phonological Awareness*. Austin, Tex.: PRO-ED, 2000.

Torgesen, J., S. T. Morgan, and C. Davis, "Effects of two types of phonological awareness training on word learning in kindergarten children." *Journal of Educational Psychology, 84* (1992): 364–370.

Torgesen, J., R. Wagner, and C. Rashotte, "Longitudinal studies of phonological processing and reading." *Journal of Learning Disabilities, 27* (1994): 276–286.

Torgesen, J., R. Wagner, C. Rashotte, A. Alexander, and T. Conway, "Preventative and remedial interventions for children with severe reading disabilities." *Learning Disabilities: An Interdisciplinary Journal, 81* (1997): 51–62.

Treiman, R. "The structure of spoken syllables: Evidence from novel word games." *Cognition, 15* (1983): 49–74.

Treiman, R. "Onsets and rimes as units of spoken syllables: Evidence from children." *Journal of Experimental Child Psychology, 39* (1985): 161–181.

Treiman, R., and J. Baron, "Segmental analysis ability: Development and relation to reading ability." In G. E. MacKinnon and T.G. Waller (Eds.), *Reading Research: Advances in Theory and Practice (Vol. 3)* (pp. 159–197). San Diego, Calif.: Academic Press, 1981.

Treiman, R., C. A. Fowler, J. Gross, D. Berch, and S. Weatherston, "Syllable structure or word structure? Evidence for onset and rime units with disyllabic and trisyllabic stimuli." *Journal of Memory and Language, 34* (1995): 132–155.

Treiman, R., and A. Zukowski, "Toward an understanding of English syllabification." *Journal of Memory and Language, 29* (1990): 66–85.

Treiman, R., and A. Zukowski, "Children's sensitivity to syllables, onsets, rimes, and phonemes." *Journal of Experimental Child Psychology, 61* (1996): 193–215.

van Kleeck, A., "Preliteracy domains and stages: Laying the foundations for beginning reading." *Journal of Children's Communication Development, 20* (1998): 33–51.

van Kleeck, A., R. Gillam, and T. McFadden, "A study of classroom-based phonological awareness training for preschoolers with speech and/or language disorders." *American Journal of Speech-Language Pathology, 7*(3) (1998): 65–76.

van Kleeck, A., and C. M. Schuele, "Precursors to literacy: Normal development." *Topics in Language Disorders, 7*(2) (1987): 13–31.

Vandervelden, M. C., and L. S. Siegel, "Phonological recording and phoneme awareness in early literacy: A developmental approach." *Reading Research Quarterly, 30* (1995): 854–875.

Wagner, R., and J. K. Torgesen, "The nature of phonological processing and its causal role in the acquisition of reading skills." *Psychological Bulletin, 101* (1987): 192–212.

Wagner, R., J. Torgesen, and C. Rashotte, *Comprehensive Test of Phonological Processing*. Austin, Tex.: PRO-ED, 1999.

Warrick, N., and H. Rubin, "Phonological awareness: Normally developing and language delayed children." *Journal of Speech-Language Pathology and Audiology, 16*(1) (1992): 11–20.

Warrick, N., H. Rubin, and S. Rowe-Walsh, "Phoneme awareness in language-delayed children: Comparative studies and intervention." *Annals of Dyslexia, 43* (1993): 153–173.

Webster, P., and A. Plante, "Effects of phonological impairment on word, syllable, and phoneme segmentation and reading." *Language, Speech, and Hearing Services in Schools, 23* (1992): 176–182.

Webster, P., and A. Plante, "Productive phonology and phonological awareness in preschool children." *Applied Psycholinguistics, 16* (1995): 43–57.

Whitehurst, G. J., and C. J. Lonigan, "Child development and emergent literacy." *Child Development, 69* (1998): 848–872.

Yopp, H., "The validity and reliability of phonemic awareness tests." *Reading Research Quarterly, 23* (1988): 159–177.

Procedures for Teaching Sounds

Specific Instructional Techniques

As a supplement to the establishment procedures presented in Chapter 7, the following methods for teaching sounds are presented. Clinicians must be familiar not only with general approaches to the establishment of phonemes but also with specific suggestions for teaching sounds. Material presented on the following pages represents a potpourri of ideas that may be helpful to those who are beginning to develop a repertoire of techniques for evoking and establishing consonant sounds frequently in error. Sources such as Nemoy and Davis (1954) and Bosley (1981) include more extensive instruction for phonetic placement and successive approximation approaches to sound teaching. Clinicians who need word lists, pictures, and/or treatment materials are referred to CD-Rom productions such as *Articulation I: Consonant Phonemes* (Scarry-Larkin, 2001) and materials available from commercial vendors, e.g.,*Target Words for Contextual Training* (Secord and Shine, 1997); *Contrasts: The Use of Minimal Pairs in Articulation Training* (Elbert, Rockman, and Saltzman, 1980); *Phonetic Context Drill Book* (Griffith and Miner, 1979); *Articulation* (Lanza and Flahive, 2000); *Phonological Processing* (Flahive and Lanza, 1998); and *Manual of Articulation and Phonological Disorders* (Bleile, 1995).

Instructions for Correction of an Interdental Lisp

It is important to remember that /s/ may be taught by having the client place his or her tongue behind either the upper teeth or the lower teeth.

1. Instruct the client to protrude the tongue between the teeth and produce a /θ/, and then push the tip of his or her tongue inward with a thin instrument, such as a tongue blade. As a variation, instruct the client to slowly and gradually withdraw the tongue while saying /θ/ and, while still attempting to make /θ/, scrape the tongue tip along the back of the front teeth and upward.
2. Instruct the client to produce /t/ in a word like *tea*. Have him or her pronounce it with a strong aspiration after release of the /t/ prior to the vowel. Instruct the client to slowly slide the tip of the tongue backward from the alveolar ridge following a prolonged release. The result should be [ts]. Then prolong the [s] portion of [ts].

3. Instruct the client to say the following word-pairs, pointing out that the tongue is in a similar position for /t/ and /s/.

tea—sea	*teal—seal*	*tell—sell*	*told—sold*	*tame—same*	*tip—sip*
top—sop	*tight—sight*	*too—Sue*	*tub—sub*	*turf—surf*	*till—sill*

4. Instruct the client to open his or her mouth, put the tongue in position for /t/, drop the tip of the tongue slightly, and send the airstream through the passage. The client can sometimes feel the emission of air by placing a finger in front of his or her mouth.
5. Instruct the client to produce /ʃ/ and then retract his or her lips (smile) and push the tongue slightly forward.
6. Instruct the client to say /i/ and blow through the teeth to produce /s/.
7. Insert a straw in the groove of the tongue and have the client blow to produce /s/.
8. Instruct the client to use the following phonetic placement cues:
   a. Raise the tongue so that the sides are firmly in contact with the inner surface of the upper back teeth.
   b. Groove the tongue slightly along the midline.
   c. Place the tip of the tongue about a quarter of an inch behind the upper teeth.
   d. Bring the teeth together.
   e. Direct the airstream along the groove of the tongue toward the cutting edges of the lower teeth.

Instructions for Correction of a Lateral Lisp

1. Position a straw so that it protrudes from the side of the mouth. When a lateral [s] is made, the straw should resonate on the side of the mouth where the air stream is directed. When the straw is inserted into the front of the mouth and a correct /s/ is made, the straw will resonate in the front of the mouth.
2. Direct attention to a central emission of the air stream by holding a feather, a strip of paper, or a finger in front of the center of the mouth, or have the client tap the incisor gently with his or her forefinger while [s] is being produced. If the sound is being emitted through a central aperture, a break in continuity of the outflow of the breath will be noted. If the sound is being emitted laterally, no break in the continuity of the air stream will be noted. An awareness of central emission may also be developed by instructing the client to inhale air and directing his or her attention to the cool sensation from the intake of air. Then instruct the client to exhale the air through the same aperture by which air entered upon inhalation.
3. Instruct the client to put a tongue blade down the midline of the tongue in order to establish a groove for the air stream.
4. Instruct the client to retract the lips sharply and push the tongue forward, attempting to say /s/.
5. Instruct the client to make /t/, holding the release position for a relatively long time, then retract the lips and drop the jaw slightly. A [ts] should be heard if grooving was maintained properly. Then extend the duration of the [ts], gradually decreasing the release phase of [t] until /s/ is approximated. Saying a word that ends with /ts/, such as /kæts/ or /lɜts/ might be useful.

Instructions for Production of the /ɝ/

1. Instruct the client to growl like a tiger (*grrr*), crow like a rooster (*r-rr-rr*) or sound like a race car (*rrr*).
2. Instruct the client to lower the jaw, say /l/, and push the tongue back until [ɝ] is produced. One can also move from [n] to [nɚ] or [d] to [dɚ].
3. Instruct the client to produce /l/. Then, using a tongue blade, gently push the tip of the tongue back until the depressor can be inserted between the tongue tip and teeth ridge so that an /ɝ/ is produced.
4. Instruct the client to imitate a trilled tongue plus /ɝ/ sound with the tongue tip on the alveolar ridge. Stop the trill but continue producing /ɝ/.
5. Instruct the client to produce /a/ as in the word *father*. As he or she produces the [a], instruct him or her to raise the tongue tip and blade, arching the tongue toward the palate but not touching the palate.
6. Instruct the client to produce /i/ and then lift and retract the tongue tip to produce /ɝ/.
7. Instruct the client to place the tongue lightly between the incisors as in /θ/ and then retract the tip quickly into the /ɝ/. Instruct the client to keep the tip of the tongue near the alveolar ridge to avoid the intrusion of a vowel sound.
8. Instruct the client to say /z/ and to continue to do so while dropping the jaw and saying /ɝ/.
9. Instruct the client to position the tongue for /d/ and then retract it slightly, at the same time dropping the tongue tip and saying /ɝ/. Other clusters such as /tr/, /θr/, and /gr/ may also be used.
10. Spread the sides of the child's mouth with his or her finger, then ask him or her to produce a prolonged /n/ and then curl the tongue backward, continuing to make the sound.
11. Contrast pairs of words beginning with /w/ and /r/. This task may make the distinction between these two sounds more obvious for the client who substitutes /w/ for /r/.

    Practice word-pairs might include:

wipe—ripe	*wan—ran*	*woo—rue*	*wing—ring*	*way—ray*	*wake—rake*
wag—rag	*wail—rail*	*woe—roe*	*weep—reap*	*wed—red*	

Instructions for Production of /l/

1. Instruct the client to produce /l/ with the mouth open in front of a mirror.
2. Instruct the client to position the tongue for /l/ and then lower it to produce /a/. Alternate these movements. The result should be [la], [la], [la]. This procedure can be varied by using /i/ and /u/ instead of /a/.
3. Instruct the client to imitate the clinician's singing of the nonsense syllables [leɪ], [li], [laɪ].
4. Using a lollipop, peanut butter, or tongue blade, touch the place on the client's alveolar ridge where the tongue tip makes contact to produce a correct /l/. Then tell the client to place the tongue at that point and say /l/.

5. Instruct the client to pretend that the tongue is one part of a bird's beak and the roof of the mouth is the other part of the beak. Tell him or her to put the tongue directly behind the teeth and move it up and down quickly, as a bird's beak might move when it is chirping, and say /a/.

Instructions for Production of /f/ and /v/

1. Instruct the client to touch the lower lip with the upper front teeth and blow. The breath stream may be directed by placing a feather or strip of paper in front of his or her mouth while /f/ or /v/ is being produced.
2. Instruct the client to say [a], place the lower lip under the edge of the upper teeth, and blow the breath stream between the lip and teeth so that frication is audible.

Instructions for Production of /k/ and /g/

1. Press underneath the posterior portion of the child's chin and ask him or her to say [kʌ] in a whisper as the pressure is suddenly released.
2. Hold the tongue tip behind the lower teeth, using a tongue blade if necessary. Instruct the client to hump the back of the tongue and build up oral pressure. The tongue contact should be released quickly, thus releasing the pressure built up behind the constriction.
3. Instruct the client to imitate the clinician as the clinician pretends to shoot a gun, producing a lingua-fricative, as in [ka].
4. Instruct the client to alternate the raising of the back and front of the tongue in a rocking movement from [k] to [t].

Instructions for Production of /t/ and /d/

1. Instruct the client to press the tongue tip firmly against the upper dental ridge in front of a mirror. Then have him or her quickly lower the tongue; air pressure will be released, producing approximations of /t/ or /d/.
2. Instruct the client to make a /p/. Then ask him or her to place the tongue tip between the lips and again to try to say /p/. This gives the tactual sensation of a stop made with the tip of the tongue but is not the correct position for /t/ or /d/. Finally, instruct the client to make a similar sound with the tongue tip in contact with the upper lip only. Repeat with the tongue tip touching the alveolar ridge.

REFERENCES

Bleile, K. M., *Manual of Articulation and Phonological Disorders*. San Diego, Calif.: Singular Publishing Group, Inc., 1995.

Bosley, E., *Techniques for Articulatory Disorders*. Springfield, Ill.: Charles C. Thomas, 1981.

Elbert, M., B. Rockman, and D. Saltzman, *Contrasts: The Use of Minimal Pairs in Articulation Training*. Austin, Tex.: Exceptional Resources, Inc., 1980.

Flahive, L. K., and J. R. Lanza, *Phonological Processing*. East Moline, Ill.: LinguiSystems, Inc., 1998.

Griffith, J., and L. E. Miner, *Phonetic Context Drillbook*. Englewood Cliffs, N.J.: Prentice Hall, 1979.

Lanza, J. R., and L. K. Flahive, *Articulation*. East Moline, Ill.: LinguiSystems, Inc., 2000.

Nemoy, E. M., and S. F. Davis, *The Correction of Defective Consonant Sounds*. Magnolia, Mass.: Expression Company, 1954.

Scarry-Larkin, M., *Articulation I: Consonant Phonemes*. Austin, Tex.: PRO-ED, 2001.

Secord, W. A., and R. E. Shine, *Target Words for Contextual Training*. Sedona, Ariz.: Red Rock Educational Publications, 1997.

AUTHOR INDEX

SUBJECT INDEX